D0145968

NUTRITION RESEARCH AT THE LEADING EDGE

NUTRITION RESEARCH
AT THE LEADING EDGE

RUSSELL E. CASSADY
AND
ERMA I. TIDSWELL
EDITORS

Nova Biomedical Books
New York

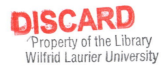
DISCARD
Property of the Library
Wilfrid Laurier University

Copyright © 2008 by Nova Science Publishers, Inc.

All rights reserved. No part of this book may be reproduced, stored in a retrieval system or transmitted in any form or by any means: electronic, electrostatic, magnetic, tape, mechanical photocopying, recording or otherwise without the written permission of the Publisher.

For permission to use material from this book please contact us:
Telephone 631-231-7269; Fax 631-231-8175
Web Site: http://www.novapublishers.com

NOTICE TO THE READER

The Publisher has taken reasonable care in the preparation of this book, but makes no expressed or implied warranty of any kind and assumes no responsibility for any errors or omissions. No liability is assumed for incidental or consequential damages in connection with or arising out of information contained in this book. The Publisher shall not be liable for any special, consequential, or exemplary damages resulting, in whole or in part, from the readers' use of, or reliance upon, this material.

Independent verification should be sought for any data, advice or recommendations contained in this book. In addition, no responsibility is assumed by the publisher for any injury and/or damage to persons or property arising from any methods, products, instructions, ideas or otherwise contained in this publication.

This publication is designed to provide accurate and authoritative information with regard to the subject matter covered herein. It is sold with the clear understanding that the Publisher is not engaged in rendering legal or any other professional services. If legal or any other expert assistance is required, the services of a competent person should be sought. FROM A DECLARATION OF PARTICIPANTS JOINTLY ADOPTED BY A COMMITTEE OF THE AMERICAN BAR ASSOCIATION AND A COMMITTEE OF PUBLISHERS.

Library of Congress Cataloging-in-Publication Data

Nutrition research at the leading edge / Russell E. Cassady and Erma I. Tidswell (editor).
    p. ; cm.
  ISBN 978-1-60456-053-4 (hardcover)
  1. Nutrition. I. Cassady, Russell E. II. Tidswell, Erma I.
  [DNLM: 1. Nutrition Physiology. QU 145 N975397 2008]
  QP141.N827 2008
  612.3--dc22

                          2007045952

Published by Nova Science Publishers, Inc. ✦ New York

Contents

Preface

Nutrition is a science that examines the relationship between diet and health. Dietitians are health professionals who specialize in this area of study, and are trained to provide safe, evidence-based dietary advice and interventions. Deficiencies, excesses and imbalances in diet can produce negative impacts on health, which may lead to diseases such as cardiovascular disease, diabetes, scurvy, obesity or osteoporosis, as well as psychological and behavioral problems. Moreover, excessive ingestion of elements that have no apparent role in health, (e.g. lead, mercury, PCBs, dioxins), may incur toxic and potentially lethal effects, depending on the dose. Many common diseases and their symptoms can often be prevented or alleviated with better nutrition. The science of nutrition attempts to understand how and why specific dietary aspects influence health.

Expert Commentary - Nutraceuticals are established food components widely consumed as supplements to the diet, either as formulated products or for fortification of foods, particularly functional foods. Over the last two decades there has been a steady growth in research into the possible health benefits. Both the general public and the media have become increasingly interested, and this has coincided with a general interest in health issues. This has resulted in increasing usage of commercially available products, as well as their food sources. It is now well understood that modern pharmaceuticals cannot successfully treat all diseases, coupled with their lack of effectiveness in certain disease states, and the possibility of marked side effects. There is logical use of a number of nutraceuticals which are endogenous nutrients from a range of food sources, as many diseases maybe caused by deficiency states.

Chapter I - Over 8,000 polyphenols have been reported to occur in plants. Polyphenols as a group include flavonoids, phenolic acids, lignans and stilbenes; and are secondary metabolites which are used in the plant response to pathogenic and environmental challenges.

Polyphenols including the catechins and procyanidins found in pomegranate, cocoa and its derivative chocolate, and cranberry, are known to be antioxidant, due to a free radical scavenging mechanism, and these are believed to be the beneficial components. In addition to widely reported antioxidant activity, a number of markers of particular disease states have been beneficially affected by these components.

Relevant scientific and medical research into these supplements is important due to the increasing media hype associated with the possible benefits of their consumption. Evidence from both clinical trials, and *in vivo* and *in vitro* research, is reported, to give a balanced view of the claimed benefits.

Chapter II - Childhood obesity is a global concern. In many countries, the prevalence has increased so rapidly that the problem is considered an epidemic. Recent data indicate that approximately 10% of children aged 2 to 5 years, and 15% of children aged 6 to 19 years, are overweight. Obese children commonly grow up to be obese adults. The co-morbid conditions associated with childhood obesity include coronary heart disease, hypertension, type 2 diabetes mellitus, polycystic ovary syndrome, hyperlipidemia, obstructive sleep apnea, increased incidence of upper respiratory tract infection, orthopedic problems, non-alcoholic fatty liver disease, cholelithiasis, renal disease, and iron deficiency. The relative risk of all-cause mortality is approximately 1.5 times greater for obese children and adolescents compared with their normal weight peers. Obese mothers are at risk for birth defects. A less acceptable body image can have a significant negative psychological and social impact. The goals of treatment should be weight stabilization and improved fitness, and improvements in psychosocial function and in the co-morbid conditions. The three primary components of therapy are decreased caloric intake, increased energy output, and behavioral modifications that include both the child and the family. Childhood obesity, once established, is notoriously difficult to treat. Good nutrition and regular physical activity help to prevent obesity. Health care professionals who care for children should promote healthy dietary and lifestyle choices. Infants should be exclusively breastfed for the first 6 months of life and mothers should be encouraged to breastfeed for as long as possible. Around 2 years of age, the intake of fat should be reduced and the intake of whole grain products, vegetables, fruit, and low-fat diary products should be increased. The consumption of juice, sweetened beverages, and soft drinks should be limited. Prevention of childhood obesity requires both family-based and school-based programs that include the promotion of physical activity, parent education and modeling, behavioral counseling, and nutrition education. Community programs should interact with school programs to provide opportunities for children to be physically active.

Chapter III - Cardiovascular diseases (CVD) which affect the heart and circulatory system are known to cause millions of deaths each year worldwide, comprising the largest contribution to mortality in Europe and North America. According to prevalence data from the National Health and Nutrition Examination Survey III, 64.4 million Americans have one or more types of CVD, of whom 25.3 million are aged 65 years or older, and accounted for 38.5% of all deaths in the US. The cost implications of this, both direct and indirect, have been estimated to be $368.4 million. Consequently much research has been aimed at developing new treatments and new methods of prevention of CVD.

Chapter IV - Many studies have associated passive smoking with an increased risk of developing certain diseases. Smoking during pregnancy increases the risk of the newborn having a low birth weight (at term or pre-term), and of suffering impaired respiratory function and ischaemic heart disease etc. In children and adolescents, environmental exposure to tobacco smoke has been associated with abnormal lipid profiles and an increased risk of atherosclerosis. Passive smoking can also be the cause of reduced female fertility in the general population. The food habits of both active and passive smokers may also be negatively affected.

The diets of smokers tend to be less adequate than those of non-smokers. Exposure to tobacco smoke modifies the sense of taste and smell, leading to changes in food preferences and food intake, and eventually to a more imbalanced diet. Matters are made worse in that smokers may have greater needs of certain nutrients such as antioxidants. Thus, even with a normal intake of these nutrients, the nutritional status of smokers can be inadequate.

As with active smokers, passive smokers may show slightly unhealthy food habits and more imbalanced diets than non-smokers – either as a consequence of living with smokers (and therefore sharing their food habits) or via the direct modification of their food choices. Passive smokers consume fewer fruits and vegetables and have lower intakes of a number of nutrients, which might be reflected at the serum level. For example, exposure to tobacco smoke is associated with reduced folate levels, via which some of the effects of active and passive smoking on health may be made manifest. Like active smokers, passive smokers may have a greater need of certain nutrients. For example, they show lower plasma concentrations of antioxidants than do non-smokers not exposed to smoke, independent of the differences in dietary antioxidant intake.

The diet of passive smokers may be an important factor in the relationship between tobacco smoke exposure and health problems. Although the cessation of smoking and the avoidance of passive smoking is the ideal goal, it cannot always be attained. Dietary intervention may therefore be a useful and indeed necessary strategy to prevent or delay smoking-related pathologies.

Chapter V - *Background.* Schools offer unique channels for youth obesity prevention. School based programs can be categorized as having an individual, environmental, or a combined (individual + environmental) focus.

Purpose. This chapter reviews the literature on school based interventions focusing on diet, physical activity, and/or sedentary behavior reporting body composition as an outcome measure, and then characterizes these programs as having an individual, environmental, or combined focus. These categories are then examined in an attempt to determine which approach appears to be more effective at promoting change in body composition within the school setting.

Method. Primary inclusionary criteria were: school based interventions; a focus on diet, physical activity, and/or sedentary behavior; reporting body composition as an outcome measure; and emphasizing prevention rather than treatment. Secondary inclusionary criteria (to enhance confidence in the inferences drawn) included having an experimental design, with school as the unit of randomization; using appropriate statistical analysis methods to account for clustering within schools; inclusion in a peer-reviewed journal; and reporting results in English

Results .Eleven interventions met all inclusionary criteria. Three of the 11 achieved significant change in body composition (27% of total). Significant group differences in body composition were reported by two of the individual focus (29%), one (50%) of the environmental focus, and none (0%) of the combined focus interventions. No consistent differences in procedures, methods, or intervention components were found among the interventions that did or did not achieve change in body composition.

Conclusion. Both individual and environmental interventions promote change in diet, physical activity, and/or sedentary behavior and have demonstrated success in impacting body composition in a school setting. More research is needed to identify the approach, procedures, and methods that are most effective at promoting body composition change in a school setting.

Chapter VI - Studies have shown elevated LDL cholesterol and other adverse responses with the addition of saturated fat to an otherwise balanced diet. Epidemiological studies have suggested that these adverse markers correlate with real adverse outcomes. There are, however, few studies documenting the effect of saturated fat intake in the face of carbohydrate restriction on markers of cardiovascular disease and, of course, there are no outcome studies. The authors will review the available data, including our own, and provide historic, epidemiological and physiologic reasons why the continuous intake of saturated fat may be needed to maximize the health benefits of a carbohydrate restricted diet.

Chapter VII - *Objective.*Coronary artery disease events have a circadian rhythmicity, clustering more in the second quartile of the day. n-3 fatty acid supplementation reduces the rate of cardiac events, but its effect on their circadian rhythmicity has not been tested.

Design. The Indo-Mediterranean Diet Heart Study was a single blind randomized study that assessed the effect of a diet rich in alpha-linolenic acid, the parent n-3 fatty acid, on the occurrence of myocardial infarction and sudden cardiac death.

Subjects. One thousand subjects of the Indo-Mediterranean Diet Heart Study, focusing on the 115 patients from both control and intervention groups in which cardiac events occurred.

Intervention. The timing of cardiac events throughout the day was compared between the intervention and control groups. The distribution of cardiac events along the four quartiles of the day was compared between groups as well as against equal distribution.

Results. The risk ratio for a cardiac event was lowest between 4:00 and 8:00 in the morning for the intervention group. The control group had a higher rate of events in the second quartile of the day, which deviated from an equal distribution, as expected ($P=0.013$). In the intervention group, events were equally distributed along the day. No statistically significant difference was found in daily event distribution between the groups.

Conclusion. A diet rich in alpha-linolenic acid may abolish the higher rate of cardiac events, normally seen in the second quartile of the day. Additional studies are needed to identify the underlying mechanism.

In: Nutrition Research at the Leading Edge
Editors: R. E. Cassady, E. I. Tidswell, pp. 1-5

ISBN: 978-1-60456-053-4
© 2008 Nova Science Publishers, Inc.

Expert Commentary

Research and Consumer Update on Nutraceuticals and Novel Antioxidant Sources

G.B. Lockwood

School of Pharmacy And Pharmaceutical Sciences,
University of Manchester,
Manchester M13 9pl, UK

Nutraceuticals are established food components widely consumed as supplements to the diet, either as formulated products or for fortification of foods, particularly functional foods. Over the last two decades there has been a steady growth in research into the possible health benefits. Both the general public and the media have become increasingly interested, and this has coincided with a general interest in health issues. This has resulted in increasing usage of commercially available products, as well as their food sources. It is now well understood that modern pharmaceuticals cannot successfully treat all diseases, coupled with their lack of effectiveness in certain disease states, and the possibility of marked side effects. There is logical use of a number of nutraceuticals which are endogenous nutrients from a range of food sources, as many diseases maybe caused by deficiency states.

The perceived health benefits, along with increasing ageing populations affected by disease states expected at increasing ages, has seen large growth in demand for the wide range of products available. In addition, it has been predicted that a number of age related ailments such as arthritis will affect most of the populations as they grow older. It is in disease states such as these where nutraceuticals are increasingly used. Health conscious consumers are also increasingly supplementing their diets with nutraceuticals, and they are becoming "life style" treatments. However, the "hype" associated with this increase in information can potentially increase the risk of individuals self medicating with nutraceuticals for serious disease states instead of seeking the correct medical attention.

Improvement in government sponsorship of clinical trials, such as the Glucosamine /chondroitin Intervention Trial (GAIT) for glucosamine and chondroitin, has taken place in tandem with more research funding for nutraceutical research, and this could significantly improve the available data, and in the long-term reduced health costs could justify the money spent. The GAIT trial used large patient numbers (1,500) and monitored effects over a long period of time in an attempt to overcome the limitations of short term trials with small patient numbers. Regulatory authorities are recently addressing the issues involved with the supply of nutraceuticals and controlling widespread use of excessive health claims. Consumer organisations are now routinely publishing detailed analytical profiles of ranges of products, which enables consumers to choose the best quality. It is believed that product conformity will improve with the introduction of official analytical monographs. These are essential for the routine quality assurance, and are now being published.The AOAC monographs for glucosamine in both raw materials and supplement formulations has been published, and monographs are expected soon for coenzyme Q10, n-3-PUFAs and chondroitin sulphate [1] .

At the same time as pharmacogenomics is being used to investigate a patient's response to medication, "nutrigenomics" may be appropriate to study the effect of nutraceuticals and dietary components on health. This latter development may allow the use of a particular individual's genetic information to predict specific personalised nutraceutical supplementation to prevent diseases and maintain health [2].

Many surveys of nutraceutical supplement use have been carried out in Western countries, and the conclusion is often that the typical patient is middle aged, middle-income, and female, but this usage profile is by no means exclusive.

The markets for nutraceuticals and functional foods are rapidly expanding, and combined they represented annual worldwide sales of $95 billion in 2001, and this was projected to grow to $127 billion by 2005, and it is expected to reach 5% of the total food bills in developed countries [3].

Problems with Available Data

Epidemiological data for foodstuffs may reveal unclear results due to the range of nutraceuticals which investigated populations may consume. This scenario is particularly pertinent with the data recorded for components of the Mediterranean Diet, which may contain different ratios of n-6: n-3 PUFAs, as well as grape and olive products containing numerous active phytochemicals. Similar problems can also occur when including data from Far Eastern populations who are known soy and tea consumers, but in addition have very different diets to Western populations, specifically in relation to the overall fat content.

Clinical trial data for nutraceuticals is often based upon relatively small numbers of subjects, with the result that there is often limited statistical significance. This problem is increasingly addressed by the use of meta analyses of the derived data. Further comparison of the derived trial data is also coming under the scrutiny of systematic reviews, particularly by the Cochrane Library, which has reported on trials of a number of widely studied nutraceuticals such as glucosamine, tea and soy.

Another problem concerns variability in composition of plant extracts used in clinical trials of nutraceuticals. Wherever possible, single chemical entities should be used to establish clear outcomes, but this of course removes the chance of recording beneficial additive or synergistic effects possibly seen with normal dietary consumption. Many of the clinical trials with specific nutraceuticals have been carried out using different protocols, resulting in incomparable results.

Another issue which may affect the overall benefits of supplementing diets with particular foods rich in nutraceuticals is demonstrated by the n PUFAs. Over the last few decades there has been a gradual substitution of saturated animal fats for polyunsaturated plant oils in foods, although many of these substitutes are of the n-6 rather than n-3 PUFAs. This causes many current diets to have an n-6:n-3 imbalance by up to 30 times in favour of n-6 which may be detrimental to health. As a result there is a suggestion that eating PUFA rich oils containing n-3 PUFAs (found in large quantities in fish oils and flaxseed) may help redress this imbalance and help in many disease states [2].

New Developments

Daidzein has for a long time been considered to be one of the major active components of soy, however, evidence that its metabolite equol is responsible for the activity has recently been published. Equol is not produced in adults who lack the intestinal bacteria that are required to metabolise diadzein in soy products, and it has been estimated that 30-50% of the population are able to produce equol. It has been proposed that the ability to make equol may hold the clue to the effectiveness of soy protein diets when employed in the treatment or prevention of hormone-dependent conditions. The failure to distinguish those subjects who are 'equol-producers' from 'non-equol producers' in most clinical studies could explain the variation seen in reported data on the health benefits of soy [4].

Clearly, the ability to produce active metabolites of other nutraceutical entities by sections of populations, could have implications in a range of therapeutic areas.

Synergistic Effects

The possibility of synergy of components in plant derived nutraceutical supplements has long been expected, but it is only recently that evidence is being reported to substantiate this. However, many products containing two or more natural sources of chemical entities are available, and often the most likely benefit is simply an additive effect. Both soy and tea components are widely quoted in these interactions.

One plant component, piperine, from the plack pepper, *Piper longum*, has been reported to improve bioavailability of certain nutraceuticals including coenzyme Q10 [2].

Although synergistic effects both within and between different nutraceuticals are possible, there appears to be no evidence to substantiate the marketing of a large number of multicomponent products currently available to consumers.

Adverse Effects

Clear evidence for toxicity of nutraceuticals is rare, but a small range of adverse effects are
documented, for the majority these are minor gastrointestinal problems, but caution has been advised with soy products as evidence of more serious effects has been found in animal studies.

Interactions of a few nutraceuticals with prescription medicines have been reported, examples include evening primrose oil with phenothiazine neuroleptics, tea with ephedrine, and cimetidine and coenzyme Q10 with warfarin. Prescription medicines have also been reported to decrease levels of nutraceuticals, for example, coenzyme Q10 levels have been depressed by certain medicines, in particular by the statins [5].

Quality of Products Available to Consumers

The content of active ingredients compared to label claims on formulated nutraceuticals and antioxidants has been reported in a number of instances. Substandard levels have often been reported. Complex whole foods and their extracts, those from tea and soy in particular, show wide variations in levels of purported active constituents, and it is to be expected that other complex plant products will show the same trend [2].

Conclusion

In other whole food supplements and complex nutraceuticals, e.g. widely available fruit extracts from pomegranate and cranberry, it is often impossible to ascertain the active constituent (s), due to their complex nature. Often a number of plant products contain the same or similar constituents, and many antioxidant components may well be responsible for the reported activity. There is also the confusion as to whether synergistic effects of the food matrix are responsible for the reported effects, possibly due to increased absorption. Grape seed proanthocyanidin extract, pycnogenol, tea and chocolate all contain catechins and procyanidins, which are most likely the cause of their activity; these components also occur widely in a number of other edible plants and their derived products.

It has been claimed that many antioxidants also have other activities, including enhancement or inhibition of Phase I and II metabolising enzymes, and modulation of DNA repair, hence their ability to interact in a number of disease states. Although dietary antioxidants are widely reported to be beneficial, excessive levels may actually be detrimental, due to their ability to generate reactive oxygen species, which can cause a number of disease states [6].

Evidence for the beneficial effects of many widely used nutraceuticals in a number of life-threatening diseases, ranges from epidemiological through to *in vitro* research and clinical trials, however a number of them show very little supporting evidence.

References

[1]   Roman, M. The AOAC validation effort for dietary supplements. *Nutraceuticals World* 2005; November: 82-86.

[2]   Lockwood, B. (2007) Nutraceuticals: A guide for healthcare professionals. Pharmaceutical Press, London, 426pp.

[3]   Iisakke, K. Nutraceuticals and functional foods demand for ingredients *NutraCos* 2003, Nov/Dec, 2-4.

[4]   Setchell, KD, Brown, NM, Lydeking-Olsen, E. The clinical importance of the metabolite equol – A clue to the effectiveness of soy and its isoflavones. *J Nutrition* 2002;132: 3577-3584.

[5]   Davies, E, Greenacre, D, Lockwood, GB. Adverse effects and toxicity of nutraceuticals. *Reviews in Food and Nutrition Toxicity* (2005), 3 165-195.

[6]   Melton, S. 2006. The antioxidant myth. New Scientist August 5, 40-43.

In: Nutrition Research at the Leading Edge
Editors: R. E. Cassady, E. I. Tidswell, pp. 7-51
ISBN: 978-1-60456-053-4
© 2008 Nova Science Publishers, Inc.

Chapter I

Health Benefits of the Polyphenols of Pomegranate, Cocoa, and Cranberry

Sarah Bickham, Kathryn Bowen, Richard Kears and Brian Lockwood
School of Pharmacy and Pharmaceutical Sciences,
University of Manchester, Manchester, M13 9PL, UK

Introduction

Over 8,000 polyphenols have been reported to occur in plants. Polyphenols as a group include flavonoids, phenolic acids, lignans and stilbenes [1]; and are secondary metabolites which are used in the plant response to pathogenic and environmental challenges.

Polyphenols including the catechins and procyanidins found in pomegranate, cocoa and its derivative chocolate, and cranberry, are known to be antioxidant, due to a free radical scavenging mechanism [2], and these are believed to be the beneficial components. In addition to widely reported antioxidant activity, a number of markers of particular disease states have been beneficially affected by these components.

Relevant scientific and medical research into these supplements is important due to the increasing media hype associated with the possible benefits of their consumption. Evidence from both clinical trials, and *in vivo* and *in vitro* research, is reported, to give a balanced view of the claimed benefits.

Pomegranate

Punica granatum L., the pomegranate tree, is an important commercial fruit in Saudi Arabia, Japan, the United States and many Mediterranean countries [3,4].

It is known to contain numerous types of polyphenols. The antioxidant activity of the polyphenols has been investigated for therapeutic effects, and pomegranate fractions have been shown to provide similar or greater antioxidant activity than a number of fruit juices, teas and wines [2-7].

Commercial pomegranate juice (PJ) is obtained by pressing the whole fruit; so many water soluble components enter the juice from other parts of the fruit, including the most abundant polyphenol in PJ, the ellagitannin (ET) punicalagin from the fruit husk [8]. Punicalagin can reach levels of 2g/L in PJ [9,10] with significant variability [11]. PJ contains many hydrolysable tannins, which account for 92% of it's antioxidant activity [12], with punicalagin alone providing 50% [10,13]. Also present is the ellagitannin hydrolysis product, ellagic acid (EA), in both free and bound forms [10].Other hydrolysable tannins present include gallotannins, and gallic/gallagic acid [2]. The contribution of antioxidant activity in PJ was found to be of the order: punicalagin > other hydrolysable tannins > anthocyanins > ellagic acids [2]. The structure of ellagic acid, the basic unit of punicalgin and other ellagitannins present in pomegranate is shown in Figure 1.

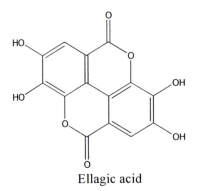

Ellagic acid

Figure 1. The structure of ellagic acid.

PJ flavonoids include the anthocyanidins cyanidin, delphinidin and pelarigenin and their glycosides [10,14], which have known antioxidant activity [15]. Also present are proanthocyanidins, anthocyanins [2], the flavonol quercetin and rutin [16]. Fermented juice (wine) has shown higher activity than fresh juice because heat during the process hydrolyzes flavonoid glycosides [16]. PJ is also rich in estrogenic flavonoids such as luteolin [17].

Pomegranate peel contains many fruit acids and phenolic compounds that are present in the juice, only in higher concentrations [16]. Although there are many flavonoids in the peel (including the flavonol quercetin [18] and the flavanone narigenin [19]) there are reportedly no anthocyanidins (although pro-anthocyanidins have been found) [16]. Also present is the flavonoid luteolin [17]. The content of anthocyanin glycosides in the peel is responsible for the red colour of the fruits [2].

The husk contains the ellagitannins punicalagin and punicalin, which are ellagic acid derivatives [8]. The distinctive yellow colour of the husks is due to the punicalagin content [13]. Commercial PJ is more active than pomegranate fruit juices used in research reports [2] because both the husk and the peel are included when the whole fruit is pressed, which extracts high levels of tannins into the juice [9,10].

During ripening, the content of pomegranate polyphenols decreases while the concentration of anthocyanins increases (this intensifies the red pigmentation of the fruits)

[1,4]. The process of ripening can be altered by light levels and numerous environmental factors, as well as the time of harvest [1]. Differences in cultivar may also affect the nutritional value of the fruit [4].

Food preparation techniques and industrial processing can alter polyphenol levels. [1]. Fermentation increases the availability of flavonoids [16], which may increase activity of pomegranate wines.

Anti-Bacterial Activity

Pomegranate extracts, usually from the rind, have demonstrated activity against many bacterial species *in vitro*. A methanolic extract (containing tannins and alkaloids) from the fruit shell inhibited completely the colony growth of the bacterial species *Staphylococcus aureus, Escherichia coli, Pseudomonas aeruginosa* and *Candida albicans* [20].

Further work analyzed the antibacterial activity of four different extracts from pomegranate fruit rind on *Staphylococcus aureus, Escherichia coli, Klebsiella pneumoniae, Proteus vulgaris, Bacillus subtilis* and *Salmonella typhi* [21]. All four extracts were found to show some antibacterial activity; EA and ET's have also shown activity against numerous micro-organisms including *Helicobacter pylori* [22].

A methanolic pomegranate extract was shown to completely eliminate the growth of *Staphylococcus aureus* (1%v/v) and also demonstrated a capacity to inhibit the organisms' production of enterotoxin A (inhibition of enterotoxin production may aid in preventing food poisoning and toxic shock caused by this organism [23]).

Interestingly, a methanolic extract from pomegranate has been shown to act synergistically with five different antibiotics against isolated strains of methicillin-resistant *Staphylococcus aureus* (MRSA) and methicillin-sensitive *Staphylococcus aureus* (MSSA) in selected cultures. A combination of extract and ampicillin reduced cell viability of MRSA by 72.5% and MSSA by 99.9%, and increased the post antibiotic effect of ampicillin from 3 to 7 hours. Thus it appears that pomegranate may have a role in enhancing the effect of certain antibiotics [24].

Pomegranate has been traditionally used in cases of dysentery, diarrhoea and abscesses [20,21]. Recent data suggests a use for this fruit in modern medicine to treat infections, although further research could identify active ingredients and mechanisms responsible [20,23].

Anti-Viral Activity

Traditional uses are for coughs and colds [23] and quercetin, a component of PJ, has shown anti-viral activity activity [25]. It was found that a mixture containing pomegranate rind extract reduced the infectivity of poliovirus, herpes simplex virus type 1 (HSV-1) and human immunodeficiency virus type 1 (HIV-1) *in vitro*, indicating a possible use in halting the spread of these diseases [26]. Anti-viral effects against HSV-2 have also been observed for a peel tannin extract [27].

A pomegranate extract was evaluated as a candidate topical microbicide against HIV-1 infection [18]. Pomegranate juice from certain geographical areas had the highest inhibitory activity against HIV-1 IIIB (X4) on cells expressing CD4 and CXCR4 compared to other fruit juices. The antimicrobial effects of pomegranate extracts could also be useful in treating AIDS associated diseases [26].

Anti-Atherosclerotic Activity

Oxidative stress is a major contributor to cardiovascular disease (CVD) [28]. Atherosclerosis is a disease of the arteries in which blood flow is compromised by fatty deposit build up on artery walls. Risk factors for the development of atherosclerosis include hypertension, increased plasma low density lipoprotein (LDL), LDL modifications (oxidation, retention, aggregation) and platelet activation [29,30]. Oxidative stress affects cellular lipids in arterial macrophages as well as LDL [7]. Oxidised LDL is taken up more readily by macrophages, whose LDL uptake rate is also increased by oxidizing its cellular lipids. These processes cause cholesterol accumulation in macrophages leading to foam cell formation, which is a characteristic of early atherosclerosis [29,31].

A link was established between the antioxidant activity of PJ polyphenols and anti-atherogenic effects, using humans and (early) atherosclerotic apolipoprotein E-deficient mice [29]. A core reason for the activity was attributed to the antioxidant capacity of PJ (and tannins in particular [30]) to reduce lipid peroxidation in lipoproteins, macrophages and platelets [9]. In mice, PJ was found to prevent oxidative modifications of LDL and lipid peroxidation in LDL and macrophages. Foam cell formation and atherosclerotic lesion size were also decreased. Platelet aggregation was reduced *in vitro*, which may have contributed to the overall anti-atherogenic effect. Human subjects showed a marked resistance of LDL to aggregation and retention and increases in serum paroxonase activity [29] (A high density lipoprotein (HDL) -associated esterase which prevents lipid oxidation in lesions using hydrolytic and peroxidative like properties [28,31]).

The use of angiotensin converting enzyme (ACE) inhibitors may reduce risk factors for atherosclerosis (blood pressure, platelet aggregation, lipid peroxidation) [30]. Using hypertensive patients, dietary PJ supplementation for 2 weeks reduced ACE activity *in vivo* and *in vitro*.

The effects of PJ (50mL) daily on atherosclerotic patients with carotid artery stenosis (CAS) were investigated over a maximum of three years [28]. A decrease in carotid intima-media thickness (IMT) by 35% and systolic BP by 12% were observed over one year compared to control (possibly by blocking reactive oxygen and nitrogen species). Total anti-oxidative status was up 130% after one year, antibodies against serum oxidised-LDL were raised, and serum paraoxonase-1 activity increased by 83% over three years. Indeed, LDL associated lipid peroxide numbers were also decreased by 90% after just 6 months of PJ treatment. This study demonstrates the anti-atherosclerotic effects of PJ in patients with CAS, by reducing serum oxidative stress and carotid IMT [28].

The effects of daily PJ consumption (240mL) on humans with ischemic coronary heart disease (CHD) were evaluated over 3 months, using a summed difference score to measure stress induced ischemia (SII). SII decreased in the treatment group over 3 months compared to control, and was accompanied by a 17% increase in myocardial perfusion compared to an 18% decrease in the control group [32]. The mechanisms responsible for this are thought to be related to those previously described for anti-atherosclerotic effects. Despite the small size of this study (45 patients), these and the above results highlight the potential of realistic daily doses of PJ in this area, and further large scale placebo controlled trials could validate these findings and identify active constituents.

Diabetes-Related Activity

Numerous studies have investigated the potential of pomegranate in the treatment of diabetes in an accepted type 2 diabetic rat model (Zucker diabetic fatty (ZDF) rats) and in humans.

A pomegranate flower (PGF) methanolic extract was found to attenuate the increase in plasma glucose in loaded ZDF rats after 6 weeks of treatment; possibly due to activation of peroxisome proliferator-activated receptor (PPAR)-γ, which increases the sensitivity of insulin receptors. PGF extract also restored down-regulated cardiac glucose transporter (GLUT)-4 mRNA (which may be regulated by PPAR-γ expression), which increases glucose transport into the heart to help avoid cardiac dysfunction and hyperglycaemia [33]. The polyphenol responsible for these effects was found to be gallic acid (GA) *in vitro*, although the mechanism of action is unknown. Atherosclerosis has been associated with decreased PPAR-γ activity in mouse macrophages, indicating that GA may have a preventative role here [33].

The effect of the methanolic flower extract on postprandial hyperglycaemia was investigated using ZDF rats, as postprandial hyperglycaemia is important in the development of type 2 diabetes and cardiovascular disease. Postprandial plasma glucose levels in sucrose loaded ZDF rats were lower compared to fasted ZDF rats after 2 weeks of treatment with PGF extract. A possible mechanism for this (at least in part) was identified *in vitro* as reduced carbohydrate digestion in the rat gastrointestinal tract through inhibition of α-glucosidase activity. Interestingly, α-glucosidase inhibitors may also prevent HIV replication *in vitro* [34].

In diabetes, a shift in cardiac metabolism results in the heart using more fatty acids (FA) as a source of ATP. Increased FA uptake and oxidation in the heart are associated with congestive heart failure and other abnormalities. PGF extract reduced excess triglyceride accumulation in ZDF rat cardiac tissues by lowering plasma FA levels, inhibiting up-regulation of cardiac fatty acid transport protein expression (which facilitates movement of FA across membranes), and suppressing cardiac over-expression of mRNA encoding for PPAR-α which is involved in mitochondrial FA uptake and oxidation. Oleanoic acid could be partly responsible for these effects as it may promote PPAR-α activation *in vitro*, which lowers circulating lipids. Cardiac TG lowering could therefore improve contractile ability in the diabetic myocardium and reverse abnormal cardiac function [35].

A persistent increase in diabetic cardiac extra-cellular matrix deposition leads to fibrosis, possible arrhythmias and congestive heart failure. Reversing this activity may improve cardiac function and mortality in diabetic patients. The extract decreased cardiac fibrosis in ZDF rats, possibly via modulation of endothelin (ET)-1 and nuclear factor (NF)-κB pathways, although a direct effect on the heart remained to be established [36]. The extract may therefore have a use as an anti-fibrinogenic agent to help prevent diabetic cardiac complications.

Trials have been conducted using PJ in type 2 diabetic patients. Consumption of 50mL PJ for 3 months caused no worsening of patient's diabetic status (despite containing sugars (10%)) [37], perhaps through similar mechanisms as seen in animals [33]. This result differs when compared to other juices (e.g. grapefruit juice), which adversely affect diabetic conditions leading to atherosclerotic complications [37]. PJ reduced serum oxidative stress (in agreement with other studies [28]), which is thought to be a major contributor to vascular pathology in type 2 diabetics, partly through increases in serum paraoxonase-1 (24%) and total sulfhydryl (12% (a marker for oxidative stress)) activity [37]. Patient serum was subsequently found to be more resistant against induced oxidation, and macrophages were found to be under a lower level of oxidative stress (with a lower oxidised-LDL uptake) *in vitro* which is important considering their influential role in early atherogenesis [37]. PJ anthocyanins and tannins were postulated as being responsible for these effects [37]. In addition, concentrated PJ (40g/day) improved the lipid profile in type 2 diabetics with hyperlipidaemia over 8 weeks by lowering numerous forms of cholesterol, which may be important in reducing the risk factors associated with heart disease [38].

These studies demonstrate the potential of PJ in modifying vascular conditions associated with diabetes such as atherosclerosis and heart disease, and form a foundation for further study into the direct effects of PJ and flower extracts on diabetic markers such as serum glucose levels, insulin sensitivity and diabetes related conditions.

Anti-Cancer Activity

Prostate Cancer

Different pomegranate fractions have shown possible synergistic, or at least supra-additive, interactions against the proliferation and invasiveness of prostate cancer cells. Pomegranate seed oil (PGO) was found to enhance the effect of both fermented PJ and pericarp polyphenols in suppressing DU 145 prostate cancer cell proliferation *in vitro*. The invasion of highly aggressive PC-3 human prostate cancer cells across Matrigel ™ was strongly inhibited by a combination of PJ polyphenols and peel polyphenols (3μg/ml total concentration – 90% inhibition), compared to 60% and 70% inhibition alone, respectively (at 3μg/ml) [16]. The addition of PGO to this mixture increased inhibition to 99% (total 3μg/ml concentration). A combination of PGO, PJ polyphenols and peel polyphenols, produced 95% inhibition of phospholipase (PLA)-2 enzyme *in vitro*, which was much greater than paired or single samples (PLA-2 may promote prostate cancer cell invasiveness) [16]. More detailed research into pomegranate components found a similar complementary inhibition of PC-3 invasion across Matrigel ™ by a combination of caffeic acid, luteolin and punicic acid (total concentration 4μg/ml) [39]. Although this data may indicate synergy, observed effects may well be due to a dose response relationship for one component rather than a definite synergistic interaction [16,39]. Thus, the possibility of synergy requires further investigation. One study considered the effect of a pomegranate fruit extract (PFE) on anthymic nude mice which were implanted with androgen sensitive CWR22Rv1 cells; and found that serum prostate specific antigen (PSA) levels were reduced along with the progression of tumour growth. The PSA level is a diagnostic marker for prostate cancer progression in humans, so these reductions could have implications for human therapy. A phase 2 clinical trial; which involved administering 8 ounces of PJ (~240mL) daily over 2 years to 46 men with rising PSA following surgery or radiation for prostate cancer was carried out. Significant prolongation of PSA doubling time was observed (15 months at baseline to 54 months) without any falls in PSA levels, suggesting a cytostatic effect. PJ intake was associated with antiproliferative (12% decrease) and proapoptotic (17% increase) effects of patient serum *in vitro* on LNCaP prostate tumour cells compared to baseline activity, although the clinical relevance of this data is unclear [9]. Changes in oxidative status/stress and anti-inflammatory mechanisms were postulated to be responsible for these effects rather than direct alterations to PSA levels. These results, coupled with increases in patient serum nitric oxide and general reductions in oxidative stress suggest that PJ may be able to delay prostate cancer re-occurrence, and in doing so postpone the need for poorly tolerable hormonal therapy. This study was conducted without the use of a placebo, so further studies are warranted that validate the potential therapeutic effects of PJ using comparisons with untreated groups.

Colon Cancer

Cancers of the colon have been linked to diets high in saturated fats, and evidence is emerging that an increased intake of polyunsaturated fats (PUFA's) reduces the risk of colorectal malignancies [40]. Conjugated linolenic acids (CLN), including punicic acid, are PUFA's present in PGO [19,41] in levels exceeding 70% [40]. A further investigation into whether dietary PGO could inhibit induced colonic adeno-carcinomas in rats when compared to conjugated linoleic acid (CLA) which has anti-cancer properties. PGO inhibited the emergence and number of colonic tumours, with no apparent side effects. In comparison, CLA only showed minor inhibitory effects. No clear dose response relationship was observed, however. These results were attributed to effects on PPAR-γ, which was elevated in the non-lesional colonic mucosa by PGO, and may protect against cancer by modification of cell growth, cyclooxygenase (COX)-2 regulation and by elevating PGO (CLN)-derived CLA levels in the colonic mucosa and liver [40]. Thus, according to these results PGO provides a chemo-preventive effect against induced colon cancer in rats. Further experiments are recommended to determine whether pre- or post-initiation administration is more effective.

Punicalagin and its hydrolysis product ellagic acid (EA) both showed arrestive properties against human colon cancer Caco-2 cell lines (including induction of apoptosis via an intrinsic mitochondrial pathway and cell cycle arrest in S phase), it was only EA that could have specific effects attributed to it as ET's were hydrolysed in the medium to EA which entered the cells to be metabolised into dimethyl-EA derivatives [42]. These results illustrate that *in vitro* activity of ET's may be due to EA and further derivatives produced by, for example, the human colonic microflora. Indeed, EA derivatives are detectable in human blood, urine and faeces after consumption of ET's.

Chronic inflammation of the colon may increase the risk of colon cancer. Inflammatory cell signalling pathways can lead to the initiation and progression of cancer by inducing DNA damage and sensitivity to growth factors [43]. PJ significantly inhibited tumour necrosis alpha (TNF-α)-induced COX-2 expression in human HT-29 colon cancer cell lines by 79%, with a total pomegranate tannin (TPT) extract producing 55% inhibition, and punicalagin 48% [43]. EA was ineffective in modulating these activities, which indicates that dissimilar fractions of pomegranate alter different pathways of colon cancer cells. Indeed, seed oil possesses chemo-preventive effects possibly through modulation of PPAR-γ and CLA concentrations [40], EA and metabolites cause apoptosis in Caco-2 cell lines [42] and PJ inhibits inflammatory cell signalling in HT-29 cells [43]. This suggests the possibility of synergy, especially in the case of the superior activity of whole PJ over TPT and punicalagin against HT-29 cells. Other studies have discussed the extent of synergy in pomegranate [16,39]. As none of the above studies are in humans, *in vivo* research could further validate these findings.

Breast Cancer

The effects of pomegranate juice (fresh and fermented), and peel and seed oil polyphenols on human breast cancer cells *in vitro* revealed multiple cancer suppressive mechanisms. All four blocked active oestrogen production (34 - 79%), and inhibited both oestrogen dependant and independent cancerous human cell lines [19]. Fermented juice polyphenols attenuated lesion formation in a murine mammary gland organ culture by 47%. Specific fractions showed superior activity in some areas compared to others, which may be a result of their different chemistries: Seed oil (comprising only ~1% polyphenols) exhibited the strongest activity against 17-β-oestradiol biosynthesis, indicating that its content of punicic acid, among others, may be responsible, as it is known to inhibit prostaglandin synthesis and the related CLA's are known anti-cancer agents [19,40]. Fermented juice polyphenols were found to be more active than fresh, although *in vivo* relationships remain to be established. Oestrogenic flavonoid components of PJ and peel (quercetin, naringenin, luteolin, coumestrol) were thought to be partly responsible for the inhibition of oestrogen dependant breast cancer cell lines through an anti-oestrogenic effect at receptors. Other constituents from PJ such as the phenolic acids (caffeic acid) and anthocyanins may also be involved [19]. Thus it appears that pomegranate fractions may possess different, if not complementary, activities against breast cancer.

Research into the potential anti-angiogenic effects of pomegranate fractions used oestrogen dependant and independent human breast cancer cell lines [17]. Fermented PJ and seed oil inhibited signalling in these cells *in vitro* by down-regulating vascular endothelial growth factor (VEGF – pro-angiogenic) in oestrogen dependant cell lines and up-regulating migration inhibitory factor (MIF) in resistant cell lines, possibly through antioxidant and anti-oestrogenic effects [17], which may result in reduced tumour growth. *In vivo* experiments using a chick embryo model showed inhibition of vascularisation by fermented PJ. These results, coupled with inhibitory activity of fermented PJ on fibroblasts and human umbilical vein endothelial cell proliferation suggest a potential anti-angiogenic activity of pomegranate against a variety of cancers.

More recently, an evaluation of the activity of a purified component of fermented PJ using a murine mammary organ culture (MMOC) containing induced lesions, and compared this against fermented PJ and seed oil activities. MMOC provides 75% predictive accuracy of *in vivo* carcinogenesis [44], which makes the results here more comparable to *in vivo* conditions. After 10 days of MMOC treatment with the extracts, the purified compound and the seed oil were more effective than fermented PJ in reducing the number of induced lesions (75-90% more effective) [44]. This suggests that there may be an individual component of PJ with greater activity than the mixture itself, and that a strategy to utilize the seed oil activity (and other fractions) in the juice would be desirable.

These *in vitro* effects of pomegranate on breast cancer warrant further investigations to identify active mechanisms responsible.

Skin Cancer

Using two groups of 30 CD-1 mice with 12-*O*-tetradecanoylphorbol 13-acetate (TPA) induced skin cancer, a topical formulation of PGO applied prior to each TPA administration reduced tumour incidence by 7% and the number of tumours per mouse from 20.8 to 16.3 when compared to a control group (TPA applied biweekly for 20 weeks) [45]. TPA-induced ornithine decarboxylase (ODC) activity was reduced by 17% after one application of PGO 1 hour prior to TPA, which is important considering that ODC activity is associated with cell proliferation and skin cancer promotion, and that it is present in many animal tumours [3,45]. A topical PFE was also found to reduce TPA-induced ODC activity in mice when applied prior to TPA (probably not through direct action on ODC), along with reduced protein expression of COX-2 [3] - an important mediator in cancer promotion.

PFE inhibited tumour growth (like PGO), potentially by multiple pathways [3]: TPA induced skin hyperplasia and oedema were inhibited by application of PFE prior to TPA, as was phosphorylation of mitogen-activated protein kinases (MAPK) and NF-κB activation (which are involved in tumour metastasis/angiogenesis and carcinogenesis, respectively) and other mediators described above. The constituents responsible for these effects, although apparently safe [8], require identification. Pomegranate appears an effective inhibitor of the markers of skin and other cancer promotion [3], which indicates that PGO and PFE could therefore be contenders for a chemo-preventive preparation such as an emollient or patch.

In addition to the reported *in vivo* activities on CD-1 mice, pomegranate extracts show *in vitro* evidence of human skin cell repair [46] and protection against ultraviolet (UV)-B-induced adverse effects [47]. PFE inhibited UV-B mediated activation of MAPK and NF-κB pathways in normal human epidermal keratinocytes when applied 24 hours before UV-B exposure [47]. By blocking these pathways, the adverse effects associated with UV-B exposure (hyperplasia, photoaging, skin cancer) could be prevented [47]. Exact mechanisms behind this activity are unclear, but may involve the antioxidant capacity of PFE neutralizing

UV-B generated reactive oxygen species (ROS) [47]. As polyphenols provide UV-B protection in plants they may also be responsible for this activity.

Aqueous extracts from pomegranate peel and juice, had stimulatory effects on human skin cells [46]. Water soluble peel extracts (which could contain ellagitannins) inhibited enzymic collagen breakdown and promoted collagen synthesis in fibroblasts, whereas the seed oil stimulated keratinocyte proliferation [46]. This observed activity is similar to the retinoid drug class, although the pomegranate fractions may need to be combined to produce a similar level of skin repair [46]. Further research could identify the active constituents and validate these studies by determining the benefits using human volunteers.

Other Activities

Chronic Obstructive Pulmonary Disease (COPD)

Considering the antioxidant activity of PJ polyphenols and that COPD pathology involves oxidative stress. It was investigated whether PJ supplementation for 5 weeks had any affect on COPD patients [48]. Results showed no observed difference between placebo and test groups, and suggested extensive metabolism of PJ polyphenols by the colonic microflora of subjects.

Neurological Protection

Neonatal hypoxic brain injury occurs in around 2 out of every 1000 babies born, and can lead to disabilities and death [49]. PJ supplementation in the mouse maternal diet was investigated for neuroprotective activity, and found significant protection against induced hypoxic-ischemic brain injury to neonatal mice when given during the peripartum period. This activity was thought to be attributable to PJ polyphenols, but the mechanism of action is still uncertain, which indicates that further research needs to be completed [49].

Erectile Dysfunction (ED)

The mechanisms that produce an erection can be disrupted by conditions such as atherosclerosis and diabetes, which involve oxidative stress. Oxidative products have been shown to accumulate in the erectile tissue of rabbits after prolonged ischemia [5]. The antioxidant capacity of PJ was compared to that of red wine and numerous fruit juices when producing penile erection in a rabbit with arteriogenic erectile dysfunction (ED) after long term administration. PJ reduced ischemia-induced cavernous fibrosis (possibly through effects on ACE), promoted smooth muscle relaxation (by restoring nitric oxide (NO) levels) and improved the erectile response, possibly due to the antioxidant capacity of PJ, which had the highest free radical scavenging activity compared to the other samples [5]. As PJ affects

ACE activity in humans and NO is implicated in human vasodilatation, human ED studies may be justifiable.

Adverse Effects

Throughout history, pomegranates have been utilized safely by humans [49,50]. The recent interest in the fruit due to reported health benefits may lead to an increase in consumption worldwide (particularly for PJ), consequently adverse effects may become evident.

There have been conflicting reports regarding the toxicity of pomegranate components. When reviewed, observations include punicalagin induced toxicity in cattle [8], a possible link between crushed pomegranate seed consumption and oesophageal cancer, and allergic reactions to pomegranate seeds [26]. In contrast, an aqueous pomegranate extract was found to be non-mutagenic in the bone marrow of mice at doses up to 2g/kg over a 3 day period [50], and punicalagin may have shown hepato-protective effects in mice [8]. However, these extracts were toxic to these animals in higher doses (4g/kg [50]) [8]. High dose toxicity was evaluated using rats, with a safety margin of punicalagin consumption equivalent to a large volume (194L) of PJ per day for a 70kg person over a 37 day period, and no toxicity to liver function or the bile duct was observed [28]. Human trials considered in this review revealed no toxicity, even over a 3 year period [11].

Drug Interactions

Grapefruit juice and other citrus fruits are known to interact with concurrent medication [14]. Upon administration to human liver microsomes, PJ ($25\mu L$) inhibited carbamazepine 10, 11-epoxidase activity of human cytochrome P450 3A (CYP3A) in a dose dependant fashion, with a similar potency as grapefruit juice [14]. The serum levels of carbamazepine were also raised in a similar fashion to grapefruit juice in rats fed with PJ when compared to control, with pre-systemic irreversible enzyme inhibition of CYP3A being responsible [14]. Indeed, digestive enzyme inhibition by punicalagin has also been postulated as a growth modulator in rats [8].

Bioavailability and Metabolism

In animals ET's are converted to EA and then to EA metabolites. These metabolites and/or small amounts of EA can be found in animal plasma and/or urine [22,51]. More recently, ET's have been shown to be hydrolyzed by the human colonic microflora to form EA *in vitro* [42]. Other constituents of pomegranate juice with antioxidant activity (Vitamin C, anthocyanins, ascorbic acid) demonstrated bioavailability after simulated *in vitro* digestion, and the levels remaining may not have been sufficient for therapeutic effects [53].

The bioavailability of PJ polyphenols was first investigated acutely using one volunteer who ingested 1L PJ, and showed no PJ polyphenols or their metabolites in subsequent plasma samples, although some urinary ET/EA derivatives were present [13] as was the case with animals [53]. In contrast, a similar study measured intact EA in the circulation up until 4-6 hours after ingestion of 180mL PJ (25mg EA, 318mg ET's - zero levels after 6 hours) [51]. However, these results should be viewed with caution, as inter-individual variation in EA absorption or metabolism was not considered and the trials were not conducted over an extended period to assess accumulation [51]. A 5 day trial involving 6 human subjects consuming 1L (16.09 mmoles EA equivalents) of PJ/day found none of the initially ingested polyphenols or their metabolites present in the plasma or urine of the volunteers [13]. Certain metabolites (as found in rat urine [53]) known as 6H-dibenzo[b,d]pyran-6-one derivatives ('urolithins'), were detected in plasma and urine, and are also thought to be produced by the human colon bacteria [11,13]. Large inter-individual differences in amount of metabolites were observed, possibly due to variant colon bacteria [13]. Recent COPD research echoed these findings [48]. No increase in serum antioxidant capacity was observed after PJ administration, with the 6H-dibenzo metabolites actually showing a lower antioxidant capacity than punicalagin [13]. Thus, any health benefits may not be attributable to PJ polyphenols or their metabolites [13].

Subsequent investigations into the bioavailability of pomegranate polyphenols found that after consumption of either two pomegranate extract capsules (800mg extract: 330.4mg ET's, 21.5mg EA) [11] or PJ (180mL of concentrate) [54] by humans EA was in fact bioavailable; reaching similar maximal levels after ~1hr [31, 59] and being completely cleared from plasma after 5 hours [51, 54]. The same 'urolithin' metabolites (A and B) were identified in either plasma [11] or both plasma and urine [54], along with dimethylellagic acid glucuronide (DMEAG) [11,54]. Urolithin metabolites have been postulated to circulate in the blood for over 24 hours [11] although this requires further study. The level of these metabolites in the subjects showed considerable inter-individual variability as previously described [13, 54]. Interestingly, the anti-oxidative capacity of plasma was increased by a maximum of 31.8% over the next 2 hours in one study, which indicates that these metabolites may be antioxidant [11]. Thus, in contrast with earlier research [13], the presence of urolithin metabolites in the plasma and tissues in human subjects makes them a candidate responsible for *in vivo* therapeutic activities [54].

As with many food phenolics [25], the evidence surrounding bioavailability of pomegranate polyphenols is clearly controversial. Research demonstrates that it is the metabolites of PJ polyphenols that may produce some of the observed effects *in vivo*. Thus, the same effects may not be documented if PJ were replaced with these metabolites *in vitro*. These 'urolithins' and possibly other undiscovered metabolites need to be identified and used *in vitro* before placebo controlled clinical trials determine their effect on disease biomarkers and the extent of individual variability.

Levels of Consumption

Estimating the consumption of polyphenols in the diet is often based on limited knowledge of their species-dependant content in foods and the influence of numerous processing or storage conditions. There appears to be a lack of information regarding effective amounts of antioxidant dietary supplements in general [11]. Much *in vitro* work described above may not be easily related to ingested amounts of PJ, as absorption efficiency and metabolism prevent many whole PJ polyphenols from reaching the cells in question. *In vivo* animal data, although useful in terms of initial activity and safety profiles, differs from man in metabolism and clearance pathways [14], suggesting that human data may be more useful here.

Some human studies noted the anti-atherosclerotic potential of PJ; with patients consuming 50mL (1.5mmol polyphenols) daily over periods from weeks to years. Beneficial vascular-related modifications were also found in diabetic patients using either concentrated PJ (40g/day over 8 weeks) or PJ (50mL/day over 3 months). Elsewhere, larger daily amounts (240mL/day) benefited CHD over 3 months [32]. However no beneficial effects of 400mL/day (2.66g polyphenols) of PJ on COPD over 5 weeks were noted, which may suggest poor penetration into some tissues. These studies highlight the need for standardized administration volumes which would allow reliable comparison between studies.

It appears that a realistic amount of PJ consumed orally per day could provide therapeutic activity, irrespective of concerns over bioavailability. However, inter-individual variability in polyphenol metabolism and absorption requires further study, as those who have a greater digestive capacity for PJ may need to consume more to experience an equivalent therapeutic effect. Polyphenol content differences between cultivars also require further investigation, as the same variety was not always used for the studies in this review. Considering a lack of reported adverse effects the consumption of as little as 50mL PJ per day may be appropriate to provide adequate polyphenols for therapeutic benefit, although long-term safety evaluations are recommended.

Conclusion

Polyphenolic constituents of pomegranate fruits have been studied by *in vitro* or *in vivo* animal research, with some areas having been investigated using only these methods (e.g. breast/colon/skin cancer anti-bacterial/viral), and this research suggests use in topical formulation for a number of conditions.

Research has already been carried out which investigates anti-carcinogenic (prostate), anti-diabetic and particularly anti-atherosclerotic (and related CAS and CHD) effects using pomegranate in man. With the exception of COPD all these trials yielded positive results with regards to disease modification; with evidence of reductions in factors leading to atherosclerosis and prostate cancer. This demonstrates the apparent clinical benefits of PJ, and supports a role as a dietary health supplement.

The safe use of pomegranate throughout history and the lack of adverse effects during clinical trials promote its use as a dietary adjunct. It has been shown that EA and EA derivatives ('urolithins', DMEAG) were present in human plasma and urine after PJ consumption, and that these substances may be responsible for some *in vivo* antioxidant effects. Progress has been made to produce food supplements containing mainly EA (as ellagitannins) [55]. However, a high EA content has been questioned [56] as the most appropriate amount of EA for optimal benefit may be quite low, and the role of synergy between pomegranate constituents may exist based on *in vitro* evidence and the possibility of this activity arising from uncharacterized PJ derivatives. Thus, a full metabolite profile is necessary before PJ can be accepted as an effective and acceptable method of providing therapeutic benefits attributed to pomegranate.

Cocoa/Chocolate

Cocoa, in the form of chocolate and cocoa beverage, has gained much interest in recent years for its potential contribution to health and, in particular, for its positive effects on the cardiovascular system in that it might protect against cardiovascular disease. Cocoa is prepared from the seeds of *Cocoa theobroma*, a tree that is native to South America [57]. The use of cocoa as a medicine originates back to ancient Mayan and Aztec civilizations, where it was also used for ceremonial rituals and considered a divine food. During this period, cocoa was prepared as a beverage [57] and was not processed into chocolate until after its arrival into Europe [58].

Chocolate is made up of varying amounts of sugar, milk and cocoa butter [59], in addition to cocoa liquor, the ingredient considered to be responsible for the proposed health benefits [60]. Cocoa liquor is produced from the seeds of *Cocoa theobroma* by various processes including fermentation and roasting [60]. There is a complex array of compounds present in cocoa seeds including caffeine and theobromine [61], but of particular interest are the polyphenol flavanoids that compose sixty per cent of the seed [62]. Examples of flavanoids present in cocoa include quercetin, condensed tannins and anthocyanidins [59]. The major flavanoids present are epicatechin and catechin, which are known as flavanols, a subset of flavanoids. It is considered that epicatechin, catechin and their oligomers, known as procyanidins, are primarily responsible for the proposed health benefits offered by cocoa and chocolate [63]. However, many studies have investigated the *in vitro* properties of only epicatechin and its oligomers. Nevertheless, it is important to note that other polyphenols in chocolate may have important contributions to the health benefits. For example, catechin is known for its antioxidant activities and the results of a survey found that chocolate contributed twenty per cent of catechin monomers to the total catechin intake in the diet of a Dutch population, of which tea contributed fifty five per cent of this total intake [64]. Similarly, quercetin, which is present in chocolate, has been found to exhibit antioxidant properties [65]. The structures of the two major flavonoids found in cocoa are shown in Figure 2.

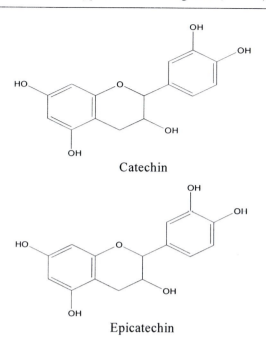

Figure 2. The structures of the two major cocoa flavonoids.

The polyphenol content can vary considerably between different types of chocolate as a result of the manufacturing processes employed [60]. Many of the studies investigating the health benefits of chocolate use specially manufactured procyanidin rich chocolate with procyanidin concentrations up to 688mg procyanidins per 100g chocolate [66]. Commercially available dark chocolate contains up to 365mg procyanidins per 100g of chocolate [67], and has been shown to inhibit platelet coagulation [68]. In contrast, commercially available milk chocolate has not shown any significant health benefits, and only contains up to 70mg procyanidins per 100g chocolate [59]. White chocolate is not composed of cocoa liquor and thus does not contain any procyanidins [69].

Bioavailability and Metabolism

The polyphenols are a significant component in chocolate, and must reach sufficient quantities in the plasma in order to have a positive effect on the health status [61,66]. The plasma levels of epicatechin monomers have been demonstrated to reach a peak concentration of 0.7µmol/L two hours after the consumption of 80g dark chocolate [61]. Furthermore, epicatechin is mostly cleared from the plasma after eight hours [61,66,70]. The epicatechin dimer has also been detected in the plasma after chocolate ingestion, however, the bioavailability of higher epicatechin oligomers is not known [58]. The levels of epicatechin and its oligomers in the plasma are governed by their absorption across the gastrointestinal membrane and subsequent metabolism and elimination from the body. Firstly, the absorption of epicatechin across the gastrointestinal wall depends on the amount present in chocolate and hence, the type of chocolate ingested is an important factor as previously described. Furthermore, a query remains whether milk, either present in chocolate or taken in addition with chocolate, reduces the absorption of epicatechin, possibly by the formation of bonds between milk proteins and epicatechin [71]. Other studies suggest that milk has no affect on the absorption of epicatechin from chocolate [61,72]. It is clearly possible that other dietary components may influence the absorption of epicatechin from chocolate.

Secondly, the metabolism of epicatechin can affect its plasma levels [61,70]. Epicatechin is metabolised to glucuronide conjugates in the gastrointestinal mucosa, to glucuronide and sulphate conjugates in the liver [70], and is also broken down by bacteria in the colon [61]. So far, there have not been any studies conducted on the activity of epicatechin metabolites. However, it is worth noting that the methods used to assess epicatechin plasma levels make no distinction between epicatechin in its pure form and as glucuronide and sulphate conjugates [70]. Finally, many studies agree that the elimination of epicatechin from the body is rapid; the plasma is cleared within eight hours after the ingestion of chocolate [61,66,70]. In line with this, it has been suggested that flavanols should be consumed frequently in order to get the most health benefits [70]. However, ingesting large amounts of chocolate poses obvious health implications; thus fruit, vegetables and green tea should be relied upon as other dietary sources of flavanols [69]. Many studies support the fact that the bioavailability of epicatechin after the ingestion of dark chocolate is sufficient to produce a physiological response, for instance, plasma epicatechin levels have been demonstrated to rise in association with an increased plasma antioxidant capacity [70] and an improved endothelial function [73]. Further investigations are required to see whether the physiological responses caused by epicatechin have any relevance on overall health status.

Cardiac Activity

Many *in vitro* and *in vivo* investigations support the fact that chocolate may have a positive influence on cardiovascular health, but no epidemiological studies have yet been conducted to assess the relationship between the ingestion of chocolate and the risk of coronary heart disease [59]. A major mechanism through which chocolate may offer protection against cardiovascular disease is through its antioxidant activity [66]. Reactive oxidant species cause cellular damage and can oxidise low density lipoproteins (LDL) within the body, these processes have a role in the onset of atherosclerosis [58]. The antioxidant properties of chocolate have been demonstrated in healthy individuals by an increase in antioxidant status [70] and inhibition of LDL oxidation [74]. Similarly, the ability of cocoa procyanidins to protect against the oxidation by peroxynitrite has been demonstrated *in vitro* [75]. Other contributing factors to cardiovascular disease, atherosclerosis and thrombosis are endothelial dysfunction, inflammatory responses and activated platelets [59]. Chocolate has been shown to improve endothelial function *in vivo* [73], inhibit platelet activation and aggregation [76,77] and affect the modulation of cytokines to favour an anti-inflammatory state *in vitro* [78,79].

It has been postulated that the antioxidant activity of chocolate might offer protection against coronary heart disease and other chronic disease states [66]. For instance, the progression of atherosclerosis is associated with the oxidation of LDL particles in the body [74], and this process has been inhibited *in vitro* by procyanidins isolated from cocoa [74,80] and *in vivo* by dark chocolate [81]. Similarly, *in vitro* studies have demonstrated that cocoa procyanidin oligomers can provide protection against the action of peroxynitrite, which is a potent oxidising and nitrating agent responsible for causing tissue damage associated with some disease states [75,82]. In addition, the ability of chocolate to modulate immune function [83] and inhibit platelet activation [77] has been suggested to have antioxidant involvement.

An *in vivo* study demonstrated that the ingestion of dark chocolate was followed by an increase in plasma levels of epicatechin to sufficient quantities to produce an associated increase in plasma oxidant capacity [70]. However, it is recognised that the contribution of cocoa procyanidins to the antioxidant defence system needs to be determined in order to know the significance of its antioxidant activity [66]. Furthermore, it has been suggested that to determine the clinical importance that this increase in oxidation status by epicatechin has on the health status of an individual, other markers need to be examined. One such marker that has been investigated is the susceptibility of LDL to oxidation, which is known to play a role in atherosclerosis [66,74,81].

Chocolate has demonstrated an ability to inhibit LDL oxidation in humans. A four week study of chocolate and cocoa ingestion reported a decrease in LDL oxidation susceptibility [81]. Therefore, these studies suggest that chocolate ingestion may have the potential to reduce the risk of atherosclerosis, only in the case where LDL oxidation is a contributing factor to atherosclerosis.

The ability of chocolate to inhibit LDL oxidation has also been reported *in vitro*, using artificial LDL particles and oxidation models [74,80]. These studies have been helpful to identify specific procyanidins involved in the response, in addition to identifying the possible mechanisms of action. In particular, a study measured the time of onset of LDL oxidation, which depends on the antioxidant activity in the particle [80]. The results of this study showed that epicatechin and catechin monomers inhibited LDL oxidation significantly by prolonging the time of onset of oxidation. Another study reported that cocoa procyanidins caused significant inhibition of copper catalysed LDL oxidation [74]. This was shown as a reduction in oxidation products within the LDL particle. The results of this study are suggested to support the metal ion chelating mechanism, due to an increase in antioxidant activity as the number of procyanidin monomers increased. Additionally, the study also suggests that procyanidins may evoke a response by a free radical mechanism [74].

The precise mechanism by which chocolate procyanidins may function as antioxidants is unknown, but there are several postulations in addition to the metal ion chelating and free radical scavenging previously described. Firstly, the procyanidins may have a sparing effect on antioxidants already within the particle. This has been demonstrated *in vitro* where a mixture of epicatechin and catechin effectively delayed the depletion of the antioxidant α-tocopherol within the LDL particle [80]. Therefore, procyanidins are able to protect LDL particles from oxidation indirectly by maintaining levels of antioxidants present in the particle. The author suggests that procyanidins, being hydrophilic, do not enter the hydrophobic core of the LDL particle, but rather adsorbs to the outer surface where they are able to restrict the movement of radical ions into the particle [80]. A further mechanism to explain the antioxidant activity of procyanidins is by exposing the LDL particles to procyanidins for long periods of time, which may change the composition of the LDL particles making them less susceptible to oxidation [81].

The concentrations used in these *in vitro* studies are consistent with the plasma epicatechin levels that have been observed after the ingestion of dark chocolate *in vivo*, suggesting that levels are sufficient to evoke similar responses. For instance, two hours after the consumption of 80g dark chocolate, plasma epicatechin levels reach 0.7μM [61] The concentrations of epicatechin from the *in vitro* studies to give the observed effects were 1.0μM, which inhibited production of oxidation products from copper catalysed LDL oxidation by thirty three per cent [74]. Similarly, 0.5μM of epicatechin and catechin monomers were able to significantly prolong the onset of LDL oxidation and effectively delay the consumption of the antioxidant α-tocopherol [80]. Thus, the concentrations which are able to demonstrate antioxidant potential *in vitro* are similar to those that have been observed in the plasma.

Effects on Endothelial Function

Another mechanism by which chocolate may reduce the progression of atherosclerosis and, hence, reduce the risk of coronary heart disease, is through its ability to improve endothelial function. This has been demonstrated in a number of studies conducted in healthy individuals [73,84,85], and also in individuals who have known impaired endothelial function, including the elderly [86], smokers [87], and individuals with hypertension [88]. Furthermore, dark chocolate can significantly increase insulin sensitivity in healthy volunteers, which might prove to be beneficial in the prevention of obesity and hypertension, two conditions that are affected by insulin resistance [88,89].

Endothelial dysfunction occurs when the endothelium looses its ability to control thrombosis and vascular tone [84]. Such dysfunction is an early manifestation of atherosclerosis and coronary heart disease [84]. It is thought to be present in individuals who have diabetes, hypertension, hypercholestelemia, and also occurs with increased age and cigarette smoking [84,89]. Endothelial dysfunction arises from a reduction of nitric oxide and is, indeed, characterised by a reduced nitric oxide bioavailability and a reduced vasodilatory ability [73,85]. Various causative factors may contribute to a reduction in nitric oxide bioavailability in endothelial dysfunction. Studies have suggested that endothelial dysfunction is reversible [90]; probably by increasing nitric oxide bioavailability by interfering with one or more of the above processes [84,85,89].

Dark chocolate is postulated to improve endothelial function in healthy individuals by inducing vasodilation, as shown by an increase in flow mediated dilation [73,84,85]. Furthermore, this observed vasodilation has been associated with an increase in epicatechin plasma levels [73]. Many *in vitro* and *in vivo* studies suggest that epicatechin may evoke vasodilation, and thus improve endothelial function, by increasing the bioavailability of the vasodilator, nitric oxide [84,85,89]. This mechanism is supported by the fact that flow mediated dilation is primarily dependent upon the release of nitric oxide from the endothelium [84,85]. A further investigation into the effects of cocoa procyanidins on endothelial dilation *in vitro* has demonstrated that certain procyanidins evoke endothelial dependent relaxation of rabbit aortic rings precontracted with noradrenaline [91]. In particular, the tetramer to decamer oligomers, isolated from cocoa extract, produced significant relaxation of the aorta, which was reversed by N^G- nitro-L-arginine methyl ester (L-NAME). This compound is an analogue of the precursor to nitric oxide, L-arginine, and is also a specific inhibitor of NOS. Thus, this study supports the hypothesis that cocoa procyanidins evoke endothelial relaxation through increasing nitric oxide bioavailability due to an ability to activate NOS [91]. Moreover, the involvement of NOS in increasing nitric oxide availability is a proposed mechanism by which dark chocolate may improve endothelial function in humans. This mechanism is deduced from the fact that the increase in flow mediated dilation induced by dark chocolate was abolished after the infusion of a NOS inhibitor [85].

In addition to activating NOS, cocoa procyanidins may increase the levels of nitric oxide and evoke endothelial relaxation through an antioxidant mechanism. For instance, chocolate may prevent the degradation of nitric oxide to peroxynitrite by inhibiting its oxidation by superoxide [88].

In addition to increasing endothelial function of healthy individuals, chocolate has also shown to be beneficial in individuals with known endothelial impairment including smokers [87], the elderly [86], and individuals with high blood pressure [88]. It is considered that the bioavailability of nitric oxide reduces with age, possibly due to a decrease in concentrations of the precursor L-arginine or the accumulation of a NOS inhibitor within the body [86]. Smoking is also associated with a reduced bioavailability of nitric oxide. This is because smoking increases oxidative stress in the body, which damages the endothelium and reduces the production of nitric oxide from the endothelium [87]. In a similar manner, endothelial dysfunction is a common feature in hypertensive patients. As a result, the endothelium looses its ability to produce nitric oxide and, thus, its ability to control blood pressure diminishes [88].

Research also indicates that dark chocolate has promising effects in improving insulin sensitivity. It is suggested that a decline in endothelial function can lead to insulin resistance, which results in a reduction of insulin-mediated glucose uptake [88]. Insulin resistance is associated with conditions such as obesity and hypertension [88,89]. Insulin sensitivity is considered to be dependent on the availability of nitric oxide [89]. Studies have investigated the effects of dark chocolate on insulin sensitivity in healthy individuals by assessing two markers of insulin sensitivity: the quantitative insulin sensitivity check index and insulin sensitivity index. One marker for insulin sensitivity has been assessed - homeostasis model assessment of insulin resistance. All of these markers are obtained from an oral glucose tolerance test [89]. Two studies showed that after 15 days of ingesting dark chocolate insulin sensitivity was increased and insulin resistance was decreased significantly [88,89]. Furthermore, this improvement in insulin sensitivity has been correlated with an improvement in endothelial function, suggesting an association between the two events [88].

The studies that have investigated the effects of chocolate on endothelial function are short term, and thus, the long term effects of chocolate on endothelial function are unknown [73]. Therefore, long term studies are required to assess the prospect that dark chocolate may prevent the progression of cardiovascular disease through improving endothelial function and insulin sensitivity.

Effects on Platelet Function

Another mechanism by which chocolate may reduce atherosclerosis, and also prevent the progression of thromboembolism, is by modulating platelet activity.

Studies have demonstrated that chocolate may have anti aggregating properties by inhibiting platelet activation [76,77,92] and decreasing platelet function [68,76,77]. Firstly, the inhibition of platelet activation after the ingestion of a cocoa beverage has been shown by a decreased PAC-1 binding on adrenaline and ADP induced platelets [76,92]. PAC-1 is a ligand for the active conformation of glycoprotein IIb-IIIa and so is a useful marker for platelet activation [76]. Other markers of activation include the expression of P-Selectin and microparticles, which are formed on activated platelets [76]. Cocoa has been shown to suppress the expression of ADP induced P Selectin [76,92], but not adrenaline induced expression [76,77,92]. Similarly, a reduction in the formation of microparticles has been demonstrated after cocoa ingestion [76]. The ability of cocoa to inhibit the activation of platelets is attributed to epicatechin and its oligomers since plasma epicatechin levels increase in association with activity [77]. The involvement of epicatechin and its oligomers is supported by an *in vitro* study, which incubated cocoa trimer and pentamer procyanidins with whole blood. The result was a reduction in platelet activation by decreasing the binding of PAC-1 and the expression P-Selectin in adrenaline stimulated platelets [92].

Cocoa was shown to reduce the time of clot formation in platelets stimulated with collagen-adrenaline [76,77] and collagen-ADP [77]. Chocolate was shown to reduce aggregation of platelets when stimulated with collagen, but not ADP [68]. There are two important conclusions that can be obtained from these results, firstly, that chocolate may have anti-aggregation properties through its ability to inhibit platelet function, an important event in the thrombus formation. Secondly, chocolate may inhibit platelet aggregation through a mechanism similar to aspirin [68,77]. In fact, the consumption of dark chocolate was shown to have only slightly lower effect than that of aspirin [77]

One possible mechanism by which procyanidins may inhibit platelet aggregation is by modulating the synthesis of eicosanoids [93]. This was demonstrated by a study in which cocoa procyanidins increased the production of prostacyclin and decreased the production of leukotrienes [93]. Thus, cocoa procyanidins shifted the balance of eicosanoid to favour an anti-aggregatory state. Another suggested mechanism is through antioxidation whereby chocolate reduces the levels of superoxide anion, which in turn prevents the oxidation of nitric oxide to peroxynitrite. As a result, nitric oxide levels in the body are maintained which promotes the anti-aggregation effects of nitric oxide [77].

Effects on Immune Response

Some *in vitro* studies have reported that cocoa procyanidins may have the ability to modulate cytokines that are involved in the inflammatory response. In particular, certain cocoa procyanidin fractions and cocoa extract have been demonstrated to modulate the production and secretion of the cytokines interleukin (IL)-1β, IL-2, and IL-4 from T lymphocytes or peripheral blood mononuclear cells (PBMC). In addition, cocoa extract and epicatechin have been shown to reduce the expression of the IL-2 receptor subunit, IL-2Rα, on T Lymphocytes. These cytokines have a role in the onset of inflammation, and the findings suggest that cocoa procyanidins may possess anti-inflammatory activity, which could potentially be helpful in disease states that involve an activated immune system, such as arthritis, psoriasis and eczema [78,79].

Cocoa procyanidins have demonstrated variable activity on the production and secretion of these cytokines. *In vitro* studies have demonstrated that cocoa procyanidins can significantly modulate the transcription and subsequent secretion of IL-1β in PBMC to varying degrees depending on the size of the procyanidin oligomer [79,94]. It was generally shown that monomer to tetramer procyanidin oligomers suppressed gene transcription in stimulated PBMC and reduced the secretion of IL-1β . In contrast, the pentamer to decamer procyanidin oligomers increased gene transcription in stimulated PBMC with a resulting increase in IL-1β secretion [79,94]. Since IL-1β is involved in initiating the immune response, the results suggest that smaller procyanidins may have anti-inflammatory activity whereas the larger oligomers may promote inflammation when exclusively taking IL-1β modulation into consideration. However, the actual ability of these procyanidins to regulate immune function *in vivo* is uncertain since the immune response is regulated by a number of cytokines. Furthermore, the cocoa procyanidins were investigated as individual fractions in these studies, and so the overall affect of these procyanidins on the inflammatory response may depend on synergistic reactions [79]. The affect on inflammatory response also depends on the bioavailability of these procyanidin oligomers in the body and the ability to reach sufficient concentrations at the site of action. Up until now, only epicatechin and catechin monomers and dimers have been detected in the plasma [58,61]. Interestingly, a study, which involved six weeks of cocoa beverage ingestion, showed that concentrations of IL-1β did not change, which suggesting that immune response is not regulated by chocolate through IL-1β modulation [95].

In vitro studies have reported that the transcription and secretion of the cytokine IL-2 from PBMC may also be modulated by cocoa procyanidins [78,79]. In particular, the pentamer to heptamer oligomers demonstrated a significant inhibition of IL-2 transcription in stimulated PBMC [79]. This finding is supported by a study in which isolated epicatechin and cocoa extract were able to reduce the secretion of IL-2 from stimulated T lymphocytes [78]. These results demonstrate that cocoa procyanidins may have anti-inflammatory activity by reducing the levels of IL-2, which are required for the subsequent activation of T lymphocytes. Furthermore, it has been demonstrated that cocoa extract and isolated epicatechin significantly reduce the expression of IL-2Rα on stimulated T lymphocyte cells [78]. Conflicting opinions exist on the relationship between IL-2 secretion and IL-2Rα expression. One viewpoint is that IL-2 enhances its own expression of the receptor. Another perspective is that there is no link between IL-2 secretion and IL-2Rα expression. Nevertheless, the results show that a decrease in IL-2Rα expression by cocoa procyanidins renders the T lymphocyte less sensitive to the effects of IL-2 in eliciting an immune response [78].

Conflicting results have appeared on the effects of cocoa procyanidins on the transcription and secretion of IL-4 [78,79]. The oligomer procyanidins have been shown to inhibit gene transcription and secretion of this cytokine in stimulated PBMC, with the hexamer, decamer and octamer having a greater activity [79]. In contrast, a different study reported an increase in IL-4 secretion from T lymphocytes after incubation with epicatechin and cocoa extract [78]. The cocoa extract takes into account synergistic reactions and so may give a greater indication of the modulation of IL-4 *in vitro* by cocoa. If this is the case, an increase in IL-4 levels results in anti-inflammatory activity. However, if IL-4 levels decrease then it suggests cocoa may induce an inflammatory response.

The precise mechanism of action by which cocoa is able to modulation the production and secretion of cytokines is unknown, although it has been suggested that the opposite effects of IL-2 and IL-4 secretion indicate that cocoa procyanidins may act through a variety of pathways [78]. It is postulated that procyanidins modulate the cytokine at a level of transcription by an antioxidant mechanism [78,79]. Reactive oxygen species are responsible for upregulating transcription of the cytokine gene by activating the nuclear transcription factor κB, a process that might be inhibited by procyanidins [78,79]. This mechanism is supported by a study that shows a greater inhibition of IL-2 secretion by cocoa procyanidins when they were added two hours before the T lymphocytes were stimulated, than when added simultaneously. It suggested that this two hours might be essential in order for the procyanidins to enter the cell and modulate gene expression [78].

Further investigations are required to determine whether the reported ability of cocoa procyanidins to modulate the synthesis and secretion of immunoregulatory cytokines *in vitro,* are reflected in humans. Studies that have investigated the effects of isolated cocoa procyanidins *in vitro* have been useful to observe specific procyanidins that exhibit activity, and in investigating the mechanism by which they might modulate the inflammatory response. However, there are limitations to these *in vitro* studies that highlight the necessity of *in vivo* investigations using chocolate. Firstly, synergistic or antagonistic interactions may exist between procyanidin oligomers and so the activity observed when present together in chocolate might be different from that when in isolation [72]. Secondly, the immune response is a complex process with the involvement of many different cytokines and other components [78,79.94]. Hence, the *in vitro* models that are used to assess the effect of cocoa procyanidins on cytokines in isolation do truly represent the human physiology. Thirdly, the bioavailability of epicatechin and its oligomers from chocolate and the appearance of relevant quantities of these compounds at the site of action are important considerations. Finally, it is necessary to assess clinical markers of inflammation *in vivo* to ascertain whether the observed regulatory activity on specific cytokines has the potential to contribute to immune status as a whole. Furthermore, the effect of chocolate could be investigated in individuals with inflammatory disease states, such as arthritis, to determine whether there is a potential role of cocoa in this context.

Conclusion

Studies conducted in human volunteers support the fact that chocolate may have the potential to reduce the risk of atherosclerosis through antioxidant mechanisms in addition to inhibiting platelet activation, improving endothelial function and modulating the inflammatory response.

The major flavanoids in cocoa that are considered to be responsible for these observed effects are epicatechin and its oligomers.

In order for chocolate to also be considered as a therapeutic source of flavanoids, the activity of other components present in chocolate must also be considered. The cocoa seed contains caffeine, which is a weak competitive antagonist of various adenosine receptors. Caffeine has the potential to promote the anti-aggregatory effects of cocoa procyandins as demonstrated by a delay in clot formation by collagen-ADP stimulated platelets [76]. Similarly, cocoa seed contains high levels theobromine, which, like cocoa procyanidins, inhibit platelet aggregation [76]. Epicatechin is cleared from the body within eight hours and thus frequent cocoa flavanoid intake is suggested in order to maintain plasma levels at a concentration necessary for cardioprotective activity to occur [93]. Confectionary chocolate contains high levels of fat and so excessive chocolate consumption may contribute to obesity and have a detrimental effect on cardiovascular health [59]. However, the primary form of fat in dark chocolate is the saturated fat, stearic acid [96,97] which has been shown to have neutral effects on cholesterol and is actually considered to offer protection against cardiovascular disease [97].

Existing studies have investigated the health benefits derived from chocolate following short term consumption, either as a single ingestion or over several weeks. Therefore, further studies are necessary in order to determine whether the potential of chocolate to act as an antioxidant, inhibit the activation and function of platelets, improve endothelial function and modulate inflammatory cytokines have any long term significance in preventing cardiovascular disease. Clinical markers, such as the susceptibility of LDL oxidation, flow mediated dilation and platelet coagulation, are useful to measure the effects of chocolate in the body. Further investigation is required to determine the involvement of these markers in cardiovascular disease in order to assess the contribution of chocolate in protecting against disease. Additionally, there should be further investigation into the effects of chocolate in different disease states, such as the effect of chocolate on endothelial function in hypertenstives. Finally, an epidemiological study would be of benefit to determine the association between chocolate consumption and cardiovascular disease.

Cranberry

The American cranberry, *Vaccinium macrocarpon*, the fruit of small woody plants [98] is indigenous to North America. Cranberries are extremely sour, the pH of the single-strength juice is approximately 2.5 [99] on account of the berries being low in sugar and having a high acid content. Thus, cranberry is commonly delivered as a juice, developed in the early 1950s [100] consisting of single strength cranberry juice, diluted and sweetened to remove the astringency. The astringency is the result of the high tannin content present. [101]

Cranberry fruit is rich in polyphenolics. Analysis of cranberry juice compounds [102] found that one sample consisted of 56% flavonoids and 44% phenolic acids. Of eleven common fruits analysed, cranberry had the highest total phenolic content [103] but, the concentrations found in food varies depending on environmental, genetic and technological factors. However, the health benefits of polyphenols depends on sufficient intake and bioavailability *in vivo*. Isolation and quantification of individual components in cranberry is complicated because of the diversity of the compounds present and the extensive difference in levels.

Three flavonoid classes have been identified in cranberry; the anthocyanins, the flavonols, for example quercetin and myricetin, which often occur as flavonol glycosides, and the flavan-3-ols, which consist of monomer forms of catechin and their respective oligomers and polymers producing proanthocyanidins [104] or condensed tannins [101] Proanthocyanidins were found to be predominantly made up of epicatechin extender units with the molecular weight depending on the number of flavan-3-ol monomers that make up the structure. The dominant entities where found to be tetramers, degree of polymerisation of 4 (Dp4) and pentamers (Dp5). Hexamers and heptamers were also identified. Each entity consisted of at least one A-type linkage. The interflavonoid bond that links proanthocyanidin units can be either the A-, B- or C-type [105].

Additionally, a large molecular weight, non-dialysable material known as NDM, with a molecular weight greater than 15,000, prepared from cranberry juice has also been shown to have anti-adhesive activity [106] NDM inhibits the adhesion of *Helicobacter pylori in vitro,* [107,108] prevents co-aggregation of oral bacteria [109,110,111] and inhibits influenza virus adhesion [106] NDM, is composed of 61.5% proanthocyanidins [110] Although it has been proposed to be the cranberry proanthocyanidins that are one of the active anti-adhesion agents [112] results and unpublished data show that NDM is 4 – 6 times more potent than proanthocyanidins in preventing adhesion and co-aggregation of bacteria [106].

Cranberry is also beneficial in atherosclerosis, that can lead to the development of cardiovascular disease (CVD). In particular it was the proanthocyanidins, oligomers of catechin and epicatechin linked by A- and B-type interflavan bonds, that inhibited LDL oxidation, thus preventing the onset of atherosclerosis [113]. Larger oligomers, containing gallocatechin and/or epigallocatechin have also been reported. Additional studies also indicate that cranberry could prevent cardiovascular disease via interfering with other processes that lead to the chronic disease [114,115,116] It has been demonstrated that there is a direct relationship between phenolic content and antioxidant activity [103].

Cranberry having one of the highest concentrations of quercetin, has many health benefits [104] It was found that quercetin was solely present in the hydrolysed cranberry juices, where it accounted for 42% of the total phenolics and 75% of the total flavonoids [102]. Quercetin is usually found conjugatedas glycosides, the major flavonol glycoside being quercetin-3-β-galactoside [104] Cranberry and particular flavonoids present, including quercetin, have been shown to inhibit tumour cell proliferation *in vitro* [103,117-119] A fraction known as fraction 6, elucidated using acidified methanol, contained flavonoids that demonstrated anti-proliferative activity [117,118] Quercetin, myricetin and resveratrol all found in cranberry may contribute to the activity of fraction 6. Further analysis of cranberry using bioactivity-guided fractionation found that quercetin and the phenolic acid, ursolic acid, inhibited proliferation of HepG$_2$ human liver cancer and MCF-7 breast cancer cells *in vitro* [118] Additionally, a study previously conducted in 2003 [119] further identified that two triterpenoid esters derived from cranberry inhibited the proliferation of the ME180 cervical, MCF-7 breast and the PC3 prostate tumour cell lines, and hence tumour cell growth. These were the cis- and tran- isomers of 3-O-*p*-hydroxycinnamoyl ursolic acid. This evidence indicates the potential anticancer effects of phytochemicals, particularly the polyphenols, found in cranberry. The structures of ursolic acid, quercetin and resveratrol are shown in Figure 3.

glucoside and galactoside.

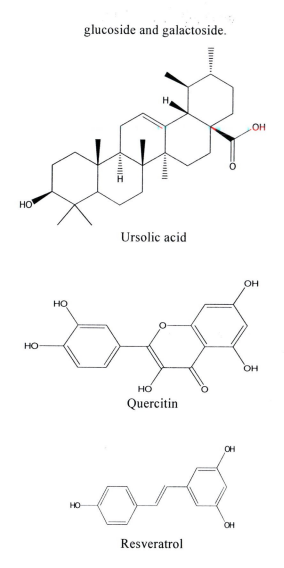

Ursolic acid

Quercitin

Resveratrol

Figure 3.

Results indicate that the anti-adhesion mechanism offered by polyphenolic compounds of cranberry could act to prevent infections, in the urinary tract, the gastrointestinal tract, the oral cavity, and influenza outbreaks. Furthermore, cranberry has demonstrated that health benefits in the development of cardiovascular disease and cancer could also be achieved.

It has been suggested that it is the low molecular weight constituents that are the active anti-adhesion agents in cranberry [112]

Unique anti-bacterial activity of cranberry [120], may be a result of a different composition of polyphenols compared to other fruits, in particular the presence of the unique

A-type linkage in the proanthocyanidins. A health benefit exhibited by cranberry, particularly of the proanthocyanidins, has been shown to be the anti-adhesion activity towards P-fimbriated *E.coli* on uroepithelial cells [112,120] Analysis of the proanthocyanidins found them to be composed of the repeating unit of epicatechin, with one or more A-type interflavanyl linkage [120].

Pathogenic Adhesion and Resulting Infections

Adherence of pathogenic bacteria to eukaryotic cells is the initial step in the establishment of an infection, allowing greater capability of bacteria colonising the host [121] This has been amply demonstrated in clinical studies showing that bacterial attachment to uroepithelial cells, predominantly *Escherichia coli,* results in urinary tract infections (UTIs) [122,123]. Once attachment has taken place, bacteria can proliferate and synthesise toxins that mediate tissue damage without being removed by shear forces that cleanse mucosal surfaces, such as urinary and salivary flow in the oral cavity.

It has been demonstrated that it is usually fimbriae that are the organs of adhesion, allowing initiation of an infection [124] . Fimbriae are described as stable filaments of proteinaceous subunits. The surface lectins show specific recognition and complementarily bind to sugar moieties on the surface of mucosal and endothelial cells [121]. Therefore therapies, particularly the consumption of products containing carbohydrates and lectins, that may interfere with the fimbrial attachment and result in anti-adhesion, have the potential to eradicate the causative pathogens that result in various infections.

Urinary Tract Infections (UTIs)

UTIs affect 20% of women aged between 20 and 56 years per annum [125] UTIs can also
occur in men however, they are approximately 50 times more common in women. This is probably due to the extra urethral length in men resulting in bacteria ascending less easily. Furthermore, children are a group with a high probability of UTIs. Boys between the age of 6 and 12 months frequently suffer UTIs but on the whole girls endure UTIs three times more often [126]

Symptomatic UTIs are diagnosed when bacteria in the urine reaches a threshold number of approximately 100 colony-forming units (CFU)/ml. This stage being identified as bacteriuria [125] UTIs consist of cystitis, urethral syndrome and pyelonephritis. Symptoms include dysuria, frequency and urgency to urinate, cloudy urine and occasionally haematuria. Faecal flora is a source of organisms that can instigate UTIs. They colonise the periurethral tissues and subsequently pass through the urethra, proliferating in the sterile urinary tract [126]. The uropathogen most commonly detected, in 70 – 95% [125] of cases, is *Escherichia coli.* There is anecdotal evidence supporting this from the 2002 longitudinal study performed where of the 235 women with UTIs, 69% were infected with *E.coli* and additionally, *E.coli* was accountable for a further 2.4% of infections in combination with other pathogens [127].

The consumption of cranberries has been linked to the treatment of UTIs for decades. However, epidemiological evidence and randomized controlled trials now show a positive link between ingestion of cranberries and prevention of UTIs [122,123] One study of volunteers dosed with a single serving of cranberry juice and the results illustrated that the anti-adhesion activity of cranberry was present and continued to exist in the uroepithelium 8 hours post-consumption [120]. It was thought until the 1970s [98] that cranberry's anti-adhesive effect was due to acidification of urine. This mechanism was not substantiated in a study in 2005 [120] in which urine samples showing bacterial anti-adhesion activity had a pH of 6.5. The current theory is that particular compounds in cranberry juice prevent adherence of *E.coli*, via their fimbriae, to the uroepithelium and hence prevent the establishment of infection.

There are two common fimbrial types abundant on the *E.coli* cell surface, the best characterized type 1 and the P-type, distinguished by their specific antigenic binding and varying sites of attachment on cell surfaces [105]. The majority of *E.coli* strains express the uniformly distributed type 1 fimbriae, present in numbers between 100 and 400 per cell [124] Type 1 fimbriae are further known as mannose-specific fimbriae as they reversibly and specifically bind to D-mannose residues, common constituents on the cell surface of eukaryotes [124,128]. The P-type fimbriae, additionally described as mannose-resistant fimbriae, attach to the oligosaccharide receptor sequences (α – Gal(1→4)β – Gal), abbreviated to Gal-Gal [120].

Cranberry has two inhibitors that have been identified as preventing adhesion via both type 1 and type P fimbriae of *E.coli*. These are fructose and a polymeric compound of unknown nature, respectively [121]

One report concluded that although both the type 1 and type P fimbriated *E.coli* result in UTIs it is the P-fimbriated bacterium that are essential and responsible for colonisation of the upper and lower urinary tract of humans [120]. It has been shown that the condensed tannins (proanthocyanidins), rather than the hydrolysable tannins, that are accountable for preventing the P-fimbriated *E.coli* from adhering to the urinary tract [129]. Proanthocyanidin units are linked via interflavonoid bonds comprising of either the single B-type linkages, the more common dimeric B-type or trimeric C-type linkages or the less common double A-type linkage [105]. To date, no antibacterial activity has been found in other tannin-rich fruits which possess the B-linked proanthocyanidins, rather than the A-type linkage found in cranberries. This signifies that proanthocyanidins with the B-type linkage and/or their metabolites are either not bioavailable or do not fabricate bacterial anti-adhesion activity [120]. Therefore, the prerequisite for anti-adhesion activity, particularly in urine, perhaps is the A-type linkage present in cranberry components explaining why cranberry consumption prevents UTIs while other fruits do not. A recent study [120] analysed the structure of proanthocyanidins of cranberry juice in greater depth compared to those of other fruits. Proanthocyanidins are heterogeneous structures mainly composed of oligomers, based on a repetitive unit structure of epicatechin containing at least one, but often multiple, interflavan A-type linkages within the oligomeric series. Consequentially, the A-linked dimers have greater conformational rigidity than proanthocyanidins with B-linkages, which may have a role in the formation of the bioactive urine metabolite, and therefore the beneficial effects in UTIs [112].

Potent anti-adherence activity towards uropathogenic phenotypes of P-fimbriated *E.coli* is exhibited by proanthocyanidin fractions at a concentration as low as 75µg/ml [112]. Cranberry juice has demonstrated positive results *in vivo,* demonstrating that it has a definite benefit in preventing urinary tract infections. In a double-blind, placebo-controlled study in which 376 elderly patients in hospital were given 150 millilitres twice daily of cranberry juice, there were fewer infections as result of the bacterium *E.coli*; 4 infections in the cranberry group compared to 13 infections in the placebo group [122]. The effect of cranberry juice in reducing bacteriuria and pyuria in elderly patients was also studied [123]. A controlled study using 153 randomised women given 300 millilitres daily of cranberry juice. It was concluded that cranberry moved individuals from being in an infected state and therefore, reduced their risk of contracting a urinary tract infection. A most recent study involving spinal cord injured patients, who also suffered from UTIs, was conducted, dosing with 250ml three times daily, over 15 days. A reduction in adhesion of both gram-negative, particularly *E. coli,* and gram-positive bacteria was observed. This particular patient population are highly susceptible to morbidity and mortality associated with drug resistant uropathogens, and large scale trials are required to demonstrate effectiveness over a longer time period [130].

Adhesion of Helicobacter Pylori

Helicobacter pylori is a Gram negative, spiral, microaerophilic bacterium that resides in the duodenum and stomach, and is considered a human-specific inhabitant [108]. Species of *Helicobacter* are resident in the stomach of more than 50% of the population. However, many infections are asymptomatic, with symptoms only appearing in 15% - 20% of the infected individuals [131].

Cranberry consumption may inhibit *H.pylori* from adhering to new sites either on the epithelium or in the mucus. *H.pylori* resembles other pathogens, such as *E.coli,* in the respect that adhesion to the epithelium is a fundamental step in colonisation and initiation of an infection. The major consequence of *H.pylori* infections has been numerous gastrointestinal diseases, such as gastric cancer and peptic ulcer [131]. To cause gastrointestinal disorders *H.pylori* must break away from its common environment, the gastric mucus layer, and adhere to the underlying epithelium [108]. Currently, about ten adhesins of *H.pylori* have been identified that allow the pathogen to attach to erythrocytes and epithelial cells. These consist of adhesions specific for sialic acid, sialyllactose and the sulphated glycosaminoglycans, to name but a few [107]. Moreover, one theory exists that states that the diversity in the host and *H.pylori* results in different combinations of attachments between them, and determines whether *H.pylori* remains in the gastric mucus layer or attaches to the underlying epithelium [108]. Therefore, the adhesins have fine-tuned specificities for interacting with cell-surface carbohydrates and proteins. Numerous studies have proven that adhesion of different strains of *H.pylori* to gastric cells and human gastric mucus *in vitro* is preventable by using NDM [108,131]. It was confirmed, using an *in vitro* study, that bacteria and not mucus is the target for NDM action and confirmed that the sialic acid-specific adhesin of *H.pylori* that binds to sialic acid glycoconjugates in the gastric mucus is inhibited by NDM in a dose dependent fashion [108]. However, the anti-adhesion activity of NDM is strain specific. A review [107] of this investigation indicated that 0.2mg/ml NDM strongly inhibited the adhesion of 12 strains of *H.pylori* however, the other strains were only partially or not at all inhibited from adhering. Cranberry has been reported to have the highest antimicrobial action against *H.pylori* compared to blueberry and grape seed extracts indicating that the anti-adhesive activity is a defined property of cranberry [131]. Anti-*H.pylori* activity also increased in a hyperbolic fashion with increase in dose of cranberry. This may suggest that cranberry polyphenols may have a synergistic mode of action against *H.pylori* adhesion.

Consumption of cranberry juice, may prevent *de novo* sialic acid-specific adhesion and other adhesions of *H.pylori* to the epithelium or the mucus, thus preventing gastrointestinal disorders as a result of *H.pylori*.

Adhesion of Pathogens in the Oral Cavity

NDM, may also have a beneficial effect in preventing infections of the oral cavity and controlling periodontal diseases. Dental plaque is a reservoir of many proliferating bacterial species, attached to teeth, which instigate the development of caries and periodontal diseases. Approximately 51,000 individual bacteria, from over 500 different families, have been detected in the gingival crevice, with the microflora differing from one person to another [109]. However, it is primarily the Gram-negative anaerobes that initiate periodontal diseases. They include *Porphyromonas gingivalis, Actinomomyces* species and *Streptococci* species [109].

The formation of a dental biofilm involves many stages and is coupled to the development of periodontal disease and tooth decay [109]. The primary surface of the teeth exterior is a layer of enzymes and salivary proteins. Two of the most prevalent enzymes are fructosyltransferase (FTF) and glucosyltransferase (GTF). They synthesize fructans and glucans, respectively, via a sucrose-dependent mechanism. They are secreted by the prominent early colonisers of tooth surfaces, which are generally oral streptococci and actinomyces, which constitute greater than 90% of the viable cells of plaque formed early on [132]. They attach via adhesin-receptors or hydrophobic interactions to macromolecules adsorbed to the enamel, and generate microcolonies [109]. The fructans and glucans then provide binding sites for successive bacteria to adhere to [111]. Further aggregation (co-aggregation) of predominantly Gram-negative bacterium occurs, generally between strains belonging to a different genra. This is generally mediated by lectin-like adhesions that specifically recognise complementary receptors, such as lactose and other galactosides, on the partner pathogen [133]. Co-aggregation prevents plaque being disengaged from the tooth surface by salivary flow and mechanical force [109]. The late colonisers play a pivotal role in establishment of periodontal diseases [133].

Anti-adhesive therapy may prevent the co-aggregation of bacteria, which would hinder the development of dental plaque and potentially enhance oral hygiene. Many studies have been conducted that show that NDM has the potential to eradicate causative bacterium from the gingival cavity, and prevent subsequent damage [109-111,134]. NDM has a extensive spectrum of action in inhibiting co-aggregation [133] and reducing growth and virulence of periodontal pathogens, such as the inhibition of protease enzymes of oral bacteria [134] responsible for the degradation of the gingival tissue, the enzyme inhibition of FTF and GTF [111], preventing co-aggregation of bacteria in both the sucrose environment [109,134] and the sucrose-free environment [135] and enhancing bacterial clearance via the saliva-induced bacterial clearance mechanism [109].

The results of the *in vitro* investigation [134] indicate the cranberry NDM fraction inhibiting protease enzymes, produced by *Porphyromonas gingivalis, Treponema denticola* and *Tanneralla forsythia,* that are critical for their survival, as they are responsible for the degradation of periodontal tissue [134]. This specific group of Gram-negative anaerobic bacteria contribute to the pathogenesis of periodontitis. The degradation of type 1 collagen and transferrin, which provides substances such as iron for the periodontopathogens, by proteases produced by *P. gingivalis* was affected by NDM from cranberry. Furthermore, an *in vitro* study involving the bacterium *Streptococcus sobrinus,* showed that NDM affects the formation of the biofilm by affecting the action of pathogenic enzymes subsequently interfering with co-aggregation of the biofilm [111]. NDM had up to a 90% inhibitory effect on GTF and FTF, the enzymes primarily responsible for the synthesis of specific polysaccharides that allow co-aggregation of the late colonisers in the gingival cavity via a sucrose-dependent mechanism. By reducing the quantity of glucans and frucans produced there is nothing to mediate the adhesion of *S.sobrinus* to the biofilm. Also, although NDM showed a less significant effect in the sucrose-free environment, by preventing adherence of bacterium to the tooth surface using such properties as hydrophobicity [134], it implies that NDM can affect more than one mechanism of bacterial adhesion.

An *in vitro* study conducted showed an additional mechanism of action of NDM, in preventing co-aggregation of different pairs of bacterium. Co-aggregation was reversed in practically 90% of the pairs, when higher concentrations of NDM were tested, acting preferentially when either one or both pairs of bacteria were Gram-negative [109]. Therefore, one of the main mechanisms by which NDM improves oral hygiene is by inhibiting or reversing co-aggregation of interspecies interactions. The review of this study [133] proposes that NDM is not as effective in dissociating preformed co-aggregates as it is in inhibiting co-aggregation. The cranberry fraction did not desorb a preformed *P. gingivalis* biofilm [110]. However, the report concluded that NDM, dose-dependently, reduced the growth and adherence of *P. gingivalis* to the biofilm. It appears that co-aggregation is a unique benefit of cranberry alone, as other fruit juices had weak or no co-aggregation inhibitory activity in the oral cavity [109]. The effect of saliva in a mixture with NDM was investigated. Saliva contains a high number of viable bacteria and so could modify the nature of plaque. Results indicated that when both saliva and NDM were present, aggregation of bacterial strains was induced. It was postulated that this could enhance bacterial clearance via the saliva-induced bacterial clearance mechanism, therefore improving oral hygiene. Thus suggesting a further mechanism of action of NDM found in cranberry [109]. A clinical trial was later undertaken [109] in which 30 volunteers used a mouthwash containing NDM. There was a reduction of *S.mutans* in the saliva counts of those that had used the mouthwash supplemented with NDM compared to the placebo group.

The mechanism of action, in the gingival cavity, of NDM has not yet been elucidated. However, the promising results, of NDM in dental plaque control warrants further studies.

Inhibiting co-aggregation can disturb the formation and development of dental plaque and so may benefit in the treatment of periodontitis and other periodontal diseases.

Influenza Virus Adhesion

One study has been conducted which indicated that the NDM component can also inhibit influenza virus adhesion and infectivity. Results indicated that NDM significantly inhibited the infectivity of all the virus strains tested, and reduced or inhibited *in vitro* viral replication, at concentrations of NDM much lower than those found in commercial cranberry juice [106]. Therefore, NDM may be a natural antiviral substance and have therapeutic potential. It interacts directly with the virus, prevents adsorption of the virus onto cells, so suppressing viral multiplication, and prevents subsequent infection of new cells, and it may also inhibit bacterial infections that are secondary to viral infections.

Antioxidant Activity

It has been hypothesized for many years that risk of chronic diseases, such as cardiovascular diseases (CVD) and cancer, can be reduced by consumption of fruit and vegetables containing anti-oxidants. From eleven fruit extracts the most potent antioxidant activity was found in the cranberry phytochemical extract, which had a direct relationship with the total phenolic content [103]. Evidence exists that it may actually be the flavonoids that are the strong antioxidants [118] Four flavonoids with different sugar moieties attached showed potent antioxidant activity, all compounds contained the flavonol quercetin.

Cardiovascular Health

CVD is the principal cause of death in the majority of industrialised countries, diet and hereditary factors being the primary contributors [114]. Atherosclerosis, an inflammatory disease, is the principal cause of CVD. It is characterised by the formation of atherosclerotic plaque, in the subendothelial space known as the intima, which consists of lipids and cholesterol [113]. Obstruction of blood flow can lead to myocardial infarction and stroke.

Cranberry polyphenolics may affect the development of atherosclerosis and CVD by exerting an antioxidant action and reducing cholesterol. In particular it is thought to be the cranberry monomeric and oligomeric flavonoids that are absorbed and are thought to have a therapeutic effect, for example in preventing LDL oxidation and aiding blood flow via vasodilation [113]. However, the polymers are thought not to be absorbed but could inhibit the development of atherosclerosis by affecting the clearance of cholesterol from the plasma via the liver. It has been concluded that it is the proanthocyanidins in cranberry that associate with LDL and inhibit its oxidation. The proanthocyanidins have been identified which prevented *E.coli* from adhering to uroepithelium cells *in vitro* were identified as trimers of the oligomers of catechin and epi-catechin, linked together by at least one A-type interflavan bond [112]. Preliminary results indicate that cranberry also has oligomers containing gallocatechin and/or epigallocatechin [113]. Greater antioxidant capacity and affinity for LDL appears to be with the oligomers consisting of 5 to 9 catechin units. It was found that flavonoids inhibited LDL oxidation, which is performed by macrophages [136]. This was demonstrated in an *ex vivo* experiment [116], where the cranberry extract largely containing anthocyanidins and the flavonols quercetin and myrecetin inhibited *in vitro* LDL oxidation. Therefore, antioxidants, from cranberry, that operate in the intima and distinctively act on LDL will possibly protect against atherosclerosis and importantly prevent the development of CVD.

Oxidized LDL plays a significant role in the atherosclerotic process, as it is more atherogenic than native LDL. Numerous studies and clinical research have proposed many theories in which cranberry could prevent atherosclerosis. A study to determine whether cranberry bore an antioxidant effect towards LDL oxidation and, whether cranberry altered the expression of LDL receptors in HepG$_2$ human liver cancer cells *in vitro*. Analysis of the results indicates that LDL oxidation was completely inhibited at the highest dose of 10mg/ml of cranberry extract. Partial inhibition was demonstrated at lower doses. Furthermore, HepG$_2$ hepatocytes expressed a significant up-regulation of their LDL receptor with 15 and 30mg/ml of cranberry extract. Induction was observed in a dose-dependent manner. Similarly, increased uptake of cholesterol by the human liver cancer cells was also observed with equivalent doses of the cranberry extract [114]. These results indicate that cranberry could be a potent antioxidant and could further reduce hypercholesterolemia by up-regulating the expression of LDL receptors in liver cells.

Two essential factors that influence whether an individual suffers from hypercholes - terolemia is the balance between liver cholesterol absorption, synthesis and excretion, and the action of the hepatocyte LDL receptor that clears LDL from the blood. In the majority of cases familial hypercholesterolemia is the result of a defective LDL receptor [113]. Cranberry juice has been investigated for its beneficial effect on hypercholesterolemia. A recent study explored whether short-term cranberry juice consumption, for 14 consecutive days, would have an impact on the antioxidant capacity and the oxidised LDL concentration in the plasma of twenty-one healthy males [115]. The results supported the theory that consumption of foods high in antioxidants, particularly those containing flavonoids such as cranberry, could lessen the risk of CVD [137]. On average there was a 6% increase in the antioxidant capacity and a reduction in the oxidised LDL concentration of the plasma. Later a 12 week investigation was carried out, by the same individuals, to assess whether cranberry juice effected the lipoprotein concentration in plasma, particularly of HDL cholesterol, of abdominally obese men [138]. The intervention yielded a significant decrease in the ratio of total cholesterol to HDL-cholesterol, probably attributed to the significant HDL cholesterol increase of about 8%. Therefore, the plasma antioxidant capacity of these individuals changed extensively with cranberry juice consumption.

Moreover, CVD can impair vasodilation, which is controlled by the release of NO from endothelial cells. *In vitro* research indicates that oligomeric proanthocyanidins present in other foods and beverages [139] can improve vasodilation by up-regulating the production of NO by endothelial cells.

Cancer Prevention

Cancer is a major cause of death with environmental factors, such as diet, being a large contributing factor [98]. Increased consumption of fruit and vegetables containing a rich source of polyphenolics, such as flavonoids, may prevent cancer development. The antiproliferative activities were investigated *in vitro* using HepG$_2$ human liver cancer cells. Cranberry demonstrated the most potent antiproliferative effect, in a dose-dependent manner, indicated by the lowest EC$_{50}$ value. However, the antiproliferative activity did not correlate with the total phenolic content and antioxidant activity of the fruits, thus suggesting that it may be a particular phenolic compound or class of phenolics present in the fruit accountable for the antiproliferative activity. The cranberry phytochemicals most likely to have antiproliferative activity would be the polyphenolic class of flavonoids [117]. This family of compounds has three main groups found in cranberry: flavonols, flavan-3-ols (catechins), which make up the proanthocyanidins, and the anthocyanins. However, it is not solely this class that has been shown to have anticancer activity [119]. Three compounds were identified that inhibited the proliferation of the HepG$_2$ cell growth in a dose-dependent manner and without toxicity. These compounds were identified as a derivative of the triterpenoids named ursolic acid, the flavonol quercetin, and quercetin glucoside [118]. These compounds also inhibited the proliferation of human breast cancer cells, MCF-7 cells. However, urosolic acid displayed cytotoxicity towards the MCF-7 cells. The flavonoids in cranberry that are independently known to affect tumour cell growth include the flavonols myricetin, quercetin and resveratrol, compounds known also to have potent anti-oxidant activity [116], and the flavan-3-ols. The flavan-3-ol that appears to have the greatest antiproliferative activity is epigallocatechin (EGCG), made up of the monomers catechin and epicatechin, which constitute about 7% of cranberry's proanthocyanins. Cranberry consists of polymers of these flavan-3-ols and a cranberry fraction enriched with proanthocyanidins consisting primarily of epicatechin units joined by A-type linkages, with degrees of polymerisation (Dp) of 4 and 5 showed anticancer activity [120]. Proliferation was inhibited in the KB and CAL27 oral cancer cells by 41% and 37.6% respectively. Also, significant activity was shown towards prostate cell lines and a small degree of activity towards two colon cancer cell lines.

Preliminary evidence found that when mice bearing the human breast tumour cells MDA-MB-435, oestrogen-receptor negative breast carcinomas, were given cranberry presscake the growth and metastasis of the cells was inhibited [117]. Fraction 6, of unknown constitution, was the only fraction that consistently demonstrated antiproliferative activity towards all cell types, in a dose-dependent manner.

Two phenolic compounds from fraction 6 were identified from cranberry, and both inhibited the *in vitro* proliferation of tumour cells. These triterpenoid esters, were identified as the *cis-* and *trans-* isomers of 3-O-p-hydroxycinnamoyl ursolic acid.

In addition to the major phenolic constituents, cranberry is also known to contain salicylates, and salicylic acid is found in serum and urine after ingestion of the juice, in levels comparable to those of low dose aspirin. Regular intake of aspirin has been shown to cause reduced incidence of a number of cancers, particularly colorectal adenomas, which has increased the interest in cranberry as a protective agent. Salicylic acid levels up to 7mg/L have been reported in the juice, and subjects have been dosed with up to 1800ml daily [140].

Conclusion

Cranberry has been shown to have a range of potential beneficial health effects, especially by interfering with microbial adhesion. Evidence is seen particularly in the urinary tract, of E.coli, in the gastrointestinal tract, of H.pylori, and the adhesion of the influenza virus. Inhibition of adhesion is an appealing area for developing innovative therapies. The action of NDM on the pathogenicity of H.pylori has of yet been solely examined in vitro, but it may be possible that it could be inhibited from adhering in vivo and prevent the development of stomach ulcers. Also, NDM can inhibit the co-aggregation of various oral bacteria in the gingival cavity. Manipulation of the ecology of bacteria in the gingival cavity by applying anti-adhesion agents could be a more effective approach in controlling periodontal diseases.

By inhibiting bacterial adhesion to host cells thus preventing the propagation of infections and disease represents a novel, yet attractive approach. The theory of using a cranberry drink to prevent urinary tract infections is appealing and well accepted by both the patient and the physicians. Cranberry acceptability and tolerability, thus resulting in compliance with the therapy, is demonstrated with both elderly people [122] and children [141], where compliance exceeded that of long-term prophylaxis using anti-microbials.

Cranberry and its compounds have also been illustrated to exhibit potent antioxidant activity by protecting against LDL oxidation and decreasing cholesterol levels, thus possibly reducing the risk of cardiovascular disease.

Tumour cell proliferation has also been shown to be prevented by specific phytochemicals that are known to exist in cranberry, but this activity has been shown to be enhanced by a possible additive mode of action between flavonoids present in cranberry. Therefore, further investigations are required in this area of research to discover any possible in vivo activity.

However, the bioavailability of cranberry and its components are important if beneficial results are to be achieved. Few in vivo studies demonstrate the quantity of cranberry juice required to have a beneficial effect. Clinical investigations examining the health benefits of cranberry juice on urinary tract health have used differing dosing schedules and quantities. Bacterial anti-adhesion activity was found in the urine of individuals whom had consumed a 240 millilitre single serving of cranberry juice. However, a beneficial effect of cranberry juice preventing UTIs in elderly people when administration persisted over days, 150 millilitres of cranberry juice twice daily for 16 days and 300 millilitres daily for 6 months, respectively, was found.

Studies revealing the beneficial cardiovascular effects of cranberry also incorporate differing doses of cranberry juice. Therefore, the variation and limitations of these studies emphasize the necessity for long term, comparative investigations to be conducted.

Very few adverse effects have been reported following cranberry consumption, however, there are a few reports on the possible increase in formation of kidney stones [142]. Markers of stone formation were variably affected, suggesting that it would be sensible to limit consumption to realistic levels.

As the majority of research that has been carried out on a single component of cranberry or a class of flavonoids it is difficult to extrapolate the results of the intake of individual compounds to the intake of the whole cranberry and its beverages, as many compounds may have a synergistic effect, as have been demonstrated. Therefore, there is a need for further investigations, in vivo and epidemiological studies, to thoroughly understand the health effects in vivo, structure-activity relations and the dose of particular compounds, and cranberry juice, to have a beneficial response. Nevertheless, substantial evidence exists to warrant the incorporation of cranberry, and the phytochemicals it contains, into a balanced diet.

Overall Conclusion

These three increasingly popular food sources of polyphenols have been shown to demonstrate a wide variety of effects, particularly cardiovascular and anticancer activity, but also antibacterial and antibacterial effects, and cranberry shows promise in the areas of UTIs and oral hygiene.

As polyphenols, specifically tannins, are able to bind and precipitate carbohydrates, protein and dietary enzymes present in foodstuffs, they may inhibit the digestion of food, and therefore reduce the bioavailability of nutrients.

The overall effects seen after administration of these food sources of polyphenols may be caused by other components present, or by combination or synergistic effects.

Further research into their beneficial effects will undoubtedly be carried out, and probably the most important progress can be made by running large scale clinical trials, to study their effects in a number of therapeutic areas indicated by current results. As with research into the effects of all nutraceutical supplements, the use of standardised extracts and individual components will produce more detailed information concerning their role in specific disease states.

References

[1]   Manach C, Scalbert A, Morand C, Rémésy C, Jiménez L. Polyphenols: food sources and bioavailability. *American Journal of Clinical Nutrition* 2004; 79: 727-47.

[2]   Gil MI, Tomás-Barberán F.A, Hess-Pierce B, Holcroft DM, Kader AA. Antioxidant activity of pomegranate juice and its relationship with phenolic composition and processing. *Journal of Agricultural and Food Chemistry* 2000; 48: 4581-4589.

[3]   Afaq F, Saleem M, Krueger CG, Reed JD, Mukhtar H. Anthocyanin- and hydrolyzable tannin-rich pomegranate fruit extract modulates MAPK and NF-κB pathways and inhibits skin tumorigenesis in CD-1 mice. *International Journal of Cancer* 2005; 113: 423-433.

[4]   Al-Maiman SA, Ahmad D. Changes in physical and chemical properties during pomegranate (*Punica granatum* L.) fruit maturation. Food Chemistry 2002; 76: 437-441.

[5]   Azadzoi KM, Schulman RN, Aviram M, Siroky MB. Oxidative stress in atreriogenic erectile dysfunction: prophylactic role of antioxidants. *Journal of Urology* 2005; 174: 386-393.

[6]   Schubert SY, Lansky EP, Neeman I. Antioxidant and eicosanoid enzyme inhibition properties of pomegranate seed oil and fermented juice flavonoids. *Journal of Ethnopharmacology* 1999; 66: 11-17.

[7]   Fuhrman B, Volkova N, Aviram M. Pomegranate juice inhibits oxidized LDL uptake and cholesterol biosynthesis in macrophages. *Journal of Nutritional Biochemistry* 2005; 16: 570-576.

[8]   Cerdá B, Cerón JJ, Tomás-Barberán FA, Espín JC. Repeated oral administration of high doses of the pomegranate ellagitannin punicalagin to rats for 37 days is not toxic. *Journal of Agricultural and Food Chemistry* 2003; 51: 3493-3501.

[9]   Pantuck AJ, Leppert JT, Zomorodian N, Aronson W, Hong J, Barnard RJ, Seeram N, Liker H, Wang H, Elashoff R, Heber D, Aviram M, Ignarro L, Belldegrun A. Phase II study of pomegranate juice for men with rising prostate-specific antigen following surgery or radiation for prostate cancer. *Clinical Cancer Research* 2006; 12: 4018-4026.

[10]   Seeram NP, Adams LS, Henning SM, Niu Y, Zhang Y, Nair MG, Heber D. In vitro antiproliferative, apoptotic and antioxidant activities of punicalagin, ellagic acid and a total pomegranate tannin extract are enhanced in combination with other polyphenols as found in pomegranate juice. *Journal of Nutritional Biochemistry* 2005; 16: 360-367.

[11]   Mertens-Talcott SU, Jilma-Stohlawetz P, Rios J, Hingorani L, Derendorf H. Absorption, metabolism, and antioxidant effects of pomegranate (*Punica granatum* L.) polyphenols after ingestion of a standardized extract in healthy human volunteers. *Journal of Agricultural and Food Chemistry* 2006; 54: 8956-8961.

[12]   Malik A, Afaq F, Sarfaraz S, Adhami VM, Syed DN, Mukhtar H. Pomegranate fruit juice for the chemoprevention and chemotherapy of prostate cancer. *Proceedings of the National Academy of Sciences of the United States of America* 2005; 102: 14813-14818.

[13]   Cerdá B, Espín JC, Parra S, Martínez P, Tomás-Barberán FA. The potent in vitro antioxidant ellagitannins from pomegranate juice are metabolised into bioavailable but poor antioxidant hydroxyl-6H-dibenzopyran-6-one derivatives by the colonic microflora of healthy humans. *European Journal of Nutrition* 2004; 43: 205-220.

[14]   Hidaka M, Okumura M, Fujita K, Ogikubo T, Yamasaki K, Iwakiri T, Setoguchi N, Arimori K. Effects of pomegranate juice on human cytochrome P450 3A (CYP3A) and carbamazepine pharmacokinetics in rats. *Drug Metabolism and Disposition* 2005; 33: 644-648.

[15]   Noda Y, Kaneyuki T, Mori A, Packer L. Antioxidant activities of pomegranate Fruit extract and its anthocyanidins: delphinidin, cyanidin, and pelargonidin. *Journal of Agricultural and Food Chemistry* 2002; 50: 166-171.

[16]   Lansky EP, Jiang W, Mo H, Bravo L, Froom P, Yu W, Harris NM, Neeman I, Campbell MJ. Possible synergistic prostate cancer suppression by anatomically discrete pomegranate fractions. *Investigational New Drugs* 2005; 23: 11-20.

[17] Toi M, Bando H, Ramachandran C, Melnick SJ, Imai A, Fife RS, Carr RE, Oikawa T, Lansky EP. Preliminary studies on the anti-angiogenic potential of pomegranate fractions *in vitro* and *in vivo*. *Angiogenesis* 2003; 6: 121-128.

[18] Neurath AR, Strick N, Li Y, Debnath AK. Punica granatum (Pomegranate) juice provides an HIV-1 entry inhibitor and candidate topical microbicide. *BMC Infectious Diseases* 2004; 4: 41.

[19] Kim ND, Mehta R, Yu W, Neeman I, Livney T, Amichay A, Poirier D, Nicholls P, Kirby A, Jiang W, Mansel R, Ramachandran C, Rabi T, Kaplan B, Lansky E. Chemopreventive and adjuvant therapeutic potential of pomegranate (*Punica granatum*) for human breast cancer. *Breast Cancer Research and Treatment* 2002; 71: 203-217.

[20] Navarro V, Villarreal ML, Rojas G, Lozoya X. Antimicrobial evaluation of some plants used in Mexican traditional medicine for the treatment of infectious diseases. *Journal of Ethnopharmacology* 1996; 53: 143-147.

[21] Prashanth D, Asha MK, Amit A. Antibacterial activity of *Punica granatum*. *Fitoterapia* 2001; 72: 171-173.

[22] Clifford MN, Scalbert A. Review: Ellagitannins – nature, occurrence and dietary burden. *Journal of the Science of Food and Agriculture* 2000; 80: 1118-1125.

[23] Braga LC, Shupp JW, Cummings C, Jett M, Takahashi JA, Carmo LS, Chartone-Souza E, Nascimento AMA. Pomegranate extract inhibits *Staphylococcus aureus* growth and subsequent enterotoxin production. *Journal of Ethnopharmacology* 2005; 96: 335-339.

[24] Braga LC, Leite AAM, Xavier KGS, Takahashi JA, Bemquerer MP, Chartone-Souza E, Nascimento AMA. Synergic interaction between pomegranate extract and antibiotics against Staphylococcus aureus. *Canadian Journal of Microbiology* 2005; 51: 541-547.

[25] Shahidi F, Naczk M. Nutritional and Pharmacological Effects of Food Phenolics, in Phenolics in Food and Nutraceuticals, CRC Press LLC,*Boca Raton, Fla.* 2003, 331-402.

[26] Lee J, Watson RR. Pomegranate: a role in health promotion and AIDS? In Nutrients and Foods in AIDS. Edited by Watson, R.R. CRC Press LLC, *Boca Raton, Fla.* 1998,213-216.

[27] Zhang J, Zhan B, Yao X, Gao Y, Shong J. Antiviral activity of tannin from the pericarp of Punica granatum L. against genital Herpes virus in vitro. Zhongguo Zhong Yao Za Zhi 1995; 20: 556-8, 576. (ABSTRACT)

[28] Aviram M, Rosenblat M, Gaitini D, Nitecki S, Hoffman A, Dornfeld L, Volkova N, Presser D, Attias J, Liker H, Hayek T. Poemgranate juice consumption for 3 years by patients with carotid artery stenosis reduces common carotid intima-media thickness, blood pressure and LDL oxidation. *Clinicial Nutrition* 2004; 23: 423-433.

[29] Aviram M, Dornfeld L, Rosenblat M, Volkova N, Kaplan M, Coleman R, Hayek T, Presser D, Fuhrman B. Pomegranate juice consumption reduces oxidative stress, atherogenic modifications to LDL, and platelet aggregation: studies in humans and atherosclerotic apolipoprotein E-deficient mice. *American Journal of Clinical Nutrition* 2000; 71: 1062-76.

[30] Aviram M, Dornfeld L. Pomegranate juice consumption inhibits serum angiotensin converting enzyme activity and reduces systolic blood pressure. *Atherosclerosis* 2001; 158: 195-198.

[31] Kaplan M, Hayek T, Raz A, Coleman R, Dornfeld L, Vaya J, Aviram M. Pomegranate juice supplementation to atherosclerotic mice reduces macrophage lipid peroxidation, cellular cholesterol accumulation and development of atherosclerosis. *Journal of Nutrition* 2001; 131: 2082-2089.

[32] Sumner MD, Elliott-Eller M, Weidner G, Daubenmier JJ, Chew MH, Marlin R, Raisin CJ, Ornish D. Effects of pomegranate juice consumption on myocardial perfusion in patients with coronary heart disease. *American Journal of Cardiology* 2005; 96: 810-814.

[33] Huang TH-W, Peng G, Kota BP, Li GQ, Yamahara J, Roufogalis BD, Li Y. Anti-diabetic action of Punica granatum flower extract: Activation of PPAR-γ and identification of an active component. *Toxicology and Applied Pharmacology* 2005; 207: 160-169.

[34] Li Y, Wen S, Kota BP, Peng G, Li GQ, Yamahara J, Roufogalis BD. *Punica granatum* flower extract, a potent α-glucosidase inhibitor, improves postprandial hyperglycemia in Zucker diabetic fatty rats. *Journal of Ethnopharmacology* 2005; 99: 239-244.

[35] Huang TH-W, Peng G, Kota BP, Li GQ, Yamahara J, Roufogalis BD, Li Y. Pomegranate flower improves cardiac lipid metabolism in a diabetic rat model: role of lowering circulating lipids. *British Journal of Pharmacology* 2005; 145: 767-774.

[36] Huang TH-W, Yang Q, Harada M, Li GQ, Yamahara J, Roufogalis BD, Li Y. Pomegranate flower extract diminishes cardiac fibrosis in Zucker diabetic fatty rats: Modulation of cardiac Endothelin-1 and Nuclear Factor-kappaB pathways. *Journal of Cardiovascular Pharmacology* 2005, 46, 856-862

[37] Rosenblat M, Hayek T, Aviram M. Anti-oxidative effects of pomegranate juice (PJ) consumption by diabetic patients on serum and on macrophages. *Atherosclerosis* 2006; 187: 363-371.

[38] Esmaillzadeh A, Tahbaz F, Gaieni I, Alavi-Majd H, Azadbakht L. Concentrated pomegranate juice improves lipid profiles in diabetic patients with hyperlipidemia. *Journal of Medicinal Food* 2004; 7: 305-308.

[39] Lansky EP, Harrison G, Froom P, Jiang WG. Pomegranate (Punica granatum) pure chemicals show possible synergistic inhibition of human PC-3 prostate cancer cell invasion across Matrigel™. *Investigational New Drugs* 2005; 23: 121-122.

[40] Kohno H, Suzuki R, Yasui Y, Hosokawa M, Miyashita K, Tanaka T. Pomegranate seed oil rich in conjugated linolenic acid suppresses chemically induced colon carcinogenesis in rats. *Cancer Science* 2004; 95: 481-486.

[41] Longtin R. The Pomegranate: Nature's Power Fruit? *Journal of the National Cancer Institute* 2003; 95: 346-348.

[42] Larrosa M, Tomás-Barberán FA, Espín JC. The dietary hydrolysable tannin punicalagin releases ellagic acid that induces apoptosis in human colon adenocarcinoma Caco-2 cells by using the mitochondrial pathway. *Journal of Nutritional Biochemistry* 2006; 17: 611-625.

[43] Adams LS, Seeram NP, Aggarwal BB, Takada Y, Sand D, Heber D. Pomegranate juice, total pomegranate ellagitannins, and punicalagin suppress inflammatory cell signalling in colon cancer cells. *Journal of Agricultural and Food Chemistry* 2006; 54: 980-985.

[44] Mehta R, Lansky EP. Breast cancer chemopreventive properties of pomegranate (*Punica granatum*) fruit extracts in a mouse mammary organ culture. *European Journal of Cancer Prevention* 2004; 13: 345-348.

[45] Hora JJ, Maydew ER, Lansky EP, Dwivedi C. Chemopreventive Effects of pomegranate seed oil on skin tumor development in CD_1 mice. Journal of Medicinal Food 2003; 6: 157-161.

[46] Aslam MN, Lansky EP, Varani J. Pomegranate as a cosmeceutical source: Pomegranate fractions promote proliferation and procollagen synthesis and inhibit matrix metalloproteinase-1 production in human skin cells. *Journal of Ethnopharmacology* 2006; 103: 311-318.

[47] Afaq F, Malik A, Syed D, Maes D, Matsui MS, Mukhtar H. Pomegranate fruit extract modulates UV-B-mediated phosphorylation of mitogen-activated protein kinases and activation of Nuclear Factor Kappa B in normal human epidermal keratinocytes. *Photochemistry and Photobiology* 2005; 81: 38-45.

[48] Cerdá B, Soto C, Albaladejo MD, Martínez P, Sánchez-Gascón F, Tomás-Barberán F, Espín JC. Pomegranate juice supplementation in chronic obstructive pulmonary disease: a 5-week randomized, double blind, placebo-controlled trial. *European Journal of Clinical Nutrition* 2006; 60: 245-253.

[49] Loren DJ, Seeram NP, Schulman RN, Holtzman DM. Maternal dietary supplementation with pomegranate juice is neuroprotective in an animal model of neonatal hypoxic-ischemic brain injury. *Pediatric Research* 2005; 57: 858-864.

[50] De Amorim A, Borba HR, Armada JL. Test of mutagenesis in mice treated with aqueous extracts from *Punica granatum* L. (Pomegranate). *Revista Brasileira de Farmacia* 1995; 76: 110-111. (ABSTRACT)

[51] Seeram NP, Lee R, Heber D. Bioavailability of ellagic acid in human plasma after consumption of ellagitannins from pomegranate (Punica granatum L.) juice. *Clinica Chimica Acta* 2004; 348: 63-68.

[52] Pérez-Vicente A, Gil-Izquierdo A, García-Viguera C. In vitro gastrointestinal digestion study of pomegranate juice phenolic compounds, anthocyanins, and Vitamin C. *Journal of Agricultural and Food Chemistry* 2002; 50: 2308-2312.

[53] Cerdá B, Llorach R, Cerón JJ, Espín JC, Tomás-Barberán FA. Evaluation of the bioavailability and metabolism in the rat of punicalagin, an antioxidant polyphenol from pomegranate juice. *European Journal of Nutrition* 2003; 42: 18-28.

[54] Seeram NP, Henning SM, Zhang Y, Suchard M, Li Z, Heber D. Pomegranate juice ellagitannin metabolites are present in human plasma and some persist in urine for up to 48 hours. *Journal of Nutrition* 2006; 136: 2481-2485.

[55] Ahmad A. Ellagic acid food supplement prepared from pomegranate seed. U.S. Pat. Appl. Publ. 2006. Patent Number: 2006251753 A1 20061109.

[56] Lansky EP. Beware of pomegranates bearing 40% ellagic acid. *Journal of Medicinal Food* 2006; 9: 119-122.

[57] Dillinger TL, Barriga P, Escarcega S, Jimenez M, Lowe DS, Grivetti LE. Food of the Gods: Cure for humanity? A cultural history of the medicinal and ritual use of chocolate. *Journal of Nutrition* 2000; 130: 2057S-2072S.

[58] Keen CL, Holt RR, Polagruto JA, Wang JF, Schmitz HH. Cocoa flavanols and cardiovascular health. *Phytochemistry Reviews* 2003; 1: 231-240.

[59] Bearden MM, Keen CL. Cocoa and chocolate flavonoids: implications for cardiovascular health. *Journal of the American Dietetic Association* 2003; 103: 215-223.

[60] Sanbongi C, Osakabe N, Natsume M, Takizawa T, Gomi S, Osawa T. Antioxidative Polyphenols Isolated from *Theobroma cacao. Journal of Agricultural and Food Chemistry* 1998; 46: 454-457.

[61] Richelle M, Tavazzi I, Enslen M, Offord EA. Plasma kinetics in man of epicatechin from black chocolate. *European Journal of Clinical Nutrition* 1999; 53: 22-26.

[62] Porter LJ, Ma Z, Chan BG. Cacao procyanidins: major flavanoids and identification of some minor metabolites. *Phytochemistry* 1991; 30: 1657-1663

[63] Vinson JA, Proch J, Zubik L. Phenol antioxidant quantity and quality in foods: Cocoa, dark chocolate, and milk chocolate. *Journal of Agricultural and Food Chemistry* 1999; 47: 4821-4824.

[64] Arts ICW, Hollman PCH, Kromhout D. Chocolate as a source of tea flavonoids. *Lancet* 1999; 354: 488.

[65] Lamuela-Raventós RM, Andrés-Lacueva C. More Antioxidants in Cocoa. *Journal of Nutrition.* 2001;131: 834.

[66] Wang JF, Schramm DD, Holt RR, Ensunsa JL, Fraga CG, Schmitz HH, Keen CL. A dose-response effect from chocolate consumption on plasma epicatechin and oxidative damage. *The Journal of nutrition* 2000; 130: 2115S-2119S.

[67] Mursu J, Voutilainen S, Nurmi T; Rissanen TH, Virtanen JK, Kaikkonen J, Nyyssonen K, Salonen JT. Dark chocolate consumption increases HDL cholesterol concentration and chocolate fatty acids may inhibit lipid peroxidation in healthy humans. *Free Radical Biology and Medicine* 2004; 37: 1351-1359.

[68] Innes AJ, Kennedy G, McLaren M, Bancroft AJ, Belch JJF. Dark chocolate inhibits platelet aggregation in healthy volunteers. *Platelets* 2003; 14: 325-327.

[69] Fisher NDL, Hollenberg NK. Flavanols for cardiovascular health: the science behind the sweetness. *Journal of Hypertension* 2005; 23: 1453-1459.

[70] Rein D, Lotito S, Holt RR, Keen CL, Schmitz HH, Fraga CG. Epicatechin in human plasma: In vivo determination and effect of chocolate consumption on plasma oxidation status. *Journal of Nutrition* 2000; 130: 2109S-2114S.

[71] Serafini M, Bugianesi R, Maiani G, Valtuena S, De Santis S, Crozier A. Plasma antioxidants from chocolate. *Nature* 2003; 424: 1013.

[72] Richelle M, Tavazzi I, Offord E. Comparison of the antioxidant activity of commonly consumed polyphenolic beverages (coffee, cocoa and tea) prepared per cup serving. . *Journal of Agricultural and Food Chemistry* 2001; 49: 3438-3442.

[73] Engler MB, Engler MM, Chen CY, Malloy MJ, Browne Amanda, Chiu EY, Kwak H, Milbury Paul, Paul SM, Blumberg J, Mietus-Snyder ML. Flavonoid-rich dark chocolate

improves endothelial function and increases plasma epicatechin concentrations in healthy adults. *Journal of the American College of Nutrition* 2004; 23: 197-204.

[74] Pearson DA, Schmitz HH, Lazarus SA, Keen CL. Inhibition of *in vitro* low-density lipoprotein oxidation by oligomeric procyanidins present in chocolate and cocoas. *Methods in Enzymology* 2001; 335: 350-360.

[75] Arteel GE, Schroeder P, Sies H. Reactions of peroxynitrite with cocoa procyandin oligomers. *Journal of Nutrition* 2000; 130: 2100S-2104S.

[76] Rein D, Paglieroni TG, Wun T, Pearson DA, Schmitz HH, Gosselin R, Keen CL. Cocoa inhibits platelet activation and function. *American Journal of Clinical Nutrition* 2000; 72: 30-35.

[77] Pearson DA, Paglieroni TG, Rein D, Wun T, Schramm DD, Wang JF, Holt RR, Gosselin R, Schmitz HH, Keen CL. The effects of flavanol-rich cocoa and aspirin on ex vivo platelet function. *Thrombosis Research* 2002; 106: 191-197.

[78] Ramiro E, Franch À, Castellote C, Andrés-Lacueva C, Izquierdo-Pulido M, Castell M. Effect of *Theobroma cacao* flavanoids on immune activation of a lymphoid cell line. *British Journal of Nutrition* 2005; 93: 859-866.

[79] Mao T, Van de Water J, Keen CL, Schmitz HH, Gershwin ME. Cocoa procyanidins and human cytokine transcription and secretion. *Journal of Nutrition* 2000; 130: 2093S-2099S.

[80] Steinberg FM, Holt RR, Schmitz HH, Keen CL. Cocoa procyanidin chain length does not determine ability to protect LDL from oxidation when monomer units are controlled. *The Journal of Nutritional Biochemistry* 2002; 13: 645-652.

[81] Wan Y, Vinson JA, Etherton TD, Proch J, Lazarus SA, Kris-Etherton PM. Effects of cocoa powder and dark chocolate on LDL oxidative susceptibility and prostaglandin concentrations in humans. *American Journal of Clinical Nutrition* 2001; 74: 596-602.

[82] Arteel GE, Sies H. Protection against peroxynitrite by cocoa polyphenol oligomers. FEBS Letters 1999; 462: 167-170.

[83] Sanbongi C, Suzuki N, Sakane T. Polyphenols in chocolate, which have antioxidant activity, modulate immune functions in humans *in vitro*. *Cellular Immunology* 1997; 177: 129-136.

[84] Vlachopoulos C, Aznaouridis K, Alexopoulos N, Economou E, Andreadou I, Stefanadis C. Effect of dark chocolate on arterial function in healthy individuals. *American Journal of Hypertension* 2005; 18: 785-791.

[85] Schroeter H, Heiss C, Balzer J, Kleinbongard P, Keen CL, Hollenberg NK, Sies H, Kwik-Uribe C, Schmitz HH, Kelm M. (−)-Epicatechin mediates beneficial effects of flavanol-rich cocoa on vascular function in humans. *Proceedings of the National Academy of Sciences of the United States of America* 2006; 103: 1024-1029.

[86] Fisher NDL, Hollenberg NK. Aging and vascular responses to flavanol-rich cocoa. *Journal of Hypertension* 2006; 24: 1575-1580.

[87] Hermann F, Spieker LE, Ruschitzka F, Sudano I, Hermann M, Binggeli C, Luscher TF, Riesen W, Noll G, Corti R. Dark chocolate improves endothelial and platelet function. *Heart* 2006; 92: 119-120.

[88] Grassi D, Necozione S, Lippi C, Croce G, Valeri L, Pasqualetti P, Desideri G, Blumberg JB, Ferri C. Cocoa reduces blood pressure and insulin resistance and

improves endothelium-dependent vasodilation in hypertensives. *Hypertension* 2005; 46: 398-405.

[89]   Grassi D, Lippi C, Necozione S, Desideri G, Ferri C. Short-term administration of dark chocolate is followed by a significant increase in insulin sensitivity and a decrease in blood pressure in healthy persons. *American Journal of Clinical Nutrition* 2005; 81: 611-614.

[90]   Celermajer DS. Endothelial dysfunction: Does it matter? Is it reversible? *Journal of the American College of Cardiology* 1997; 30: 325-333.

[91]   Karim M, McCormick K, Kappagoda CT. Effects of cocoa extracts on endothelium-dependent relaxation. *Journal of Nutrition* 2000; 130: 2105S-2109S.

[92]   Rein D, Paglieroni TG, Pearson DA, Wun T, Schmitz HH, Gosselin R, Keen CL. Cocoa and wine polyphenols modulate platelet activation and function. *Journal of Nutrition* 2000; 130: 2120S-2126S.

[93]   Schramm DD, Wang JF, Holt RR, Ensunsa JL, Gonsalves JL, Lazarus SA, Schmitz HH, Keen CL. Chocolate procyanidins decrease the leukotriene-prostacyclin ratio in humans and human aortic endothelial cells. *American Journal of Clinical Nutrition* 2001; 73: 36-40.

[94]   Mao TK, Powell J, Van de Water J, Keen CL, Schmitz HH, Hammerstone JF, Gershwin ME. The effect of cocoa procyanidins on the transcription and secretion of interleukin 1 in peripheral blood mononuclear cells. *Life Sciences* 2000; 66: 1377-1386.

[95]   Mathur S, Devaraj S, Grundy SM, Jialal I. Cocoa products decrease low density lipoprotein oxidative susceptibility but do not affect biomarkers of inflammation in humans. *Journal of Nutrition* 2002; 132: 3663-3667.

[96]   Kris-Etherton P M, Keen CL. Evidence that the antioxidant flavonoids in tea and cocoa are beneficial for cardiovascular health. *Current Opinion in Lipidology* 2002; 13: 41-49.

[97]   Ding EL, Hutfless SM, Ding X, Girotra S. Chocolate and prevention of cardiovascular disease: A systematic review. *Nutrition and Metabolism* 2006; 3 (2).

[98]   Lee J, Watson RR. Cranberry: a role in health promotion. In Watson RR . *Nutrients and foods in AIDS.* CRC: 1998, 217-222.

[99]   Henig YS, Leahy MM. Cranberry juice and urinary-tract health: Science supports folklore. Nutrition 2000; 16:684-687.

[100] Lowe FC, Fagelman E. Cranberry juice and urinary tract infections: what is the evidence? *Urology* 2001; 57:407-413.

[101] Scalbert A. Antimicrobial properties of tannins. *Phytochemistry* 1991; 30:3875-3883.

[102] Chen H, Zuo Y, Deng Y. Separation and determination of flavonoids and other phenolic compounds in cranberry juice by high-performance liquid chromatography. *Journal of Chromatography* 2001; 913:387-395.

[103] Sun J, Chu Y, Wu X, Liu R. Antioxidant and antiproliferative activities of common fruits. *Journal of Agricultural and Food Chemistry* 2002; 50:7449-7454.

[104] Vvedenskaya IO, Rosen RT, Guido JE, Russell DJ, Mills KA, Vorsa N. Characterization of flavonols in cranberry (*Vaccinium macrocarpon*) powder. *Journal of Agricultural and Food Chemistry* 2004; 52:188-195.

[105] Howell AB. Cranberry proanthocyanidins and the maintenance of urinary tract health. *Critical Reviews in Food Science and Nutrition* 2002; 42(suppl.):273-278.

[106] Weiss EI, Houri-Haddad Y, Greenbaum E, Hochman N, Ofek I, Zakay-Rones. Cranberry juice constituents affect influenza virus adhesion and infectivity. *Antiviral Research* 2005; 66:9-12.

[107] Burger O, Weiss E, Sharon N, Tabak M, Neeman I, Ofek I. Inhibition of *Helicobacter pylori* adhesion to human gastric mucus by a high-molecular weight constituent of cranberry juice. *Critical Reviews in Food Science and Nutrition* 2002; 42(suppl.):279-284.

[108] Burger O, Ofek I, Tabak M, Weiss EI, Sharon N, Neeman I. A high molecular mass constituent of cranberry juice inhibits *Helicobacter pylori* adhesion to human gastric mucus. *FEMS Immunology and Medical Microbiology* 2000; 29:295-301.

[109] Weiss EI, Lev-Dor R, Sharon N, Ofek I. Inhibitory effect of a high-molecular-weight constituent of cranberry on adhesion of oral bacteria. *Critical Reviews in Food Science and Nutrition* 2002; 42(suppl.):285-292.

[110] Labreque J, Bodet C, Chandad F, Grenier D. Effects of a high-molecular-weight cranberry fraction on growth, biofilm formation and adherence of *Porphyromonas gingivalis*. *Journal of Antimicrobial Chemotherapy* 2006; 58:439-443.

[111] Steinberg D, Feldman M, Ofek I, Weiss EI. Effect of a high-molecular-weight component of cranberry on constituents of dental biofilm. *Journal of Antimicrobial Chemotherapy* 2004; 54:86-89.

[112] Foo LY, Lu Y, Howell AB, Vorsa N. The structure of cranberry proanthocyanidins which inhibit adherence to uropathogenic P-fimbriated *Escherichia coli* in vitro. *Phytochemistry* 2000; 54:173-181.

[113] Reed J. Cranberry flavonoids, atherosclerosis and cardiovascular health. *Critical Reviews in Food Science and Nutrition* 2002; 42(suppl.):301-316.

[114] Chu Y, Liu RH. Cranberries inhibit LDL oxidation and induce LDL receptor expression in hepatocytes. *Life Sciences* 2005; 77:1892-1901.

[115] Ruel G, Pomerleau S, Couture P, Lamarche B, Couillard C. Changes in plasma antioxidant capacity and oxidized low-density lipoprotein levels in men after short-term cranberry juice consumption. *Metabolism Clinical and Experimental* 2005; 54:856-861.

[116] Wilson T, Porcari JP, Harbin D. Cranberry extract inhibits low density lipoprotein oxidation. *Life Sciences* 1998; 62:381-386.

[117] Ferguson PJ, Kurowska E, Freeman DJ, Chambers AF, Koropatnick DJ. A flavonoid fraction from cranberry extract inhibits proliferation of human tumour cell lines. *The Journal of Nutrition* 2004; 134:1529-1535.

[118] He X, Liu R. Cranberry phytochemicals: Isolation, structure elucidation, and their antiproliferative and antioxidant activities. *Journal of Agricultural and Food Chemistry* 2006; 54:7069-7074.

[119] Murphy BT, MacKinnon SL, Yan X, Hammond GB, Vaisberg AJ, Neto CC. Identification of triterpene hydroxycinnamates with *in vitro* antitumor activity from whole cranberry fruit (*Vaccinium macrocarpon*). *Journal of Agricultural and Food Chemistry* 2003; 51:3541-3545.

[120] Howell AB, Reed JD, Krueger CG, Winterbottom R, Cunningham DG, Leahy M. A-type cranberry proanthocyanidins and uropathogenic bacterial anti-adhesion activity. *Phytochemisty* 2005; 66:2281-2291.

[121] Zafriri D, Ofek I, Adar R, Pocino M, Sharon N. Inhibitory activity of cranberry juice on adherence of Type 1 and Type P fimbriated *Escherichia coli* to eukaryotic cells. *Antimicrobial Agents and Chemotherapy* 1989;33:92-98.

[122] McMurdo MET, Bissett LY, Price RJG, Phillips G, Crombie IK. Does ingestion of cranberry juice reduce symptomatic urinary tract infections in older people in hospital? A double-blind, placebo-controlled trail. *Age and Ageing* 2005; 34:256-261.

[123] Avorn J, Monane M, Gurwitz JH, Glynn RJ, Choodnovskiy I, Lipsitz LA. Reduction of bacteriuria and pyuria after ingestion of cranberry juice. *JAMA* 1994; 271:751-754.

[124] Sharon N. Bacerial lectins, cell-cell recognition and infectious disease. FEBS Letters 1987; 217:145-157.

[125] Franco AV. Recurrent urinary tract infections. Best Practice and Research Clinical Obstetrics and Gynaecology 2005; 19(6):861-873.

[126] Jepson RG, Mihaljevic L, Craig J. Cranberries for preventing urinary tract infections (Review). *Cochrane Database Systematic Reviews.* 2006;(3).

[127] Vosti KL. Infections of the Urinary Tract in women: A prospective, longitudinal study of 235 women observed for 1-19 years. *Medicine* 2002; 81:369-387.

[128] Ofek I, Beachey EH. Mannose binding and epithelial cell adherence of *Escherichia coli*. *Infection and immunity* 1978; 22:247-254.

[129] Howell AB, Vorsa N. Inhibition of the adherence of P-fimbriated *Escherichia coli* to uroepithelial-cell surfaces by proanthocyanidin extracts from cranberry. New England *Journal of Medicine* 1998; 339:1085-1086.

[130] Reid G; Hsiehl J; Potter P; Mighton J; Lam D; Warren D; Stephenson J Cranberry juice consumption may reduce biofilms on uroepithelial cells: pilot study in spinal cord injured patients. *Spinal Cord* 2001; 39, 26-30.

[131] Vattem DA, Lin YT, Ghardian R, Shetty K. Cranberry synergies for dietary management of *Helicobacter pylori* infections. *Process Biochemistry* 2005; 40:1583-1592.

[132] Kolenbrander PE, London J. Adhere today, here tomorrow: oral bacterial adherence. *Journal of Bacteriology* 1993; 175:3247-3252.

[133] Weiss EI, Lev-Dor R, Kashamn Y, Goldhar J, Sharon N, Ofek I. Inhibiting interspecies coaggregation of plaque bacteria with a cranberry juice constituent. *Journal of the American Dental Association* 1998; 129:1719-1723.

[134] Bodet C, Piche M, Chandad F, Grenier D. Inhibition of periodontopathogen-derived proteolytic enzymes by a high-molecular-weight fraction isolated from cranberry. *Journal of Antimicrobial Chemotherapy* 2006; 57:685-690.

[135] Temple NJ. Antioxidants and disease: more questions than answers. *Nutrition Research* 2000; 20:449-459.

[136] De Whalley C, Rankin S, Hoult JRS, Jessup W, Leake DS. Flavonoids inhibit the oxidative modification of low density lipoproteins by macrophages. *Biochemical Pharmacology* 1990; 39:1743-1750.

[137] Duthie GG, Bellizzi MC. Effects of antioxidants on vascular health. *British Medical Bulletin* 1999; 55:568-577.

[138] Ruel G, Pomerleau S, Couture P, Lemieux S, Lamarche B, Couillard C. Favourable impact of low-calorie cranberry juice consumption on plasma HDL-cholesterol concentrations in men. *British Journal of Nutrition* 2006; 96:357-364.

[139] Andriambeloson E, Kleschyov A, Muller B, Beretz A, Stoclet J, Andriantsitohaina R. Nitric oxide production and endothelium-dependent vasorelaxation induced by wine polyphenols in rat aorta. *British Journal of Pharmacology* 1997; 120:1053-1058.

[140] Seeram NP, Adams LS, Hardy ML, Heber D. Total cranberry extract versus its phytochemical constituents: antiproliferative and synergistic effects against human tumor cell lines. *Journal of Agricultural and Food Chemistry* 2004; 52:2512-2517.

[141] Duthie, Garry G.; Kyle, Janet A. M.; Jenkinson, Alison McE.; Duthie, Susan J.; Baxter, Gwen J.; Paterson, John R. Increased salicylate concentrations in urine of human volunteers after consumption of cranberry juice. *Journal of Agricultural and Food Chemistry* 2005; 53, 2897-2900.

[142] Kontiokari T, Salo J, Eerola E, Uhari M. Cranberry juice and bacterial colonization in children – A placebo-controlled randomized trial. *Clinical Nutrition* 2005; 24:1065-1072.

[143] Gettman, Matthew T.; Ogan, Kenneth; Brinkley, Linda J.; Adams-Huet, Beverley; Pak, Charles Y. C.; Pearle, Margaret S. Effect of cranberry juice consumption on urinary stone risk factors. *Journal of Urology* 2005; 174: 590-594.

In: Nutrition Research at the Leading Edge
Editors: R. E. Cassady, E. I. Tidswell, pp. 53-93

ISBN: 978-1-60456-053-4
© 2008 Nova Science Publishers, Inc.

Chapter II

Childhood Obesity

Alexander K.C. Leung[1] and Wm. Lane M. Robson

University of Calgary, the Alberta Children's Hospital, #200, 233 - 16th Avenue NW,
Calgary, Alberta, T2M 0H5, Canada
Childrens' Clinic, #111, 4411 16th Avenue NW,
Calgary, Alberta, T3B 0M3, Canada

Abstract

Childhood obesity is a global concern. In many countries, the prevalence has increased so rapidly that the problem is considered an epidemic. Recent data indicate that approximately 10% of children aged 2 to 5 years, and 15% of children aged 6 to 19 years, are overweight. Obese children commonly grow up to be obese adults. The co-morbid conditions associated with childhood obesity include coronary heart disease, hypertension, type 2 diabetes mellitus, polycystic ovary syndrome, hyperlipidemia, obstructive sleep apnea, increased incidence of upper respiratory tract infection, orthopedic problems, non-alcoholic fatty liver disease, cholelithiasis, renal disease, and iron deficiency. The relative risk of all-cause mortality is approximately 1.5 times greater for obese children and adolescents compared with their normal weight peers. Obese mothers are at risk for birth defects. A less acceptable body image can have a significant negative psychological and social impact. The goals of treatment should be weight stabilization and improved fitness, and improvements in psychosocial function and in the co-morbid conditions. The three primary components of therapy are decreased caloric intake, increased energy output, and behavioral modifications that include both the child and the family. Childhood obesity, once established, is notoriously difficult to treat. Good nutrition and regular physical activity help to prevent obesity. Health care professionals who care for children should promote healthy dietary and lifestyle choices. Infants should be exclusively breastfed for the first 6 months of life and mothers should be encouraged to breastfeed for as long as possible. Around 2 years of age, the intake of fat should be reduced and the intake of whole grain products, vegetables, fruit, and low-

1 Correspondence to: Dr. Alexander K.C. Leung #200, 233 - 16th Avenue NW Calgary, Alberta, Canada T2M 0H5
Telefax: (403) 230-3322 e-mail: aleung@ucalgary.ca.

fat diary products should be increased. The consumption of juice, sweetened beverages, and soft drinks should be limited. Prevention of childhood obesity requires both family-based and school-based programs that include the promotion of physical activity, parent education and modeling, behavioral counseling, and nutrition education. Community programs should interact with school programs to provide opportunities for children to be physically active.

Keywords: obesity, complications, diet, exercise, behavioral modification.

Introduction

The prevalence of obesity has increased at an alarming rate [1]. The prevalence has increased two- to three-fold over the last three decades [2,3] and the prevalence of adult obesity has doubled in the past 20 years [4]. Since obese children often grow up to be obese adults, the prevalence of adult obesity will likely continue to increase [5]. The morbidity and mortality associated with obesity continues to increase and the economic burden is substantial [6]. Despite the high prevalence, there is considerable confusion about the definition of obesity, the significance of childhood obesity, which group of children requires treatment, and the best therapy. There are not enough evidenced-based strategies on the prevention of obesity and further research is needed.

Definitions and Methods of Assessing Obesity

Obesity is characterized by an excess of adipose tissue in relation to lean body mass [7]. Acceptable levels of body fat are 17 to 18% for prepubertal children [8]. At the age of 18 years, the normal body fat level for a male is 15 to 18% and for a female 20 to 25% [8]. The body fat can be measured directly by hydrodensitometry, by measurement of the absorption of gases by adipose tissue, or by the measurement of the level of intracellular potassium [7]. These methods are impractical in a clinical setting, but data obtained with these methods establishes the standards against which indirect methods are compared.

Indirect methods to assess obesity are less precise but less invasive. The body mass index (BMI), calculated by dividing the weight in kilograms by the height in meters squared (kg/m^2), is a widely accepted measure of adiposity, is considered simple and reliable, and correlates well with measures of adult obesity [9-11]. BMI has replaced body weight or the weight to height ratio as a measure of obesity. The mean value, standard deviation, and the degree of skewness of BMI changes with age, and differs between sexes, such that the measurement must be interpreted with the use of specific percentile charts or by the calculation of either a standard deviation or a z score relative to reference data for a specific population [12,13]. The growth charts provided by the Centers for Disease Control and Prevention (CDC) now include the BMI values for age and gender [14]. Validity testing of BMI as a measure of adiposity shows a strong association between BMI and body fat [15,16]. In adults, BMI values of > 25 kg/m^2 but < 30 kg/m^2 are considered as overweight and > 30 kg/m^2 are considered as obese [17]. In children, there are many definitions of overweight and obesity. According to the CDC, International Life Sciences Institute, and the American Academy of Pediatrics, children with a BMI between the 85th and 95th percentile are classified as at risk for overweight and those with a BMI > 95th percentile are classified as overweight [18,19]. In this regard, a z score > 2 correlates to the 95th percentile that defines overweight in children. The term overweight is often used in place of obese for individuals in the highest category because there is less of a stigma associated with this term [10]. Overweight and obesity are often used interchangeably in the literature. In the United Kingdom the definitions used for research and for clinical practice are different and this has resulted in considerable confusion. For research and epidemiological purposes in the United Kingdom, overweight and obesity are defined as a BMI ≥ 85th and ≥ 95th percentiles, respectively, [13]. However in clinical practice, the commonly used charts in the United Kingdom provide the 91st and 98th percentiles, and these are used for the definitions of overweight and obesity, respectively [13]. The International Obesity Task Force (IOTF) has developed a definition of overweight based on pooled data from six international BMI references from the United States, United Kingdom, Netherlands, Hong Kong, Singapore, and Brazil. The definitions for overweight and obesity are based on the BMI for age percentile curves to ensure that at age 18 they match the adult definitions of 25 and 30 kg/m^2, respectively [11].

The BMI might not be reliable in individuals with extremely high or low percentages of body fat. An extremely high percentage of fat might lead to a false negative BMI and an extremely low percentage might lead to a false positive BMI [20]. In most cases, a physician should be able to clinically distinguish an obese child from an extremely muscular child.

Other indirect methods to assess obesity include estimation of body fat by dual-energy X-ray absorptiometry or by bioelectric impedance [8,21]. The latter is based on the principle that fat and bone are poor conductors compared with muscle [8]. Measurement of skin-fold thickness with a suitable caliper is a practical method that has published standards [7]. Fat is correlated with caliper measurement in the range of 0.7 to 0.8. Limitations include the biologic variation in the distribution of fat in the body, the inability to palpate the fat-muscle interface, variation in skin-fold compressibility, and variation in the site of measurement between examiners [7]. Measurement of waist circumference is a good measure of visceral fat while BMI is not [6,22]. The waist-to-hip ratio is a better predictor of myocardial infarction than BMI [22,23]. Yusuf et al preformed a large case-control study on risk factors for myocardial infarction in 52 countries [23]. The authors investigated the relation of four different measures of obesity that included BMI, waist measure, hip measure, and waist-to-hip ratio for the risk of myocardial infarction. In all ethnic groups, waist-to-hip ratio was the best predictor of myocardial infarction.

Epidemiology

According to the data of the National Health and Nutritional Examination Surveys conducted between 1971 and 1974, and between 1999 and 2002, the prevalence of overweight males aged 12 to 19 years increased from 5.4% to 16.7% and for females from 6.4% to 15.4% [24]. For males aged 6 to 11 years the prevalence increased from 3.8% to

16.8%, and for females from 3.6% to 15.1% [24]. For male children aged 2 to 5 years, the prevalence increased from 5% to 10.3% and for females from 5% to 10.7. The prevalence among Hispanic and African American individuals exceeds that of white individuals [2]. According to the 2004 Canadian Community Health survey, the rate of obesity increased dramatically in the last 15 years from 2% to 10% among boys, and from 2% to 9% among girls [25,26]. The health survey for England in 2004 showed that 14% of 2 to 11 year-old children and 25% of 11 to 15 year-old children were obese [27]. The prevalence has increased in almost all countries and secular trends vary considerably within countries [27,28]. The increase in prevalence is more dramatic in economically developed countries and in urbanized populations [28].

In developed countries, obesity is more prevalent among those with lower socioeconomic status [29,30]. In a study of 4,298 grade 5 students, children in high-income neighborhoods were half as likely to be obese as their peers who lived in low-income neighborhoods (odds ratio: 0.5; 95% confidence interval: 0.36 to 0.7) [30]. The paradoxical relationship between food insecurity and the development of obesity might be related to consumption of low-cost energy-dense foods and over-eating when food is available [8,31,32]. In contrast, in developing countries, obesity is more prevalent among those with higher socioeconomic status [29].

Parental obesity is an important risk factor for childhood obesity [33,34]. Agras et al prospectively followed 150 children from birth to 9.5 year of age [33]. The authors found that the most common independent risk factor for childhood obesity was parental overweight. Danielzik et al did a cross-sectional study on 2,631 5 to 7 year-old German children and their parents [34]. The prevalence of overweight individuals was 9.2% in boys and 11.2% in girls. In multivariate analysis, parental overweight, a low socioeconomic status, and a high birth weight were the strongest independent risk factors for childhood obesity. Parental obesity constitutes both genetic and family environmental influences for childhood obesity [33,35]. The odds ratio of childhood obesity increases to 3 if one parent is obese and to 10 if both parents are obese [6,35]. Children with obese parents are more likely to experience an early adiposity rebound which is a risk factor for obesity [9,36]. Learning within the family environment might affect food preference, caloric intake, and activity levels [33].

Family size is inversely associated with childhood obesity [8]. The relative risk that an only child will be overweight is 1.5 times greater than a child in a family of two children and 2.2 times greater than a child in a family of four children [8].

Breastfeeding reduces the risk of childhood obesity to a moderate extent [37-41]. Breastfeeding affects the intake of protein and calories, secretion of insulin, modulation of fat deposition, and development of adipose tissue [40,42]. Breastfed infants have a lower caloric intake compared with formula-fed infants, and have a lower weight gain during the critical period of early infancy [43]. The concept that early nutrition has a long-term effect on growth, metabolism, and health is referred to as "nutritional programming" [44]. Dewey analyzed 11 studies that examined the prevalence of obesity in children over 3 years of age and that had a sample size of ≥100 children per feeding group [37]. After controlling for potential confounders, 8 of the studies showed a lower risk of obesity in children who had been breastfed [37]. The three studies that did not show a lower risk of obesity lacked information on the exclusivity of breastfeeding [37]. Owen et al performed a meta-analysis of

28 high quality studies that reported on the relationship of infant feeding to obesity in later life and that provided odds ratio estimates (n=298,900) [40]. The authors found that breastfeeding was associated with a reduced risk of obesity compared with formula-feeding (odds ratio: 0.87; 95% confidence interval: 0.85 to 0.89). Important confounding factors such as low socioeconomic class, maternal obesity, and the size of the infant at birth were not controlled in many of the studies. There might be a dose-dependent association between breastfeeding and the risk of obesity [43]. Harder et al performed a meta-analysis on 17 studies that examined the effect of the duration of breastfeeding on the risk that a child will be obese [43]. The authors found that the duration of breastfeeding was inversely associated with the risk that a child will be obese (regression coefficient: 0.94; 95% confidence interval: 0.89 to 0.98). Categorical analysis confirmed the dose-dependent association. The odds ratios were 1 for less than 1 month of breastfeeding (95% confidence interval: 0.65 to 1.55), 0.81 for 1 to 3 months (95% confidence interval: 0.74 to 0.88), 0.76 for 4 to 6 months (95% confidence interval: 0.67 to 0.86), 0.67 for 7 to 9 months (95% confidence interval: 0.55 to 0.82), and 0.68 for over 9 months (95% confidence interval: 0.5 to 0.91). One month of breastfeeding was associated with a 4% decrease in risk (odds ratio: 0.96/month of breastfeeding; 95% confidence interval: 0.94 to 0.98).

Large for gestational age infants such as those born to mothers with maternal diabetes, and small for gestational age infants such as those born with intrauterine growth retardation are at increased risk for obesity in childhood [5,8]. Intrauterine malnutrition might affect the development of the appetite center in the hypothalamus [20]. Other risk factors include parental neglect, parental over-involvement, and persistent temper tantrums over food [33,45].

Etiology and Pathogenesis

Obesity might be the result of high caloric intake, more efficient uptake of calories, low energy output, or a combination of these factors. An environment that favors high caloric intake and a sedentary lifestyle is considered the most likely explanation for the recent rapid increase in the prevalence of obesity.

Most investigators cite excessive caloric intake as an important cause of obesity at every age [5,7,46]. However, the relationship between caloric intake and obesity in children has been difficult to demonstrate in clinical studies. Janssen et al performed a cross-sectional study on 5,890 11 to 16 year-old Canadian youths and found no relation between dietary habits and overweight [47]. The study employed a self-report questionnaire that assessed only differences in frequency of feeding for various foods and did not assess portion sizes, which might have made detections of dietary differences difficult. In many studies, data were obtained by recall, a notoriously inaccurate method of nutritional review, which is subject to recall errors or under-reporting. Investigators that employed direct observation found a positive correlation between weight gain and dietary intake [48]. Bunch found that 58 (78%) of 74 boys and 59 (68%) of 86 girls who were assessed in her obesity clinic were large eaters [48]. Stunkard et al performed a prospective, longitudinal study on 40 infants of obese mothers and 38 infants of lean mothers to determine the risk factors for weight gain [49]. The authors found that energy intake, and not energy expenditure, was the determinant of body size at 1 and 2 years of age. Portion sizes have grown both at home and in restaurants, and children tend to eat more in the presence of large portions.

Nutritive sucking behavior during a test meal positively contributed to the weight gain (p=0.003) in the Nutrition and Growth Laboratory of the Children's Hospital of Philadelphia [50]. Barkeling et al observed that obese children ate lunch significantly faster and did not decelerate their eating toward the end of the lunch compared to children of normal weight [50]. The authors suggested that the lack of deceleration might indicate a deficient satiation signal or an impaired behavioral response to the satiation signal.

The frequency of visits to a fast food restaurant by children has increased and increased fast food consumption can lead to obesity [46,51]. Thompson et al prospectively studied 101 girls aged 8 to 12 years. The authors found that consumption of two or more fast food meals per week correlated with a high BMI in adolescence, although eating restaurant meals did not [51]. Bowman et al studied 6,212 children and adolescents 4 to 19 years of age who lived in the United States and who were participants in the nation-wide Continuing Survey of Food Intake by Individuals conducted from 1994 to 1996 and the Supplemental Children's Survey conducted in 1998 [46]. On a typical day, 30.3% of the total sample reported that they consumed fast food. Children who ate fast food, compared with those who did not, consumed more energy (187 kcal; 95% confidence interval: 109 to 265), more energy per gram of food (0.29 kcal/kg; 95% confidence interval: 0.25 to 0.33), more total fat (9 g; 95% confidence interval: 5 to 13), more total carbohydrate (24 g; 95% confidence interval: 12.6 to 35.4), more added sugars (26 g; 95% confidence interval: 18.2 to 34.6), more sugar-sweetened beverages (228 g; 95% confidence interval: 184 to 272), less fibre (-1.1 g; 95% confidence interval: -1.8 to -0.4), less milk (-65 g; 95% confidence interval: -95 to -30), and fewer fruit and non-starchy vegetables (-45 g; 95% confidence interval: -58.6 to -31.4). Taveras et al performed a cross-sectional study on 240 parents of children 2 to 5.9 years of age [52]. Twenty two percent of parents reported that their child ate at a fast food restaurant at least once a week. After adjusting for confounding factors, the odds ratio for consumption of fast food ≥ once per week was 1.55 (95% confidence interval: 1.04 to 2.31). The dietary factors inherent in fast food that might increase energy intake and the risk for obesity, include large portion size, high caloric density, increased palatability, high content of saturated and trans fat, high glycemic load, and low fibre content [46].

Excessive consumption of sugar-sweetened beverages is an important risk factor for childhood obesity [5,53]. Ludwig et al prospectively followed 548 children aged 11 to 12 years for 19 months [53]. The authors found that soft drink consumption increased by 57% and obesity increased by 9.3%. When confounding factors were controlled, for each soft drink that was consumed daily, the risk of obesity increased by 60%. The consumption of soft drinks has markedly increased in recent years [54]. Striegel-Moore et al prospectively followed 2,371 girls who participated in the National Heart, Lung, and Blood Institute Growth and Health Study [54]. Three-day food diaries were recorded annually from the age of 9 or 10 years until 19 years of age. During this 10-year study, the consumption of milk decreased by > 25%, while the consumption of soft drinks increased almost 3-fold. Data from the Feeding Infant and Toddlers Study showed that infants and toddlers are not eating enough fruit and vegetables and are consuming too many sweetened drinks and too many sweet and salty energy-dense snacks, and that these foods are being introduced too early into their diets [55].

Obesity can be caused by reduced energy expenditure, which can result from lack of physical activity [8,56,57]. Obese children tend to be less active than their non-obese peers [7]. Lack of physical activity might be a cause or a consequence of obesity [7]. Regardless of whether inactivity is a cause or a consequence of obesity, inactivity plays an important role in the maintenance of obesity [7]. Patrick et al studied 878 adolescents aged 11 to 15 years [56]. Overall, 45.7% of the studied population had a BMI at the 85th percentile or higher. Insufficient vigorous physical activity was the only risk factor for higher BMI for these adolescent boys (odds ratio: 0.92; 95% confidence interval: 0.89 to 0.95) and girls (odds ratio: 0.93; 95% confidence interval: 0.89 to 0.97). Kimm et al examined changes in activity in relation to changes in BMI and adiposity in a cohort of 1,152 African American and 1,135 white girls from three distinct regions of the USA [58]. The subjects were followed prospectively from the age of 9 to 10 years to the age of 18 to 19 years. Kimm et al found that for African American girls, for each decline in activity of 10 metabolic equivalent-times per week, there was an associated increase in BMI of 0.14 ± 0.03 kg/m^2, and in the sum of skin-fold thickness of 0.62 ± 0.17 mm [58]. For white girls the increase in BMI was 0.09 ± 0.02 kg/m^2 and the increase in the sum of skin-fold thickness was 0.63 ± 0.13 mm . At ages 18 or 19 years, BMI differences between active and inactive girls were 2.98 kg/m^2 ($p < 0.0001$) for African American girls, and 2.1 kg/m^2 ($p < 0.0001$) for white girls. Similar results were apparent for the sum of skin-fold thickness. In the National Health and Nutrition Examination Survey 1999 to 2002 dataset, the percentage of children aged 6 to 17 years with health problems that limit their ability to walk or run was 4.1% [59]. Children with these physical activity limitations were significantly more likely to be at risk for overweight than those without physical activity limitations (50.9% versus 30.6%, $p < 0.001$). These children were also more likely to be overweight (29.7% versus 15.7%, $p < 0.01$) [59].

In recent years, children have become less physically active, rely more on mechanical modes of transportation, and spend more time in sedentary activities such as television viewing and video or computer games [60]. A meta-analysis of 30 studies showed a statistically significant association between television viewing and childhood obesity [61]. There is a relationship between the rate of obesity and the number of hours that a child watches television [62]. In the Framingham Children's Study, the rate of obesity was 8.3 times greater in children who watched over 5 hours of television per day compared with those who watched only 2 hours or less per day [62]. Television viewing promotes both inactivity and the consumption of high caloric snacks such as those that are commonly advertised on television [63].

Leptin and adiponectin participate in the pathogenesis of obesity. Leptin, which is secreted by adipose tissue and perhaps also by cells in the stomach, provides a signal that links fat stores to food intake and energy expenditure [6,20,64]. Obese individuals usually have leptin resistance with elevated levels of leptin rather than leptin deficiency with low levels of leptin [10,64]. Leptin also interacts with growth hormone and the hypothalamic-pituitary-adrenal axis [6]. The leptin level is increased as fat stores rise, which signals the hypothalamus to suppress appetite [6]. Adiponectin, which is secreted by adipose tissue, increases the oxidation of fatty acids and improves post-prandial insulin-mediated suppression of hepatic glucose output via the enhancement of insulin signaling [65]. Diamond et al measured serum concentrations of leptin and adiponectin in 14 obese children and 25 non-obese children [65]. Serum adiponectin concentrations were significantly lower in obese children compared to non-obese children (9.1 ± 3.7 µg/ml versus 17.1 ± 12.3 µg/ml; $p < 0.05$). In contrast, serum leptin concentrations were greater in obese children compared to non-obese children (31.8 ± 11.1 ng/ml versus 8.2 ± 5.7 ng/ml; $p < 0.001$). Serum adiponectin concentrations correlated inversely with body weight ($r = -0.33$; $p < 0.05$) and BMI ($r = -0.35$; $p < 0.05$). The serum leptin/adiponectin ratio was eight-fold greater in the obese children compared to the non-obese children, and correlated more strongly with BMI ($r = 0.779$; $p < 0.0001$). The serum leptin/adiponectin ratio also correlated significantly with triceps skin-fold thickness ($r = 0.77$; $p < 0.001$) and percent body fat ($r = 0.79$; $p < 0.0001$) in non-obese children.

There is a genetic predisposition to obesity [10,66,67]. Genetic factors likely interact with environmental factors to cause obesity in a susceptible individual [68]. This might explain why some individuals who are genetically predisposed to obesity become obese despite relatively low levels of caloric intake. These individuals might gain weight because they store calories more efficiently. Twin and adoption studies indicate that the heritability for BMI is approximately 65 to 80% [67,69]. The concordance rate is 0.7 to 0.9 for monozygotic twins and 0.35 to 0.45 for dizygotic twins [60,66,69]. Adoption studies reveal a closer relation between the weights of adopted children with their biological parents rather than with their adoptive parents [66,70]. Feeding behavior, responsiveness to food cues, food preference, sensitivity to internal signals of hunger and satiety, decreased postabsorptive thermogenesis, low resting energy expenditure, low ratio of fat to carbohydrate oxidation at rest, and high insulin sensitivity might be genetically determined [7,68,69,71].

The most common forms of heritable obesity are polygenic in origin, in which each gene contributes a small amount to the variation in weight [60,72]. Over 600 genes, markers, and chromosome regions have been identified that might contribute to obesity [10,60,73]. Rare families have been identified in which mutations in leptin, leptin receptors, neuropeptide Y (NPY), pro-opiomelanocortin (POMC), prohormone convertase subtilisin/kexin type1 (PCSK1), and melanocortin-4 receptor (MC4R) might result in obesity [10,60,73]. Obesity is a major phenotypic trait in genetic syndromes such as Prader-Willi syndrome, Bardet-Biedl syndrome, Beckwith-Wiedenmann syndrome, and Cohen syndrome (vide infra) [73-79].

Environmental influences are also important. Obesity tends to run in families. A logical explanation is that in addition to genetic factors, family members share common attitudes toward food, eating habits, and exercise [7]. The evidence that obese individuals tend to have obese dogs can also be interpreted in this way.

The vast majority of obese children have exogenous obesity, which is the result of excessive caloric intake relative to energy requirements [7,10]. Less than 10% of obese children have an underlying disease as the cause (Table 1) [7].

Natural History

Until recently the rate that obesity in infants persists into later life was considered to be low [68]. A review of the literature shows this to be otherwise [80,81]. Ong et al performed a systemic review of 21 articles with data on the association between rapid weight gain in the first two years of life and subsequent risk of obesity [80]. All studies uniformly reported significant positive associations (odd ratios: 1.17 to 5.7) with either a U- or a J- shaped relationship. Higher odds ratios were reported from studies with longer duration of weight gain, younger age when the outcome was measured, and less or no adjustment for potential confounding factors.

Table 1. Pathological causes of obesity

Endocrinopathies
Hypothyroidism
Cushing syndrome
Exogenous corticosteroid therapy
Growth hormone deficiency
Hyperinsulinism
Brittle diabetes mellitus (Mauriac syndrome)
Pseudohypoparathyroidism
Pseudopseudohypoparathyroidism
Central nervous system lesions
Hypothalamic tumor
Head injury
Infection
Genetic syndromes
Prader-Willi syndrome
Bardet-Biedl syndrome
Carpenter syndrome
Alström syndrome
Cohen syndrome
Single gene mutations
Leptin
Leptin receptor
Neuropeptide Y
Pro-opiomelanocortin
Prohormone convertase subtilisin / kexin
type 1
Melanocortin- 4 receptor

Modified from: Leung, AK; Robson WL. Childhood obesity. Postgrad Med 1990;87:125 [7].

Mijailović et al examined 1,451 obese adults with childhood or adolescent onset of obesity [82]. Significantly higher values for BMI and waist circumference were found in subjects with earlier onset of obesity. Kinra et al followed a cohort of 1,335 full-term infants

[83]. The authors found that BMI at the age of 7 years positively associated with z scores for weight at all ages.

Nader et al analyzed growth data from the National Institute of Child Health and Human Development Study of Early Child Care and Youth Development, a longitudinal sample of 1,042 healthy children in 10 locations in the USA [84]. The authors found that children who had an overweight measurement (>85th percentile) more than once at the ages of 24, 36, or 54 months were > 5 times as likely to be overweight at 12 years of age than those who were consistently below the 85th percentile for BMI. At the ages of 7, 9, and 11 years, the more times a child was overweight, the greater the odds of being overweight at 12 years of age relative to a child who was never overweight. Sixty percent of children who were overweight at any time during the preschool period and 80% of children who were overweight at any time during the elementary school period were overweight at 12 years of age.

Must et al explored the role of childhood overweight and maturational timing in the development of adult overweight and obesity [85]. Of the 448 women in the Newton Girls Study who participated in the adult follow-up at an age of 42.1 ± 0.76 years, 307 had childhood data sufficient to characterize premenarcheal and menarcheal weight status, and the age of menarche. After a follow-up of 30.1 ± 1.4 years, the reported BMI was 23.4 ± 4.8 kg/m^2. Twenty-eight percent of the subjects were overweight and 9% were obese. Girls who were overweight before menarche were 7.7 times more likely to be overweight as adults (95% confidence interval: 2.3 to 25.8) whereas early menarche (≤ 12 years of age) did not increase the risk (odds ratio: 1.3; 95% confidence interval: 0.66 to 2.43). In contrast, Garn et al found that girls with menarche at age ≤ 11 years were twice as likely to become obese adults as those with menarche ≥ 14 years of age [86]. Girls are particularly prone to develop persistent obesity during adolescence [68]. During puberty, the lean body mass increases and the amount of body fat decreases by approximately 40% in an average male, whereas in an average female the amount of body fat increases by approximately 40% [68].

Obesity in childhood is strongly associated with obesity in adulthood. The later the onset of childhood obesity, the more likely the problem will persist into adult life [87-89]. Freedman et al followed 2,610 children aged 2 to 17 years for a mean of 17.6 years. The authors found that childhood levels of both BMI and the triceps skin-fold measurement were associated with adult levels of BMI and adiposity. The magnitude of these associations increased with childhood age, but the BMI levels of even the youngest children (aged 2 to 5 years) were moderately associated ($r = 0.33$ to 0.41) with adult adiposity. Laitinen et al found that BMI at 14 years of age was a better predictor of adult obesity than the birth weight or BMI at 1 year of age [88]. Serdula et al also found that the risk of adult obesity was greater among children who were obese at or around puberty [89]. In general, approximately 33% of obese preschool children, 50% of obese school-aged children, and 75% of obese teenagers grow up to be obese adults [35,89].

Obesity can result from an increase in the size of adipocytes, an increase in the number of adipocytes, or a combination of these factors [7]. Adipocytes reach adult size by the end of the first year of life. Once maximal cell size is reached, further fat deposition occurs by formation of new adipocytes. The attainment of a predetermined maximal cell size might be a factor that signals adipocytes to change from hypertrophic to hyperplastic growth [7]. Once adipocytes are formed, their number cannot be reduced. The persistence of a raised number of adipocytes has been related to the difficulty to maintain weight loss that is experienced by individuals with childhood-onset obesity. The periods during childhood which are critical for the development of obesity include the prenatal period, the adiposity rebound period around 5 to 7 years of age, and the pubertal period [90]. During these periods, multiplication of adipocytes is most likely influenced by nutritional factors. Children are least likely to outgrow their obesity when the obesity is more severe and when they have at least one obese parent [27].

Clinical Manifestations

Although obesity appears most often in the first year of life and during adolescence, the problem can become evident at any age [7]. Advanced bone age is common in children with exogenous obesity [91]. Children with exogenous obesity are usually tall for their age, although they are only slightly taller than average as adults [7]. In contrast, children with endogenous obesity are often shorter than average. Obese children often have accelerated dental development [92].

The facial features of obese children often appear disproportionately fine. Obese children commonly have a double chin. The abdomen tends to be pendulous, and white or purple striae might be present on the abdomen or legs. The collection of fat in the mammary region of boys might simulate breast development, but palpation does not reveal true mammary gland tissue.

Hypogenitalism is often suspected in obese boys because their genitalia can be buried in fat. Displacing the fat during a clinical examination reveals normal genital anatomy. The external genitalia have a normal appearance in obese girls, but obese girls usually begin menses at a younger age than non-obese girls [93]. While obese girls are more likely to experience early puberty, obese boys usually do not start puberty early [93,94]. Wang et al analyzed the data from the National Health and Nutritional Examination Survey and found that the odds ratio for overweight was 0.65 (95% confidence interval: 0.44 to 0.98) for boys with early pubertal development compared to those with normal development [94].

Complications

Health and social consequences of childhood obesity are a major health problem not only in childhood and adolescence, but also in adulthood, and even if the childhood obesity does not persist [20,95]. Several long-term cohort studies have shown relative risk estimates for obese children and adolescents compared with their normal weight peers to be approximately 1.5 for all-cause mortality and 2 for mortality from coronary heart disease [96]. About 1 in 10 premature deaths among Canadian adults aged 20 to 64 years is attributable to obesity [97]. Health care expenditures are significantly higher for children with obesity than for those without [98]. The potential complications of childhood obesity are listed in Table 2. Many complications of obesity, once recognized mostly in adults, are now present in childhood [99].

Psychosocial

Psychosocial disturbances are the most common consequences of childhood obesity [96]. Obese children are often teased and ridiculed. They are often the targets of abuse by peers and are often left out of games and social activities [100,101]. Social marginalization can lead to reduced self-esteem and depression [101]. Obese children are often involved in disturbed family interactions. These children can have a poor self-image, a sense of failure, and a passive external approach to life situations, and they might express feelings of inferiority and rejection [7]. Obese children are often perceived to be less competent in sports, less physically attractive, and less successful with peer engagement [102]. Depressive disorders and oppositional defiant disorder are more common in obese children [103-105]. Overweight concerns and body dissatisfaction are also more common and are risk factors for the development of eating disorders such as anorexia nervosa and bulimia nervosa [106,107]. Obese high school students might be discriminated against when they apply for college acceptance [108]. Obesity is associated with lack of sexual desire, lack of enjoyment of sexual activity, difficulties with sexual performance, and avoidance of sexual encounters [109]. The sexual impairment is usually more severe in women than in men [109].

Table 2. Complications of childhood obesity

Psychosocial
Cardiovascular
Endocrinologic
Respiratory
Orthopedic
Gastrointestinal
Dermatologic
Renal
Hematologic
Surgical
Oncologic
Dental
Teratogenic

Cardiovascular

Data from both the Framingham Heart Study and the Bogalusa Study report an increased incidence of cardiovascular events in obese individuals [110,111]. Steinberger et al followed 31 children aged 13.3 ± 0.3 years and re-evaluated them at age 21.8 ± 0.3 years [112]. The authors found that BMI in childhood (22.6 ± 0.6 kg/m²) was highly correlated with BMI in young adulthood (26.9 ± 0.9 kg/m²). Childhood BMI was also inversely correlated with young adult glucose utilization (r = -0.5; p=0.006) and positively correlated with total cholesterol (r = 0.37; p = 0.05) and low-density lipoprotein cholesterol (r = 0.48; p = 0.01). Since diabetes mellitus and hypercholesterolemia are risk factors for cardiovascular disease, the study suggests that cardiovascular risk in adulthood is highly related to the degree of adiposity in childhood. For children with a BMI $\geq$ 99th percentile, 59% will have at least two cardiovascular risk factors [113].

Dyslipidemia is a common co-morbid problem in obese children [10]. The abnormal lipid profiles include elevated levels of serum triglyceride and low-density lipoprotein cholesterol, and low levels of high-density lipoprotein cholesterol [10]. Boyd et al performed a retrospective case-control study on 497 patients (226 boys, 271 girls) 2 to 18 years of age [114]. These children were all overweight and were assessed at the Nemours Weight Management Clinic at the duPont Hospital for Children. Elevated low-density lipoprotein cholesterol and triglyceride, and low high-density lipoprotein cholesterol were found in approximately 15%, 19.1%, and 28.2% of these children, respectively. Others studies have confirmed that obese individuals are at increased risk for dyslipidemia [112,115,116].

The association of dyslipidemia and atherosclerosis is well documented [10,117]. Newman et al analyzed the autopsy findings of 35 individuals (mean age at death, 18 years) who had previously been examined as part of the Bogalusa Heart Study [117]. The authors found that fatty streaks in the aorta were strongly related to ante-mortem levels of both total and low-density lipoprotein cholesterol (r = 0.67; p < 0.0001 for each association) and were inversely correlated with the ratio of high-density lipoprotein cholesterol to low-density plus very-low-density lipoprotein cholesterol (r = -0.35; p = 0.06). Fatty streaks in the coronary arteries were correlated with very-low-density lipoprotein cholesterol (r = 0.41; p = 0.04). Berenson et al analyzed the autopsy findings on 93 persons, 2 to 39 years of age, who had died from trauma [118]. BMI, blood pressure, and serum concentration of total cholesterol, triglyceride, and low-density lipoprotein cholesterol were strongly associated with the extent of fatty streaks and fibrous plaques in the aorta and coronary arteries (canonical correlation: r = 0.7; p < 0.001). The Bogalusa Heart Study confirmed that childhood measures of low-density lipoprotein cholesterol, waist measurement, and BMI predict carotid intima-media thickness in young adults [119, 120]. These studies suggest that the atherosclerotic process is active in youth and is accelerated appreciably in the setting of obesity and the associated clustering of cardiovascular risk factors [121].

Obese children are at risk for hypertension. In the study by Boyd et al of 497 patients seen at the Nemours Weight Management Clinic of duPont Hospital for Children (vide supra), 34 (6.8%) had hypertension [114]. Sorof et al [2004] measured blood pressure on 5,102 children aged 13.5 $\pm$ 1.7 years [122]. Those with blood pressure > 95th percentile on the first screening underwent a second screening 1 to 2 weeks later, and then a third screening if the blood pressure was still elevated. The prevalence of elevated blood pressure after the first, second, and third screening was 19.4%, 9.5%, and 4.5%, respectively. The prevalence of hypertension increased progressively as the BMI percentile increased from $\leq$ 5th percentile (2%) to $\geq$ 95th percentile (11%). After adjustment for confounding factors, the relative risk of hypertension for overweight was 3.26 (95% confidence interval: 2.5 to 4.24). Falkner et al analyzed electronic medical record data from primary care practices on 18,618 children 2 to 19 years of age [123]. The authors found that 16.7% of the children were at risk of overweight and 20.2% were overweight. Overall, 7.2% of the studied population had systolic or diastolic blood pressure values $\geq$ 95th percentile. With increasing BMI status, there was a significant increase in both systolic blood pressure (p < 0.001) and diastolic blood pressure (p < 0.001). Other studies have confirmed the strong positive correlation between obesity and elevated systolic and diastolic blood pressure [112,116]. Hypertension and dyslipidemia might independently contribute to increased oxidative stress with production of greater amounts of oxygen free radicals in childhood obesity [124]. Free radicals contribute to endothelial dysfunction and are involved in the pathogenesis and development of a variety of cardiovascular diseases [124-126].

Studies on the effect of obesity on peak heart rate have yielded inconsistent results. Loftin et al measured the peak heart rate in 88 female youths (43 obese, 45 normal weight) with a treadmill test [127]. The peak heart rate was significantly lower in the obese group compared to the normal weight group (192.3 ± 9.3 versus 203.4 ± 7.6; p ≤ 0.05). Bivariate correlations for peak heart rate and body weight, percent fat, and BMI were -0.53, -0.54, and -0.57, respectively. Either reduced secretion or response to epinephrine and norepinephrine might account for the reduced peak heart rate [128]. Other investigators found no significant difference in peak heart rate when obese individuals were compared to non-obese individuals [129,130].

Left ventricular hypertrophy is more prevalent in obese individuals [131]. Chinali et al examined left ventricular geometry and function in 460 adolescents (114 normal weight, 113 overweight, and 223 obese) who participated in the Strong Heart Study [131]. Left ventricular hypertrophy demonstrated by Doppler echocardiography was more prevalent in the obese (33.5%) and overweight (12.4%), compared with normal weight participants (3.5%; p<0.001).

Endocrinologic

Childhood obesity predisposes to insulin resistance and type 2 diabetes mellitus [91,132]. Tumor necrosis factor-α (TNF-α), interleukin-6 (IL-6), and resistin are overexpressed in the adipose tissue of obese individuals, especially the visceral adipose tissue [91,133]. TNF-α and resistin inhibit insulin-mediated glucose and free fatty acid uptake, and triglyceride synthesis in adipose tissue [91]. TNF-α and resistin also induce lipolysis and release of free fatty acids from adipose stores. The lipolytic effects are potentiated by IL-6 [91]. Increased exposure of the liver to free fatty acids results in increased triglyceride synthesis and storage in the liver, increased hepatic glucose production, and impaired insulin uptake and clearance, which leads to circulating hyperinsulinism [10,91]. Adiponectin concentrations are low in obese individuals [10]. Together with direct effects of TNF-α, IL-6, and resistin, this might exacerbate hepatic insulin resistance [91]. Accumulation of lipids in muscle cells might interfere with insulin signaling and glucose transport [10]. The accumulation of lipids in muscle cells and insulin resistance might be mediated by visceral fat and adiponectin [134]. Visceral adiposity promotes insulin resistance to a greater extent than subcutaneous adiposity [133].

Insulin resistance can lead to impaired glucose tolerance. In the presence of insulin resistance, there is a compensatory pancreatic β-cell response, which results in hyperinsulinemia. Free fatty acids, cytokines, and glucose can promote β-cell dysfunction in genetically predisposed individuals [135,136]. When β-cells fail, diabetes mellitus ensues.

The lack of insulin in patients with type 2 diabetes mellitus can lead to ketoacidosis [133]. Until recently, only 2 to 3% children with diabetes mellitus were thought to have type 2 diabetes [132]. Due to the increase in the prevalence of childhood obesity, about 30% of diabetes mellitus in childhood is now due to type 2 diabetes [137]. The transition of impaired glucose tolerance to type 2 diabetes is usually a gradual process that occurs over 5 to 10 years [138]. Weiss et al followed 102 obese children and adolescents from a pediatric weight management clinic [139]. Seventy-one had normal glucose tolerance and 31 had impaired glucose tolerance. Oral glucose tolerance tests were repeated after 18 to 24 months. Six (8.4%) of the 71 patients with normal glucose tolerance became impaired. Ten (32.3%) of 31 with impaired glucose tolerance developed type 2 diabetes mellitus, 10 (32.3%) converted to normal glucose tolerance, and 11 (36.4%) remained impaired. Transition from normal to impaired glucose tolerance and from impaired glucose tolerance to diabetes mellitus was associated with significant increases in weight, while conversion from impaired to normal glucose tolerance was associated with the least amount of weight gain [139]. Insulin resistance does not necessarily lead to frank glucose intolerance [91]. The majority of obese insulin-resistant subjects never develop type 2 diabetes [91]. The development of type 2 diabetes requires β-cell dysfunction and loss of glucose-dependent insulin secretion.

Poor glycemic control over a long duration can lead to significant morbidity, including macrovascular complications such as peripheral vascular disease, coronary artery disease, and stroke, and microvascular complications such as retinopathy, neuropathy, and nephropathy [132]. Metabolic syndrome, also known as "syndrome X," which is characterized by insulin resistance, type 2 diabetes, hypertension, and dyslipidemia, was once thought to confer increased cardiovascular risk [6]. A recent joint statement from the American Diabetes Association and European Association for the Study of Diabetes suggests that the concept of metabolic syndrome is largely irrelevant since collectively these problems do not provide additional predictive value beyond the risk factors for each individual problem [140].

Polycystic ovary syndrome is the most common endocrine disorder in women during their reproductive years [141]. The syndrome is characterized by irregular menses, acne, hirsutism, and polycystic ovaries. Insulin resistance associated with obesity is the underlying mechanism for the hyperandrogenism characteristic of the syndrome [141,142]. Hyperinsulinemia leads to increased stimulation of the activity of the cytochrome P450c 17α in the ovarian thecal cells with increased production of lutenizing hormone, which stimulates androgen production [10]. Insulin also suppresses sex hormone binding globulin production in the liver, which results in a further increase of free androgens [10].

Increased free androgens might cause an advance in bone age and premature adrenarche in prepubertal children [143,144]. Premature adrenarche and precocious puberty have been associated with insulin resistance [145,146]. The conversion of androgen to estrone in adipose tissue can lead to gynecomastia in adolescent boys [10,147].

Respiratory

Childhood obesity is associated with an increased incidence of acute respiratory infection [7,148]. One explanation is that hypoventilation together with impairment of coughing and in the clearance of secretions, which are noted with obesity, might increase the incidence and severity of respiratory infections.

The work of breathing is increased in obese children. Children with severe obesity can develop chronic hypoxemia. In some of these children, ventilation fails to increase sufficiently to normalize PCO_2 values. These children have Pickwickian (obesity-hypoventilation) syndrome, named after "the fat and red-faced boy" in Charles Dickens' "The Pickwick Papers."

Obstructive sleep apnea is more common in obese children [149]. Obstructive sleep apnea is especially prevalent among obese children with habitual snoring, and insulin resistance is independently associated with this condition [150]. Li et al studied 94 consecutive obese children with habitual snoring [150]. Sixty of the children had obstructive sleep apnea, of whom the problem was considered mild in 47 and moderate to severe in 13. Multiple logistic regression analysis revealed that the PO_2 saturation nadir (odds ratio: 0.001; 95% confidence interval: 0 to 0.244); p = 0.013) and insulin levels (odds ratio: 1.077; 95% confidence interval: 1.011 to 1.048; p =0.022) were significantly associated with obstructive sleep apnea. Li et al suggest that intermittent hypoxia can trigger a cascade of pathophysiological events that include autonomic activation, alterations in neuroendocrine function, release of pro-inflammatory mediators such as TNF-α and IL-6, and insulin resistance [150].

Studies on the association between obesity and asthma have yielded inconsistent results. Several investigators have reported a positive association [151-154] while other investigators have found no association [155,156]. Some of the studies that reported a positive association were not population-based [151,152,154] or relied on reports of respiratory symptoms to define asthma [153]. The latter is problematic in that obesity can predispose to respiratory symptoms that are similar to the symptoms of asthma [156]. To et al performed a cross-sectional study on 11,199 children aged 4 to 11 years whose biological mothers reported data on asthma, height, and weight [156]. These children were participants in the Canadian National Longitudinal Survey of Children and Youth (NLSCY). The authors found that 11.6% of boys and 8% of girls had asthma diagnosed by a health professional. The odds ratio for asthma, when the highest and lowest BMI categories were compared, was 1.02 (99% confidence interval: 0.7 to 1.46) for boys and 1.06 (99% confidence interval: 0.67 to 1.69) for girls. The study suggests that there is no statistical association between obesity and asthma.

Orthopedic

Obesity increases the stress on weight-bearing joints [7]. The incidence of slipped femoral capital epiphyses, Legg-Calvé-Perthes disease, tibia vara (Blount disease), genu valgum, genu recurvatum, knee pain, lower back pain, osteoarthritis, and tight quadriceps is increased in obese children [157]. Obese children are often clumsy, and many learn to walk late [7]. Taylor et al reviewed the medical records of 227 overweight and 128 non-overweight children and adolescents who were enrolled in pediatric clinical studies at the National Institutes of Health [158]. Compared with non-overweight children, overweight children reported a greater prevalence of fractures and musculoskeletal discomfort. The most common self-reported joint complaint was knee pain (21.4% of overweight children versus 16.7% of non-overweight children). Overweight children reported greater impairment in mobility than non-overweight children (mobility score: 17 ± 6.8 versus 11.7 ± 2.8). Both metaphyseal-diaphyseal and anatomic tibio-femoral angle measurements showed greater malalignment in overweight children compared with non-overweight children.

Gastrointestinal

Non-alcoholic fatty liver disease (NAFLD) is the most common cause of liver disease in children [159]. Obesity and insulin resistance are major established risk factors for NAFLD [160]. Only a subset of obese children will develop NAFLD. The condition is more common in boys and is associated with visceral fat deposition [160]. Free fatty acids derived from visceral fat are transported via the portal circulation to the liver for triglyceride synthesis. Excess amount of free fatty acids will lead to fatty infiltration of the liver. The spectrum of NAFLD ranges from steatosis, which is fatty infiltration of the liver without inflammation, to non-alcoholic steatohepatitis, which is also known as NASH, to fibrosis, and even to cirrhosis. NASH is characterized by elevation of serum alanine aminotransferase (ALT) levels, a fatty liver on abdominal ultrasonography, and variable degrees of microvascular and macrovascular steatosis and periportal fibrosis [161]. In a study of 475 non-overweight and 517 overweight Hispanic children, fasting serum ALT was elevated in 24% of overweight versus 4% of non-overweight children [162]. Fasting insulin, glucose, and homeostasis model-insulin resistance were higher in the overweight children with elevated ALT. In a study of 2450 children aged 12 to 18 years who were enrolled in the National Health and Examination Survey cycle III, 60% of adolescents with elevated ALT levels were either overweight or obese [163]. Conversely, 6% of overweight adolescents had elevated ALT levels (odds ratio: 3.4; 95% confidence interval: 3.5 to 12.8), while 10% of obese adolescents had elevated ALT levels (odds ratio: 6.7; 95% confidence interval: 3.5 to 12.8).

Cholelithiasis, cholecystitis, and pancreatitis occur more commonly in obese versus normal weight children [91]. Kaechele performed abdominal ultrasound on 493 (218 males, 275 females) obese children and adolescents aged 8 to 19 years to identify gallstones [164]. Gallstones were detected in 2% (2 boys, 8 girls). None of the 95 prepubertal children who were examined were found to have gallstones. Patients with gallstones were more severely obese (BMI-SDS 3.4 ± 0.5 versus 2.7 ± 0.4; p < 0.001) and older (16.1 ± 1.5 years versus 13.9 ± 2 years; p < 0.0008) than children and adolescents without gallstones. Cholelithiasis presumably results from an increased rate of biliary cholesterol excretion relative to that of bile acid or phospholipids [91]. Cholelithiasis occurs in 10 to 25% of adults who lose weight rapidly [165]. The frequency of this complication in the pediatric age group is not known. Pancreatitis in obese children might be caused by hypertriglyceridemia which accompanies obesity and insulin resistance [91].

Gastroesophageal reflux is more prevalent in obese children [96]. The reflux might be due to the increase in intra-abdominal pressure that develops consequent to increased subcutaneous and visceral fat [96]. Constipation and fecal soiling are more common in obese versus normal weight children [166]. The etiology is not known. Obese children consume less dietary fibre and are less physical active, which might lead to constipation [166]. Circulating gastrointestinal hormone abnormalities and hyperglycemia might also play a role [167,168].

Dermatologic

Cutaneous abnormalities seen in obese children include acanthosis nigricans, intertrigo, furnuculosis, and fragilitias cutis inguinalis [169].

Renal

Focal segmental glomerulosclerosis is associated with obesity in both adults and children [170-173]. Several patients have been reported in whom the proteinuria decreased or resolved after extensive reduction in body weight, without the use of any immunosuppressive therapy [172,173]. The exact etiology of focal segmental glomerulosclerosis in obesity is not known. Renal venous hypertension [174] and hyperfiltration [172,175] are possible etiologic factors. Cindek et al reported that the glomerular filtration rate increases as the BMI increases [176].

Childhood obesity might increase the risk of kidney disease as well as the progression and mortality of kidney disease [177]. The type 2 diabetes mellitus and hypertension associated with obesity increases the risk for end-stage kidney disease [177]. Overnutrition with increased nitrogenous load and physical inactivity are other potential risk factors [177].

Obesity is associated with nocturia [178]. In a mail survey of 1,663 Finnish males (43.5 ± 16.3 years) and 1,897 Finnish females (42 ± 15.7 years), the age-standardized prevalence of nocturia, which was defined as at least one void per night, was 33.4% (95% confidence interval: 28.5 to 38.3) in the non-overweight men, 35.8% (95% confidence interval: 31.4 to 40.1) in the overweight men, and 48.2% (95% confidence interval: 38.8 to 57.6) in the obese men [178]. Among women, the corresponding figures were 37.2% (95% confidence interval: 33 to 41.5), 48.3% (95% confidence interval: 42.5 to 54.2), and 53.6% (95% confidence interval: 43.9 to 63.2), respectively. The associations remained similar when nocturia was defined as two or more voids per night. The age-standardized attributable fraction (population) of increased BMI for nocturia was 17.7% for men and 18.5% for women, and corresponded to an 8.5% increase in crude prevalence of nocturia in men and a 13.9% increase in women. Nocturia can result from excessive nighttime eating and drinking. Other potential causes of nocturia in obese persons include type 2 diabetes mellitus, hypertension, and obstructive sleep apnea.

Hematologic

Obese children are at increased risk for iron deficiency [179,180]. Pinhas-Hamiel et al examined the prevalence of iron deficiency among 321 obese children and adolescents in Israel [180]. The authors found iron deficiency in 4.4%, 17.1% and 38.8% of normal weight children, children at risk for overweight, and overweight children, respectively (p < 0.001). Nead et al analyzed the data of 9,698 children aged 2 to 16 years who were participants in the National Health and Nutrition Examination Survey III (1988 to 1994) [179]. Overall, 13.7% of these children were at risk for overweight and 10.2% were overweight. The prevalence of iron deficiency increased from 2.1% for normal weight children, to 5.3% for those at risk for overweight, and to 5.5% for those who were overweight. In a multivariate regression analysis, children who were at risk for overweight and children who were overweight were approximately twice as likely to be iron deficient (odds ratio: 2; 95% confidence interval: 1.2 to 3.5; and odds ratio: 2.3; 95% confidence interval: 1.4 to 3.9; respectively) as were those who were not overweight. Dietary iron deficiency in the presence of rapid growth is likely the explanation.

Surgical

Obesity is an important risk factor for primary omental torsion. Theriot et al reviewed histopathology records at the Kosair Children's Hospital from January 1993 to March 2003 and identified 12 cases of primary omental torsion [181]. Weight percentiles were ≥ 95th in 11 (92%) of 12 patients. BMI was calculated in 9 of the 12 cases and was > 95th percentile in 8. Excess omental fat associated with obesity is the likely predisposing factor. The blood supply to the omentum might not be sufficient to supply rapidly developing fatty tissue and ischemia might develop due to torsion, or alternatively, the actual weight of the omentum might cause traction ischemia [182].

Oncologic

Obese persons are more prone to develop liver cancer, colon cancer, renal cell carcinoma, breast cancer, ovarian cancer, endometrial cancer, and cervical cancer [183,184]. Chronic exposure to insulin-like growth factor (IGF)-1 might contribute to the increased risk of malignancy in obese adults [183]. In females, early puberty increases life-time exposure to estrogen, which might increase the risk for breast cancer, and possibly ovarian cancer [185].

Dental

Several studies examined the relationship between dental carries and obesity [186,187]. Chen et al examined 5,133 3-year-old children and found no association between obesity and the prevalence of dental caries [186]. Willershausen et al examined 842 children aged 6 to 11 years of age [187]. These authors found that 36% of normal weight children had healthy teeth whereas only 28% of the overweight children and 30% of the obese children had healthy teeth. Although obesity per se might not be a good prediction of dental caries, poor dietary habits can definitely lead to dental caries. Since obesity and dental caries can be caused by diets high in sugar, further well-designed studies are needed to clarify whether there is a relationship between obesity and dental caries.

Teratogenic

Obese mothers are at risk for birth defects [188-191]. Watkins et al used data from the Atlanta Birth Defects Risk Factor Surveillance Study and conducted a population-based case-control study of several selected major birth defects [191]. Mothers who delivered an infant with and without selected birth defects in a 5-county metropolitan Atlanta area between January 1993 and August 1997 were interviewed. The authors found that obese women were more likely than average-weight women to have an infant with spina bifida (unadjusted odds ratio: 3.3; 95% confidence interval: 1.2 to 10.3), omphalocele (odds ratio: 3.3; 95% confidence interval: 1 to 10.3), heart defects (odds ratio: 2; 95% confidence interval: 1.2 to 3.4), and multiple anomalies (odds ratio: 2; 95% confidence interval: 1 to 3.8). Congenital anomalies such as esophageal atresia, Potter sequence, urogenital defects, intestinal defects, and clubfoot have been reported with increased frequency in children of obese mothers [188-191]. Coexisting maternal diabetes mellitus, metabolic derangement, and nutritional deficiency (for example, folic acid deficiency) are possible explanations.

Clinical Evaluation

A detailed history and complete physical examination are important. Table 3 lists specific features to assess [7].

A detailed dietary history should include a 24-hour dietary recall or a 3-day food diary, which will help to identify the amount and types of foods and the schedule of eating. The family eating habits such as whether the child eats in front of the television should be assessed. Information about food preferences and aversions are helpful for intervention planning [8]. The physical activity history should include school physical education, after-school activities, activities of daily living, family activities, and sedentary activities [20]. Barriers to physical activities such as walking or riding a bike to school should be explored.

A thorough functional enquiry might provide clues to the underlying cause of obesity or might suggest complications that result from obesity. Snoring, other nighttime breathing symptoms, and daytime somnolence suggest obstructive sleep apnea. Polyuria and polydipsia suggest diabetes mellitus. A history of cold intolerance, tiredness, and constipation suggests hypothyroidism. Right upper quadrant abdominal pain and fat intolerance suggest of gallstones. Menstrual irregularities, acne, and hirsutism in postpubertal girls suggest polycystic ovarian syndrome.

Anthropometric data such as weight, height, and BMI should be plotted onto standard growth charts that are specific for age and gender. Trends of the BMI over time are particularly informative. A clinical judgment about of the degree of obesity without anthropometry is not adequate, even when made by an experienced observer. Although the majority of patients have exogenous obesity, a pathologic cause should be considered. A growth rate for height above the 50th percentile, normal intelligence, normal genitalia, and lack of historical or physical evidence of an endocrine abnormality or a congenital syndrome suggests a diagnosis of exogenous obesity. Endocrine disorders such as hypothyroidism and Cushing syndrome are always associated with slow growth in height [7]. Children with exogenous obesity might have striae, but the striae in Cushing syndrome are more deeply colored, the obesity is truncal in distribution, and the buffalo hump is characteristic. Children with obesity secondary to a congenital syndrome usually present with short stature, mental retardation, early onset of severe obesity, and dysmorphic features characteristic of the specific syndrome (Table 4) [7,73,75,77-79].

Table 3. Important points in history and physical examination in evaluating childhood obesity

History
Birth weight
Age of onset of obesity and precipitating events, if any
Previous weights and heights
Early feeding history
Breastfeeding versus formula-feeding
Age when solid foods were introduced
Detailed dietary history
Physical activity level
Psychosocial history
Relationship with peers and classmates
Self-esteem
Socioeconomic status
Impact of the problem and level of support available
Readiness of the family and patient to make lifestyle changes
Family history of obesity, type 2 diabetes, dyslipidemia, and early cardiovascular disease
Past health including previously used weight loss methods and relative success of each method
Functional inquiry
Physical examination
General appearance
Weight, height, BMI
Triceps and/or subscapular skin-fold thickness if skin-fold caliper if available
Distribution of body fat
Pubertal development
Blood pressure
Visual fields
Associated signs, e.g, acanthosis nigricans and dysmorphic features

Modified from: Leung, AK; Robson, WL. Childhood obesity. Postgrad Med 1990; 87:126 [7].

Blood pressure should be measured with an appropriate size cuff. Use of a thigh cuff for the upper arm might be necessary in an obese individual. Elevated blood pressure should be confirmed on at least 3 separate occasions before a diagnosis of hypertension is established [192]. A fundoscopic examination is recommended to look for changes due to hypertension or type 2 diabetes. The intertrigionous areas and neck folds should be examined for acanthosis nigricans, which is associated with insulin resistance [169].

Table 4. Clinical features of syndromes associated with obesity

Syndrome	Phenotype
Prader-Willi	Mental retardation, hypotonia, hypogonadism, cryptorchidism, almond-shaped eyes, narrow bifrontal diameter, high-arched palate, microdentia, scoliosis, small hands and feet
Bardet-Biedl	Mental retardation, hypogonadism, postaxial polydactyly, retinitis pigmentosa
Carpenter	Mental retardation, hypogonadism, acrocephaly, lateral displacement of inner canthi, preaxial polydactyly, syndactyly
Alström	Nerve deafness, pigmentary retinal degeneration, cataracts, hypogonadism, nephropathy
Cohen	Mental retardation, short stature, microcephaly, g-shaped eyes, down-slanted palpebral eg fissure, thick eyelashes and eyebrows, pigmentary retinopathy, neutropenia
Bechwith-Wiedemann	Macroglossia, visceromegaly, omphalocele, linear creases in the ear lobes, hemihypertrophy

Laboratory Evaluation

A fasting lipid profile, including total cholesterol, low-density lipoprotein cholesterol, high-density lipoprotein cholesterol, and triglyceride concentrations as well as liver function tests should be considered [10,193]. The American Diabetes Association recommends a fasting plasma glucose test for children over 10 years of age who have a BMI $\geq$ 85th percentile and at least two risk factors, which include a family history of type 2 diabetes in a first- or second-degree relative, non-white race, and conditions associated with insulin resistance such as acanthosis nigricans, hypertension, dyslipidemia, or polycystic ovary syndrome [194]. Other tests should be considered based on the history and physical examination. A polysomnogram is helpful if obstructive sleep apnea is suspected. Thyroid function tests should be ordered if hypothyroidism is suspected.

Treatment

Long-term treatment of childhood obesity is often unsuccessful. Most treatment programs lead to a brief period of weight loss followed by rapid and almost immediate re-accumulation of the lost weight after termination of the therapy [7]. The goals of treatment should be weight stabilization and improvements in physical fitness, psychosocial function, and in any co-morbid conditions [8]. The three primary components of therapy are decreased caloric intake, increased energy output, and behavioral modification for both the patient and the family [60]. Treatment of obese children in a multidisciplinary setting is highly desirable. Weight-control interventions are unlikely to achieve long term success without alterations in the home, school, and other social environments and without cooperation of the whole family. For some children, weight loss might be undesirable [7]. Maintaining the weight or reducing the rate of weight gain and allowing the child to "grow into their weight" are acceptable strategies for some individuals [7,60]. Co-morbid conditions that do not respond to weight control should be treated.

Dietary Modification

The goal of dietary modification is to reduce the overall caloric intake and to offer foods of high nutritional value. A good strategy is to gradually decrease caloric intake until the recommended daily caloric allowance for the ideal weight is achieved. A weight reduction diet should provide enough protein, carbohydrate, fat, minerals, and vitamins to meet lean tissue growth, and should be composed of foods that the child is familiar with and in the proportions required for a normal balanced diet [7]. Less than 30% of the calories should be from fat and less than 10% of the calories should be from saturated fat [20]. Portion sizes should be reduced. Foods and drinks that are calorie-dense or have a high glycemic index should be reduced. Fruits and vegetables rather than "junk" foods should be available for snacking. Children should receive a minimum 1 gram per year of age per day of dietary fibre in fibre-rich foods [8]. All family members should alter their eating habits to conform to the needs of the child, because a double standard at the family table undermines the efforts of the child.

Excessive dietary restriction such as with a very low caloric diet or a protein-sparing modified fast is undesirable [20,96]. Growth failure and nutritional deficiency have been reported if the diet provides less than two thirds of the estimated energy needs [195]. Other complications that might follow the use of a highly restrictive diet include hypokalemia, hyperuricemia, cholelithiasis, and orthostatic hypotension [20,96].

Therapeutic Exercise

Exercise is very important in the treatment of childhood obesity. The goal is to reduce sedentary activity and to encourage physical activity. Physical exercise will increase caloric expenditure, raise metabolic rate, increase muscle mass, and reduce adipose tissue. Owens et al randomized 84 children aged 7 to 11 years into a physical training group (n=35) and a control group (n=39) [196]. The children in the intervention group attended sessions 5 days a week for 4 months. During each session the chiildren completed 20 minutes of machine exercise and played games for another 20 minutes. The authors found that children in the intervention group had a significantly greater increase in fat-free mass and a significant reduction in total fat mass and in the percent body fat compared to the control group. Studies have shown that the combination of limiting caloric intake and increasing exercise is superior to limiting caloric intake alone [7,197]. Two separate studies have shown improvements in arterial reactivity with exercise, without concomitant changes in measures of adiposity but with redistribution of body fat toward less visceral or abdominal fat [198,199]. Epstein et al [1985] compared the efficacy of aerobic exercise, calisthenics and lifestyle exercises in the weight maintenance of overweight children [197]. The authors did not find any difference in efficacy between the three different types of exercise treatment programs during the first year of treatment. However, during the second year of follow-up, children in the lifestyle exercise group maintained the weight loss while children in the other two groups gained significant amounts of weight.

The amount and type of physical activity is controversial. The CDC recommends 30 minutes of moderate-intensity exercise 7 days a week [200]. The Institute of Medicine recommends 60 minutes of moderate-intensity exercise 7 days a week [201]. Prospective studies are required to determine the relationship between specific activity patterns and changes in body weight. Integration of physical activity into daily routines and participation in structured physical activity is important. The activity prescribed should both sufficiently strenuous for the clinical circumstance and fun [97]. Family activities such as walking, swimming, and bicycle riding should be encouraged. Walking or cycling as means of transport should be encouraged.

Sedentary activities such as television viewing and internet use should be minimized [63]. The American Academy of Pediatrics recommends that television viewing should be limited to no more than 2 hours per day [2002] . Epstein et al randomized 90 families with obese children aged 8 to 12 years to groups that were provided a comprehensive family-based behavioral weight control program that included dietary and behavioral change information but differed in whether sedentary or physically active behaviors were targeted and the degree of behavioral change required [203]. Results during two years showed that either a decrease in sedentary behaviors or an increase in physical activity was associated with significant decreases in percent overweight and body fat and improvement in aerobic fitness.

Behavioral Modification

Successful weight loss is a lifelong endeavor. Greater than 90% of individuals who successfully lose weight regain their weight within one year [1]. Behavioral modification is very important. The goal is to replace unhealthy behaviors with healthier behaviors. Examples of effective tools include goal-setting with contractual agreements, environment controls, self-monitoring, positive reinforcement, and social support [60,204]. Only a properly motivated child will lose weight, and regular support and education are needed. Regular follow-up by a caring healthcare professional is important to sustain motivation. Two behavioral conditioning techniques that have been used successfully by practicing physicians are a reward system for initial conditioning followed by an educational program focused on methods to achieve alteration in food and exercise-related behavior for long-term conditioning [7]. Parents should not use food items or television to reward or discipline children. Families should learn to control environmental cues that can trigger undesired behavior. The home environment should be altered to remove high risk foods such as chips and sweets. The family should be encouraged to eat meals and exercise together. Families who do not eat together consume more fried food and soda and less fruits and vegetables than families who share meals together [205,206]. Families should not eat meals or snacks while viewing television. Children should not have television sets in their rooms. The patient should be educated to reduce vending machine snacking at school.

Children benefit the most from parents who lose the most weight in family-based behavioral treatments [207]. Parental involvement in the behavioral modification is important for the intervention to be successful. Epstein et al randomized 76 obese children aged 6 to 12 years and their parents to three groups that were provided similar diet, exercise and behavioral management training, but that differed in the reinforcement for weight loss and behavioral change [208]. The child and parent groups reinforced parent and child behavioral change and weight loss, the child group reinforced child behavioral change and weight loss, and the control group reinforced families for attendance. Children in the child and parent group showed significantly greater decreases in percent overweight after 5 and 10 years (-11.2% and -7.5%, respectively), than children in the child group (+2.7% and +4.5%, respectively), and than children in the control group (+7.9% and 14.3%, respectively).

Few studies have evaluated changes in behavioral modification as an outcome for obesity treatment. Using a randomized, 2-arm design, Faith et al tested the effects of contingent television viewing on physical activity and non-contingent television viewing in 10 obese children [209]. The intervention consisted of a cycle ergometer that electrically interfaced with a television so that pedaling was necessary to activate the television. Television viewing was not contingent on pedaling for control participants. The study was conducted over 12 weeks, and included a 2-week baseline period. During the treatment phase, the intervention group and the control group pedaled an average of 64.4 minutes and 8.3 minutes per week, respectively. The intervention group and the control group watched television for an average of 1.6 hours and 21 hours, per week, respectively. Secondary analysis indicated that the intervention group showed significantly greater reductions in total body fat and percent leg fat. Total pedaling time during intervention correlated with greater reductions in percent body fat ($r = -0.68$). The child with emotional overeating or binge eating requires a supportive treatment program composed of participants who understand the cause of the problem and who can provide regular reassurance. Emphasis on the positive aspects of their life is important when discussing their problem with these children. A referral for psychotherapy should also be considered.

Pharmacotherapy

Pharmacotherapy should be considered for adolescents who do not improve with other therapies and for those who suffer from a serious co-morbid problem. [6]. The risk of the disease and the potential side effects of pharmacotherapy should be balanced with the anticipated benefit of pharmacotherapy. Sibutramine (Meridia) acts centrally in the hypothalamus to inhibit neuronal reuptake of norepinephrine and serotonin [204]. The medication increases satiety. The medication is approved by the Food and Drug

Administration (FDA) for adolescents older than 16 years of age. In a randomized control trial of 82 adolescents aged 13 to 17 years with a BMI that ranged from 32 to 44, 63% of participants treated with sibutramine plus behavioral therapy for 6 months achieved a reduction of BMI of 5% or more, compared with 36% in those who were treated with behavioral therapy alone [210]. Side effects include hypertension, tachycardia, headache, dry mouth, insomnia, depression, and constipation [6,20]. The use of sibutramine is contraindicated in individuals with uncontrolled hypertension or cardiovascular disease and in individuals who are treated with monoamine oxidase inhibitors or other serotonin reuptake inhibitors [205].

Orlistat (Xenical) inhibits lipase activity and decreases hydrolysis and the absorption of dietary fat. The medication is approved for patients 12 years or older [6]. In a multicenter, double-blind study, Chanoine randomized 539 obese adolescents to receive 120 mg of orlistat (n=357) or placebo (n=182) three times a day for one year, a mildly hypocalorie diet (30% fat calories), exercise, and behavioral therapy [211]. At the end of the study, BMI had decreased by 0.55 kg/m^2 with orlistat but by only 0.31 kg/m^2 with placebo (p=0.001). Compared with 15.7% of the placebo group, 26.5% of subjects in the intervention group had a $\geq$ 5% decrease in BMI (p=0.05) and 4.5% and 13.3%, respectively, had a 10% or higher decrease in BMI (p=0.02). Waist circumference decreased in the intervention group but increased in the placebo group (-1.33 cm versus + 0.12 cm; p< 0.05) [211]. Side effects of orlistat therapy include loose stools, flatulence, and loss of fat soluble vitamins (A, D, E, K) in the stool [20].

Metformin (Glucophage), a biguanide, acts to increase sensitivity to insulin at both hepatic and peripheral levels [212,213]. Metformin has been approved for use in children 10 years and older with type 2 diabetes [6]. The medication might also have a role in weight reduction in obese, hyperinsulinemic, non-diabetic adolescents [213]. Kay et al randomized 24 hyperinsulinemic non-diabetic adolescents, aged 13 to 17 years, to metformin treatment or placebo [214]. After eight weeks of treatment, the metformin group had a greater weight loss compared with the placebo group (6.5 $\pm$ 0.8% versus 3.8 $\pm$ 0.4%; p=0.01). Freemark et al randomized 29 obese hyperinsulinemic non-diabetics aged 12 to 19 years to receive metformin or placebo for 6 months [215]. The authors found that metformin treatment resulted in a decline in BMI of 0.12 SD compared with a rise of 0.23 SD in the placebo group. Although the preliminary results are positive, the patient numbers are small in both studies. The medication might be particularly useful in obese adolescents with polycystic ovary syndrome or in those who are on a psychotropic medication [6]. Side effects include abdominal discomfort, electrolyte imbalances, and vitamin B deficiency [6]. Large-scale, well-designed, multicenter studies are needed to determine the safety and efficacy of pharmacotherapy in the long-term control of obesity.

Bariatric Surgery

Bariatric surgery can produce durable and substantial weight loss [96]. Guidelines for the selection of patients for bariatric surgery were established by a panel of experts who specialize in the treatment of childhood obesity [216]. Adolescents considered for bariatric surgery should have a BMI $\geq$ 40 kg/m^2 with a serious obesity-related co-morbid problem, or have a BMI ≥ 50 kg/m^2 with a less severe co-morbid problem. Other criteria include failure to lose weight after at least 6 months of organized attempts at weight management, attainment or near-attainment of physiologic (Tanner stage III or above) or skeletal maturity (generally ≥ 13 years of age for girls and ≥ 15 years of age for boys), a demonstrated commitment to comprehensive medical and psychological evaluation both before and after surgery, agreement to avoid pregnancy for at least one year postoperatively, ability and willingness to adhere to nutritional guidelines postoperatively, provision of informed assent for surgical treatment, decisional capacity, and a supportive family environment [216].

Both Roux-en-Y gastric bypass and adjustable gastric banding have been performed successfully and effectively in adolescent patients, usually with improvement of most co-morbid conditions within one year postoperatively [6,216]. Advantages of Roux-en-Y gastric bypass include substantial weight loss, deterrence to carbohydrate ingestion, and enhanced satiety after surgery [216]. For adult patients, the risk of perioperative mortality is higher with gastric bypass than with adjustable gastric banding (0.5% versus 0.05%). Other potential complications of gastric bypass include wound infection, stomal stenosis, marginal ulcers, intestinal leakage, pulmonary embolism, small bowel obstruction, incisional hernia, cholelithiasis, dumping syndrome, and nutritional deficiency [204,216].

Adjustable gastric banding is less invasive and can be performed laparoscopically. Other advantages include adjustability and less potential for nutritional deficiency [216]. Compared with gastric bypass, adjustable gastric banding is less effective. Surgical complications are significant and include port malposition or malfunction, tube leaks, band slippage, which leads to gastric prolapse, foreign body infection, and band erosion into the stomach or esophagus [216]. These mechanical devices have a finite lifetime and adolescents might require replacement of the device during their lifetimes [216].

Prevention

Childhood obesity, once established, is often refractory to treatment. As such prevention is very important. The combination of good nutrition and regular physical activity will prevent obesity. Primary care physicians should screen patients for early signs of obesity. Education on the prevention of obesity should begin with the first medical visit. Early recognition of excessive weight gain relative to linear growth should become routine in the pediatric ambulatory care setting [20]. BMI should be periodically calculated and plotted on standardized charts. If the child comes from a high-risk family with an obese parent or sibling, or if the growth chart reveals an early tendency to obesity, the family should be specifically counseled regarding methods to prevent obesity.

Obesity can be minimized by exclusive breastfeeding for six months and by delay in the introduction of solid foods until 6 months of age [39]. The average caloric requirement for a full-term infant is 110 to 120 kcal/kg during the first few months of life, and decreases to 100 kcal/kg by 1 year of age. Infants should be fed only in response to hunger. Food should not be used as a pacifier. Parents should be counseled that fat babies are not necessarily healthy babies. The primary care physician has a responsibility to identify obesity and to attempt to dissuade parents of any erroneous ideas or behaviors that might be encourage improper eating habits.

Physicians should regularly counsel families to eat well-balanced meals, to avoid junk and fast food, and to minimize the intake of saturated fat. Nutritious snacks such as fruits and vegetables, low-fat diary products, and whole grains should be offered. Gram for gram, fat has more than twice as many calories as either protein or carbohydrate. A reduction in dietary fat can be achieved by consuming low-fat milk (2% or skim), fish or lean meats with fat removed, and poultry with skin removed. However, children under two years of age should not be given skim milk because of the high solute-to-calorie ratio.

Specific instruction on the benefits of a low saturated fat and low cholesterol diet should be offered to high-risk families. The prevention of obesity and coronary artery disease is the complementary goal of regular patient education. Physicians should instill a positive attitude about healthy eating habits, offer information on preparation of healthy meals, and encourage compliance through regular office follow-up. The correct portion sizes should be specified [217]. Parents should be reminded not to use food as a reward or punishment or to make their children clean their plates. Everyone in the family should learn and follow proper nutritional practices.

Positive physical activities such as unstructured play at home, in school, and throughout the community should be promoted [218]. Use of the stairs rather than an elevator, participation in community-based sports programs, and evening walks as a family event should be encouraged. Television, video, and internet time should be limited to a maximum of 2 hours per day [218].

Parents should be made aware of the important role they can play in the prevention of obesity in their children and they should endeavor to be exemplary role models. Successful interventions are family-based. Parents should be encouraged to become involved in school and community programs that improve nutritional status and physical activity in their children [219].

The American Dietetic association suggests that childhood obesity intervention requires a combination of family-based and school-based multi-component programs that include the promotion of physical activity, parent training and modeling, behavioral counseling, and nutrition education [185]. The CDC recommends that public schools prohibit the sale and distribution of foods of minimal nutritional value and other foods of low nutritive value anywhere on the school property until after the end of the last lunch period [220]. The CDC also recommends implementation of a quality physical education program, which provides a minimum of 150 minutes each week for elementary students, and 225 minutes for students in middle and high school programs. Opportunities should be provided for children to be physically active, both during and after school hours [219]. Recently, Flodmark performed a meta-analysis on 24 studies (n=25,896) that addressed prevention of obesity in unselected children with a follow-up of at least 12 months [221]. Of the 24 studies, eight reported that prevention had a statistically positive effect on obesity, while 16 reported neutral results. One possible explanation of the neutral result is that the "dose" of dietary modification or physical activity might not be adequate to have any net impact on the BMI. The other explanation is that these children were less motivated than those children who really wanted to be treated.

Conclusion

Childhood obesity is a major health issue, which is now more prevalent, as are a range of co-morbid complications. Health costs for the treatment of obesity and the co-morbid conditions are large and continue to increase. Active intervention is necessary since spontaneous resolution is unlikely. Most treatment programs lead to a brief period of weight loss followed by rapid re-accumulation of the lost weight after termination of therapy. Strategies used to prevent obesity are equally disappointing. There are not enough evidenced-based, high-quality research studies on the treatment or prevention of childhood obesity. Prospective well-designed studies on interventions that are tailored specifically to children of various ages, and to specific ethnic and economic groups are needed to improve treatment outcomes and the maintenance of treatment results.

References

[1]   Miller, J; Rosenbloom, A; Silverstein J. Childhood obesity. *J. Clin Endocrinol Metab.* 2004;89:4211-4218.

[2]   Ogden, Cl; Flegal, KM; Carroll, MD; et al. Prevalence and trends in overweight among US children and adolescents, 1999-2000. *JAMA* 2002;288:1728-1732.

[3]   3, Xanthakos, SA; Inge, TH. Extreme pediatric obesity: weighing the health dangers. *J. Pediatr.* 2007:150:3-5.

[4]   National Center for Health Statistics. Centers for Disease Control and Prevention. Prevalence of overweight and obesity among adults: United States, 1999-2002. Available at: http://www.cdc.gov/nchs/products/pubs/pubd/hestats/obese/obse99.htm. Accessed March 20, 2007.

[5]   Philippas, NG; Lo, CW. Childhood obesity: etiology, prevention and treatment. *Nutr. Clin. Care* 2005;8:77-88.

[6]   Someshwar, J; Someshwar, S; Perkins, KC. The obese adolescent. *Pediatr. Ann.* 2006;35:180-186.

[7]   Leung, AK; Robson, WL. Childhood obesity. *Postgrad. Med.* 1990;87:123-133.

[8]   Gahagan, S. Child and adolescent obesity. *Curr. Probl. Pediatr. Adolesc. Health Care* 2004;34:6-43.

[9]   Binns, HJ; Ariza, AJ. Guidelines help clinicians identify risk factors for overweight in children. *Pediatr. Ann.* 2004;33:19-22.

[10] Chia, DJ; Boston, BA. Childhood obesity and the metabolic syndrome. *Adv. Pediatr.* 2006;53:23-53.

[11] Hall, DMB; Cole, TJ. What use is the BMI? *Arch. Dis. Child.* 2006;91:283-286.

[12] Chinn, S. Definitions of childhood obesity: current practice. *Eur. J. Clin. Nutr.* 2006;60:1189-1194.

[13] Reilly, JJ. Obesity in childhood and adolescence: evidence based clinical and public health perspectives. *Postgrad. Med. J.* 2006;82:429-437.

[14] Boys and girls BMI-for-age. Available at: http://www.cdc.gov/nchs/about/major/nhanes/ growthcharts/clincial_charts.htm. Accessed March 20, 2007.

[15]   Bass, Jl; Bhatia, A; Boas, FE; et al. Validation of a body mass index nomogram for children as an obesity screening tool in young children. *Clin. Pediatr.* 2006;45:718-724.

[16]   Pietrobelli, A; Faith, MS; Allison, DB; et al. Body mass index as a measure of adiposity among children and adolescents: a validations study. *J. Pediatr.* 1998;132:204-210.

[17]   Expert Panel on the Identification, Evaluation, and Treatment of Overweight in Adults. Clinical guidelines on the identification, evaluation, and treatment of overweight and obesity in adults: executive summary. *Am. J. Clin. Nutr.* 1998;68:899-917.

[18]   Must, A; Dallal, GE; Dietz, WM. Reference data for obesity: 85th and 95th percentiles of body mass index (wt/ht^2) and triceps skinfold thickness. *Am. J. Clin. Nutr.* 1991;53;839-846.

[19]   Troiano, RP; Flegal, KM. Overweight children and adolescents: description, epidemiology, and demographics. *Pediatrics* 1998;101:497-504.

[20]   American Academy of Pediatrics, Committee on Nutrition. Pediatric obesity. In: Kleinman, RE; ed. Pediatric Nutrition Handbook. Elk Grove Village, IL: American Academy of Pediatrics; 2004, pp 551-592.

[21]   Sopher, AB; Thornton, JC; Wang, J; et al. Measurement of percentage of body fat in 411 children and adolescents: a comparison of dual-energy X-ray absorptiometry with a four-compartment model. *Pediatrics* 2004;113:1285-1290.

[22]   Franzosi, MG. Should we continue to use BMI as a cardiovascular risk factor? *Lancet* 2006;368:624-625.

[23]   Yusuf, S; Hawken, S; Ounpuu,S; et al. Effect of potentially modifiable risk factors associated with myocardial infarction in 52 countries (the INTERHEART study): case-control study. *Lancet* 2004;365:937-952.

[24]   Hedley, AA; Ogden, CL; Johnson, CL; et al. Prevalence of overweight and obesity among US children, adolescents, and adults, 1999-2002. JAMA 2004;291:2847-2850.

[25]   Shields, M. Measured obesity: overweight Canadian children and adolescents. In: Nutrition: findings from the Canadian Community Health Survey; issue 1; 2005 (cat no 82-620-MWE2005001).   Available: www.statcan.ca/english/research/82-620-MIE/ 2005001/pdf/cobesity.pdf (accessed April 24 2007).

[26]   Willms, JD; Tremblay, MS; Katzmarzyk, PT. Geographic and demographic variation in the prevalence of overweight Canadian children. *Obes. Res.* 2003;11:668-673.

[27]   Reilly, J; Wilson, D. ABC of obesity: childhood obesity. BMJ 2006;333:1207-1210.

[28]   Wang, Y; Lobstein, T. Worldwide trends in childhood overweight and obesity. *Int. J. Pediatr. Obes.* 2006;1:11-25.

[29]   Poskitt, EME. Tackling childhood obesity: diet, physical activity or lifestyle change? *Acta Paediatr.* 2005;94:396-398.

[30]   Veugelers, PJ; Fitzgerald, AL. Prevalence of and risk factors for childhood overweight and obesity. *CMAJ* 2005;173:607-613.

[31]   Alaimo, K; Olson, CM; Frongillo, EA Jr. Low family income and food insufficiency in relation to overweight in US children: is there a paradox? *Arch. Pediatr. Adolesc. Med.* 2001:155:1161-1167.

[32] Casey, PH; Simpson, PM; Gossett, JM; et al. The association of child and household food insecurity with childhood overweight status. *Pediatrics* 2006;118:e1406-e1413.

[33] Agras, WS; Hammer, LD; McNicholas, F; et al. Risk factors for childhood overweight: a prospective study from birth to 9.5 years. *J. Pediatr.* 2004:145:20-25.

[34] Danielzik, S; Czerwinski-Mast, M; Langnäse, K; et al. Parental overweight, socioeconomic status and high birth weight are the major determinants of overweight and obesity in 5-7 y-old children: baseline data of the Kiel Obesity Prevention Study (KOPS). *Int. J. Obes.* 2004;28;1494-1502.

[35] Whitaker, RC; Wright, JA; Pepe, MS; et al. Predicting obesity in young adulthood from childhood and parental obesity. *N. Engl. J. Med*.1997;337:869-873.

[36] Dorosty, AR; Emmett, PM; Cowin, IS; et al. Factors associated with early adiposity rebound. ALSPAC Study Team. *Pediatrics* 2000;105;1115-1118.

[37] Dewey, KG. Is breastfeeding protective against child obesity? *J. Hum. Lact.* 2003;19:9-18.

[38] Grummer-Strawn, LM; Mei, Z. Does breastfeeding protect against pediatric overweight? Analysis of longitudinal data from the Centers for Disease Control and Prevention Pediatric Nutrition Surveillance System. *Pediatrics* 2004;113:e81.

[39] Leung, AK; Sauve, RS. Breast is best for babies. *J. Natl. Med. Assoc.* 2005;97:1010-1019.

[40] Owen, CG; Martin, RM; Whincup, PH; et al. Effect of infant feeding on the risk of obesity across the life course: a quantitative review of published evidence. *Pediatrics* 2005;115:1367-1377.

[41] Toschke, A; Vigerova, J; Lbotska, L; et al. Overweight and obesity in 6- to 14-year-old Czech children in 1991: protective effect of breast-feeding. *J. Pediatr.* 2002;141:764-769.

[42] von Kries, R; Koletzko, B; Sauerwald, T; et al. Breast feeding and obesity: cross sectional study. *BMJ* 1999;319:147-150.

[43] Harder, T; Bergmann, R; Kallischnigg, G; et al. Duration of breastfeeding and risk of overweight: a meta-analysis. *Am. J. Epidemiol.* 2005;162:397-403.

[44] Martin, RM; Gunnell, D; Smith, GD. Breastfeeding in infancy and blood pressure in later life: systematic review and meta-analysis. *Am. J. Epidemiol.* 2005a;161:15-26.

[45] Spruijt-Metz, D; Li, C; Cohen, E; et al. Longitudinal influence of mother's child-feeding practices on adiposity in children. *J. Pediatr.* 2006;148:314-320.

[46] Bowman, SA; Gortmaker, SL; Ebbeling, CB; et al. Effects of fast-food consumption on energy intake and diet quality among children in a national household survey. *Pediatrics* 2004;113:112-118.

[47] Janssen, I; Katzmarzyk, PT; Boyce, WF; et al. Overweight and obesity in Canadian adolescents and their associations with dietary habits and physical activity patterns. *J. Adolesc. Health* 2004;35:360-367.

[48] Bruch, H. Obesity in childhood. IV. Energy expenditure of obese children. *Am. J. Dis. Child.* 1940;60:1082-1109.

[49] Stunkard, AJ; Berkowitz, RI; Schoeller, D; et al. Predictors of body size in the first 2 y of life: a high-risk study of human obesity. *Int. J. Obes.* 2004;28:503-513.

[50] Barkeling, B; Ikman, S; Rossner, S. Eating behaviour in obese and normal weight 11-year-old children. *Int. J. Obes.* 1992;16:355-360.

[51] Thompson, OM; Ballew, C; Resnicow, K; et al. Food purchased away from home as a predictor of change in BMI z-score among girls. *Int. J. Obes.* 2004;28:282-289.

[52] Taveras, EM; Sandora, TJ; Shih, MC; et al. The association of television and video viewing with fast food intake by preschool-age children. *Obesity* 2006;14:2034-2041.

[53] Ludwig, DS; Peterson, KE; Gortmaker, SL. Relation between consumption of sugar-sweetened drinks and childhood obesity: a prospective, observational analysis. *Lancet* 2001;357:505-508.

[54] Striegel-Moore, RH; Thompson, D; Affenito, SG; et al. Correlates of beverage intake in adolescent girls: the National Heart, Lung, and Blood Institute Growth and Health Study. *J. Pediatr.* 2006;148:183-187.

[55] Fox, K; Reidy, K; Novak, T; et al. Sources of energy and nutrients in the diets of infants and toddlers. *J. Am. Diet. Assoc.* 2006;106:S23-S42.

[56] Patrick, K; Norman, GJ; Calfas, KJ; et al. Diet, physical activity, and sedentary behaviors as risk factors for overweight in adolescence. *Arch. Pediatr. Adolesc. Med.* 2004;158:385-390.

[57] Salbe, AD; Weyer, C; Harper, I; et al. Assessing risk factors for obesity between childhood and adolescence: II. Energy metabolism and physical activity. *Pediatrics* 2002;110:307-314.

[58] Kimm, SY; Glynn, NW; Obarzanek, E; et al. Relation between the changes in physical activity and body-mass index during adolescence: a multicentre longitudinal study. *Lancet* 2005;366:301-307.

[59] Bandini, LG; Curtin, C; Hamad, C; et al. Prevalence of overweight in children with developmental disorders in the continuous National Health and Nutrition Examination Survey (NHANES) 1999-2002. *J. Pediatr.* 2005:146:738-743.

[60] Schneider, MB; Brill, SR. Obesity in children and adolescents. *Pediatr. Rev.* 2005;26:155-161.

[61] Marshall, SJ; Biddle, SJH; Gorely, T; et al. Relationships between media use, body fatness and physical activity in children and youth. A meta-analysis. *Int. J. Obes.* 2004;28:1238-1246.

[62] Proctor, MH; Moore, LL; Gao, D; et al. Television viewing and change in body fat from preschool to early adolescence: The Framingham Children's Study. *Int. J. Obes. Relat.* Metab Disord 2003;27:827-833.

[63] Leung, AK; Fagan, JE; Cho, H; et al. Children and television. *Am. Fam. Physician* 1994;50:909-918.

[64] Sudi, KM; Gallistl, S; Tafeit, E; et al. The relationship between different subcutaneous adipose tissue layers, fat mass and leptin in obese children and adolescents. *J. Pediatr. Endocrinol. Metab.* 2000;13:505-512.

[65] Diamond, FB Jr; Cuthbertson, D; Hanna, S; et al. Correlates of adiponectin and the leptin/adiponectin ratio in obese and non-obese children. *J. Pediatr. Endocrinol. Metab.* 2004;17:1069-1075.

[66] Farooqi, IS; O'Rahilly, S. Recent advances in the genetics of severe childhood obesity. *Arch. Dis. Child.* 2000;83:31-34.

[67] Wardle, J. Understanding the aetiology of childhood obesity: implications for treatment. *Proc. Nutr. Soc.* 2005;64:73-79.

[68] Strauss, RS. Childhood obesity. Pediatr. *Clin. North Am.* 2002;49:175-201.

[69] Stunkard, AJ; Foch, TT; Hrubec, Z. A twin study of human obesity. *JAMA* 1986; 256: 51-54.

[70] Stunkard, AJ; Sorensen, TIA; Hanis, C; et al. An adoption stody of human obesity. *N. Engl. J. Med.* 1986;314:193-196.

[71] Sun, M; Gower, BA; Bartolucci, AA; et al. A longitudinal study of resting energy expenditure relative to body composition during puberty in African American and white children. *Am. J. Clin. Nutr.* 2001;73:308-315.

[72] Barsh, GS; Farooqi, IS; O'Rahilly, S. Genetics of body-weight regulation. *Nature* 2000;404:644-651.

[73] Martos-Moreno, GA; Argente, J. Molecular basis of human obesity. *J. Pediatr. Endocrinol. Metab.* 2005;18:1187-1197.

[74] Leung, AK; McArthur, RG; Ross, SA; et al. Thyroxine-binding globulin deficiency in Beckwith syndrome. *J. Pediatr.* 1979;95:753-754.

[75] Leung, AK; Robson, WL; McLeod, DR; et al. Prader Willi syndrome. *Int. Pediatr.* 1992;7:185-188.

[76] Leung, AK; Graham, GE. Recognizable syndromes in childhood. *Consultant* 1999;39:219-224.

[77] Leung, AK; Sauve RS. Hereditary childhood disorders. *Consultant Pediatrician* 2003;2:199-203.

[78] Leung, AK; Robson, WL. Recurrent panniculitis in an adolescent boy with Prader Willi syndrome. *J. Natl. Med. Assoc.* 2006;98:1700-1701.

[79] Leung, AK; Kao, CP. A collage of hereditary childhood disorders. *Consultant Pediatrician* 2006;5:653-657.

[80] Ong, KK; Loos, RJF. Rapid infancy weight gain and subsequent obesity: systematic reviews and hopeful suggestions. *Acta Paediatr.* 2006;95:904-908.

[81] Salsberry, PJ; Reagan, PB. Dynamics of early childhood overweight. *Pediatrics* 2005;116:1329-1338.

[82] Mijailović, M; Mijailović, V; Micić, D. Childhood onset of obesity: Does an obese child become an obese adult? *J. Pediatr. Endocrinol.* 2001;14(Suppl 5):1335-1338.

[83] Kinra, S; Baumer, JH; Davey Smith, G. Early growth and childhood obesity: a historical cohort study. *Arch. Dis. Child.* 2005;90:1122-1127.

[84] Nader, PR; O'Brien, M; Houts, R; et al. Identifying risk for obesity in early childhood. *Pediatrics* 2006;118:e594-e601.

[85] Must, A; Naumova, EN; Phillips, SM; et al. Childhood overweight and maturational timing in the development of adult overweight and fatness: The Newton Girls Study and its follow-up. *Pediatrics* 2005;116:620-627.

[86] Garn, SM; LaVelle, M; Rosenberg, KR; et al. Maturational timing as a factor in female fatness and obesity. A*m. J. Clin. Nutr.* 1986;43:879-883.

[87] Freedman, DS; Khan, LK; Serdula, MK; et al. The relation of childhood BMI to adult adiposity: the Bogalusa Heart Study. *Pediatrics* 2005;115:22-27.

[88] Laitinen, J; Power,C; Jarvelin, MR. Family social class, maternal body mass index, childhood body mass index, and age at menarche as predictors of adult obesity. *Am. J. Clin. Nutr.* 2001;74:287-294.

[89] Serdula, MK; Invery, D; Coates, RJ; et al. Do obese children become obese adults? A review of the literature. *Prev. Med.* 1993;22:167-177.

[90] Krassas, GE; Tzotzas, T. Do obese children become obese adults: childhood predictors of adult disease? *Pediatr. Endocrinol. Rev.* 2004;1(Suppl 3):433-459.

[91] Artz, E; Haqq, A; Freemark, M. Hormonal and metabolic consequences of childhood obesity. *Endocrin. Metab. Clin. North Am.* 2005;34:643-658.

[92] Hilgers, KK; Akridge, M; Scheetz, JP; et al. Childhood obesity and dental development. *Pediatr. Dent.* 2006;28:18-22.

[93] Biro, FM; Khoury, P; Morrison, JA. Influence of obesity on timing of puberty. *Int. J. Androl.* 2006;29:272-277.

[94] Wang, Y. Is obesity associated with early sexual maturation? A comparison of the association in American boys vs girls. *Pediatrics* 2002;110:903-910.

[95] Kiess, W; Reich, A; Müller, G; et al. Obesity in childhood and adolescence: clinical diagnosis and management. *J. Pediatr. Endocrinol. Metab.* 2001;14:1431-1440.

[96] Fisberg, M; Baur, L; Chen, W; et al. Obesity in children and adolescents: Working Group Report of the Second World Congress of Pediatric Gastroenterology, Hepatology, and Nutrition. *J. Pediatr. Gastroenterol. Nutr.* 2004;39:S678-S687.

[97] Lau, DC; Douketis, JD; Morrison, KM; et al. 2006 Canadian clinical practice guidelines on the management and prevention of obesity in adults and children [summary]. *CMAJ* 2007;176(8 Suppl):S1-13.

[98] Hampl, SE; Carroll, CA; Simon, SD; et al. Resource utilization and expenditures for overweight and obese children. *Arch. Pediatr. Adolesc. Med.* 2007;161:11-14.

[99] Harper, MG. Childhood obesity: strategies for prevention. *Fam. Community Health* 2006;29:288-298.

[100] Janssen I; Craig, WM; Boyce, WF; et al. Associations between overweight and obesity with bullying behaviors in school-aged children. *Pediatrics* 2004;113:1187-1194.

[101] Strauss, RS; Pollack, HA. Social marginalization of overweight children. *Arch. Pediatr. Adolesc. Med.* 2003;157:746-752.

[102] Franklin, J; Denyer, G; Steinbeck, KS; et al. Obesity and risk of low self-esteem: a statewide survey of Australian children. *Pediatrics* 2006;118:2481-2487.

[103] Erickson, SJ; Robinson, TN; Haydel, KF; et al. Are overweight children unhappy? Body mass index, depressive symptoms, and overweight concerns in elementary school children. *Arch. Pediatr. Adolesc. Med.* 2000;154:931-935.

[104] Mustillo, S; Worthman, C; Erkanli, A; et al. Obesity and psychiatric disorder: developmental trajectories. *Pediatrics* 2003;111:851-859.

[105] Richardson, LP; Davis, R; Poulton, R; et al. A longitudinal evaluation of adolescent depression and adult obesity. *Arch. Pediatr. Adolesc. Med.* 2003;157:739-745.

[106] Robinson, TN; Chang, JY; Haydel, KF; et al. Overweight concerns and body dissatisfaction among third-grade children: the impacts of ethnicity and socioeconomic status. *J. Pediatr.* 2001;138:181-187.

[107] Striegel-Moore, RH. Body image concerns among children. J Pediatr 2001;138:158-160.

[108] Canning, H; Mayer, J. Obesity: its possible effect on college acceptance. *N. Engl. J. Med.* 1966; 275:1172-1174.

[109] Kolotkin, RL; Binks, M; Crosby, RD; et al. Obesity and sexual quality of life. *Obesity* 2006;14:472-479.

[110] Freedman, DS; Khan, LK; Dietz, WH; et al. Relationship of childhood obesity to coronary heart disease risk factors in adulthood: The Bogalusa Heart Study. *Pediatrics* 2001;108:712-718.

[111] Hubert, HB; Feinleib, M; McNamara, PM; et al. Obesity as an independent risk factor for cardiovascular disease: a 26-year follow-up of participants in the Framingham Heart Study. *Circulation* 1983;67:968-977.

[112] Steinberger, J; Moran, A; Hong, CP; et al. Adiposity in childhood predicts obesity and insulin resistance in young adulthood. *J. Pediatr.* 2001;138:469-473.

[113] Freedman, DS; Mei, Z; Srinivasan, SR; et al. Cardiovascular risk factors and excess adiposity among overweight children and adolescents: The Bogalusa Heart Study. *J. Pediatr.* 2007;150:12-17.

[114] Boyd, GS; Koenigsberg, J; Falkner, B; et al. Effect of obesity and high blood pressure on plasma lipid levels in children and adolescents. *Pediatrics* 2005;116:442-446.

[115] Srinivasan, SR; Myers, L; Berenson GS. Distribution and correlates of non-high-density lipoprotein cholesterol in children: the Bogulusa Heart Study. *Pediatrics* 2002;110:e29.

[116] Thompson, DR; Obarzanek, E; Franko, DL; et al. Childhood overweight and cardiovascular disease risk factors: the National Heart, Lung, and Blood Institute Growth and Health Study. *J. Pediatr.* 2007;150:18-25.

[117] Newman, WP III; Freedman, DS; Voors, AW; et al. Relation of serum lipoprotein levels and systolic blood pressure to early atherosclerosis. The Bogalusa Heart Study. *N. Engl. J. Med.* 1986;314:138-144.

[118] Berenson, GS; Srinivasan, SR; Bao, W; et al. Association between multiple cardiovascular risk factors and atherosclerosis in children and young adults. *N. Engl. J. Med.* 1998;338:1650-1656.

[119] Berenson, GS. Childhood risk factors predict adult risk associated with subclinical cardiovascular disease. The Bogalusa Heart Study. *Am. J. Cardiol.* 2002;90:3L-7L.

[120] Li, S; Chen, W; Srinivasan, SR; et al. Childhood cardiovascular risk factors and carotid vascular changes in adulthood: the Bogalusa Heart Study. *JAMA* 2003;290:2271-2276.

[121] McCrindle, BW. Cardiovascular consequences of paediatric obesity: will there be a future epidemic of premature cardiovascular disease? *Paediatr. Child. Health.* 2007;12:175-177.

[122] Sorof, JM; Lai, D; Turner, J; et al. Overweight, ethnicity, and the prevalence of hypertension in school-aged children. *Pediatrics* 2004;113:475-482.

[123] Falkner, B; Gidding, SS; Ramirez-Garnica, G; et al. The relationship of body mass index and blood pressure in primary care pediatric patients. *J. Pediatr.* 2006;148:195-200.

[124] Atabek, ME; Vatansev, H; Erkul, I. Oxidative stress in childhood obesity. *J. Pediatr. Endocrinol. Metab.* 2004;17:1063-1068.

[125] Bauersachs, J; Fleming, I; Fraccarollo, D; et al. Prevention of endothelial dysfunction in heart failure by vitamin E: attenuation of vascular superoxide anion formation and increase in soluble guanylyl cyclase expression. *Cardiovasc. Res.* 2001;51:344-350.

[126] Doshi, SN; McDowell, IF; Moat, SJ; et al. Folate improves endothelial function in coronary artery disease: an effect mediated by reduction of intracellular superoxide? *Arterioscler. Thromb. Vasc. Biol.* 2001;21:1196-1202.

[127] Loftin, M; Sothern, M; vanVrancken, C; et al. Effect of obesity status on heart rate peak in female youth. Clin Pediatr 2003;42:505-510.

[128] Salvadori, A; Fanari, P; Palmulli, P; et al. Cardiovascular and adrenergic response to exercise in obese subjects. *J. Clin. Basic. Cardiol.* 1999;2:229-236.

[129] Maffeis, C; Schena, F; Zaccante, M; et al. Maximal aerobic power during running and cycling in obese and non-obese children. *Acta Paediatr.* 1994;83:113-116.

[130] Treuth, MS; Figueroa-Colon, R; Hunter, GR; et al. Energy expenditure and physical fitness in overweight vs non-overweight prepubertal girls. *Int. J. Obes.* 1998;22:440-447.

[131] Chinali, M; de Simone, G; Roman, MJ; et al. Impact of obesity on cardiac geometry and function in a population of adolescents: the Strong Heart Study. *J. Am. Coll. Cardiol.* 2006;47:2267-2273.

[132] Ho, J; Pacaud, D; Leung, AK. Type 2 diabetes mellitus in children: a new challenge for diagnosis and prevention. *Consultant Pediatrician* 2006;5:77-80.

[133] Hannon, TS; Rao, G; Arslanian, SA. Childhood obesity and type 2 diabetes mellitus. *Pediatrics* 2005;116:473-480.

[134] Weiss, R; Dufour, S; Groszmann, A; et al. Low adiponectin levels in adolescent obesity: a marker of increased intramyocellular lipid accumulation. *J. Clin. Endocrinol. Metab.* 2003;88:2014-2018.

[135] Boden, G; Shulman, GI. Free fatty acids in obesity and type 2 diabetes: defining their role in the development of insulin resistance and β-cell dysfunction. *Eur. J. Clin. Invest.* 2002;32(Suppl 3):14-23.

[136] Kashyap, S; Belfort, R; Gastaldelli, A; et al. A sustained increase in plasma free fatty acids impairs insulin secretion in nondiabetic subjects genetically predisposed to develop type 2 diabetes. *Diabetes* 2003;52:2461-2474.

[137] Silverstein, JH, Rosenbloom, AL. Type 2 diabetes in children. *Curr. Diab. Rep.* 2001;1:19-27.

[138] Edelstein, SL; Knowler, WC; Bain RP; et al. Predictors of progression from impaired glucose tolerance to NIDDM: an analysis of six prospective studies. *Diabetes* 1997;46:701-710.

[139] Weiss, R; Takali, SE; Tamborlane, WV; et al. Predictors of changes in glucose tolerance in obese youth. *Diabetes Care* 2005;28:902-909.

[140] Kahn, R; Buse, J; Ferannini, E; et al. The metabolic syndrome: time for a critical appraisal: joint statement from the American Diabetes Association and the European Association for the Study of Diabetes. *Diabetes Care* 2005;28:2289-2304.

[141] Ortega-González, C; Luna, S; Hernández, L; et al. Responses of serum androgen and insulin resistance to metformin and pioglitazone in obese, insulin-resistant women with polycystic ovary syndrome. *J. Clin. Endocrinol. Metab.* 2005;90:1360-1365.

[142] Dunaif, A. Insulin resistance and the polycystic ovary syndrome: mechanism and implications for pathogenesis. *Endocrinol. Rev.* 1997;18:774-800.

[143] Bideci, A; Cinaz P, Hasanoglu, A; et al. Serum levels of insulin-like growth factor-I and insulin-like growth factor binding protein-3 in obese children. *J. Pediatr. Endocrinol. Metab.* 1997;10:295-299.

[144] Witchel, SF; Smith, R; Tomboc, M; et al. Candidate gene analysis in premature pubarche and adolescent hyperandrogenism. Fertil Steril 2001;75:724-730.

[145] Chiumello, G; Brambilla, P; Guarneri, MP; et al. Precocious puberty and body composition: effects of GnRH analog treatment. *J. Pediatr. Endocrinol. Metab.* 2000;13(Suppl 1):S791-S794.

[146] Dimartino-Nardi, J. Premature adrenarche: findings in prepubertal African-American and Caribbean-Hispanic girls. *Acta Paediatr.* 1999,88 (Suppl 433):67-72.

[147] Leung, AK. Gynecomastia. *American Family Physician* 1989;39:215-222.

[148] Tracey, VV; De, NC; Harper, JR. Obesity and respiratory infection in infants and young children. *BMJ* 1971;1:16-18.

[149] Wing, YK; Hui, SH; Pak, WM; et al. A controlled study of sleep related disordered breathing in obese children. *Arch. Dis. Child* 2003;88:1043-1047.

[150] Li, AM; Chan, MHM; Chan, DFY; et al. Insulin and obstructive sleep apnea in obese Chinese children. *Pediatr. Pulmonol.* 2006;41:1175-1181.

[151] Gennuso, J; Epstein, LH; Paluch, RA; et al. The relationship between asthma and obesity in urban minority children and adolescents. *Arch. Pediatr. Adolesc. Med.* 1998;152:1197-1200.

[152] Gold, DR; Rotnitzky, A; Damokosh, AI; et al. Race and gender differences in respiratory illness prevalence and their relationship to environmental exposures in children 7 to 14 years of age. *Am. Rev. Respir. Dis.* 1993;148:10-18.

[153] Figueroa-Muñoz, JI; Chinn, S; Rona, RJ. Association between obesity and asthma in 4-11 year old children in the UK. *Thorax* 2001;56:133-137.

[154] Luder, E; Melnik, TA; DiMaio, M. Association of being overweight with greater asthma symptoms in inner city black and Hispanic children. *J. Pediatr.* 1998;132:699-703.

[155] Leung, TF; Li, CY; Lam, CWK; et al. The relation between obesity and asthmatic airway inflammation. *Pediatr. Allergy Immunol.* 2004;15:344-350.

[156] To, T; Vydykhan, TN; Dell, S; et al. Is obesity associated with asthma in young children? *J. Pediatr.* 2004;144:162-168.

[157] de Sá Pinto, A; de Barros Holanda, PM; Radu, AS; et al. Musculoskeletal findings in obese children. J Paediatr Child Health 2006;42:341-344.

[158] Taylor, ED; Theim, KR; Mirch, MC; et al. Orthopedic complications of overweight in children and adolescents. *Pediatrics* 2006;117:2167-2174.

[159] Schwimmer, JB; McGreal, N; Deutsch, R; et al. Influence of gender, race, ethnicity on suspected fatty liver in obese adolescents. *Pediatrics* 2005;115:e451-e565.

[160] Schwimmer, JB; Deutsch, R; Rauch, JB; et al. Obesity, insulin resistance, and other clinicopathological correlates of pediatric nonalcoholic fatty liver disease. *J. Pediatr.* 2003:143:500-505.

[161] Sokol, RJ. The chronic disease of childhood obesity: the sleeping giant has awakened. *J. Pediatr.* 2000;136:711-713.

[162] Quirós-Tejeira, RE; Rivera, CA; Ziba, TT; et al. Risk for nonalcoholic fatty liver disease in Hispanic youth with BMI ≥95th percentile. *J. Pediatr. Gastroenterol Nutr.* 2007;44:228-236.

[163] Strauss, RS; Barlow, SE; Dietz, WH. Prevalence of abnormal serum aminotransferase values in overweight and obese adolescents. *J. Pediatr.* 2000;136:727-733.

[164] Kaechele, V; Wabitsch, M; Thiere, D; et al. Prevalence of gallbladder stone disease in obese children and adolescents: influence of the degree of obesity, sex, and pubertal development. *J. Pediatr. Gastroenterol Nutr.* 2006;42:66-70.

[165] Everhart, JE. Contributions of obesity and weight loss to gallstone disease. *Ann. Intern. Med.* 1993;119:1029-1035.

[166] Fishman, L; Lenders, C; Fortunato, C; et al. Increased prevalence of constipation and fecal soiling in a population of obese children. *J. Pediatr.* 2004;145:253-254.

[167] Sims, MA; Hasler, WL; Chey, WD; et al. Hyperglycemia inhibits mechanorecpetor-mediated gastrocolonic responses and colonic peristaltic reflexes in healthy humans. *Gastrology* 1995;108:350-359.

[168] van der Sijp, JRM; Kamm, MA; Nightengale, JM; et al. Circulating gastrointestinal hormone abnormalities in patients with severe idiopathic constipation. *Am. J. Gastro.* 1998;93:1351-1356.

[169] Leung, AK; Kao, CP. Acanthosis nigricans. Consultant Pediatrician 2004;3:241-243.

[170] Adelman, RD; Restaino, IG; Alon, US; et al. Proteinuria and focal segmental glomerulosclerosis in severely obese adolescents. *J. Pediatr.* 2001;138:481-485.

[171] Faustinella, F; Uzoh, C; Sheikh-Hamad, D; et al. Glomerulomegaly and proteinuria in a patient with idiopathic pulmonary hypertension. *J. Am. Soc. Nephrol.* 1997;8:1966-1970.

[172] Praga, M; Morales, E; Herrero, JC; et al. Absence of hypoalbuminemia despite massive proteinuria in focal segmental glomerulosclerosis secondary to hyperfiltration. *Am. J. Kidney Dis.* 1999;33:52-58.

[173] Shimomura, Y; Murakami, M; Shimizu, H; et al. Case report: improvement of nephrotic syndrome in massively obese patient after weight loss and treatment with an anti-allergic drug. *J. Med.* 1990;21:337-347.

[174] Weisinger, JR; Kempson, RL; Eldridge, FL; et al. The nephrotic syndrome: a complication of massive obesity. *Ann. Intern. Med.* 1974;81:440-447.

[175] Welch, TR; Daniels, SR. Yet another target organ of obesity. *J. Pediatr.* 2001;138:455-456.

[176] Cindik, N; Baskin, E; Agras, PI; et al. Effect of obesity on inflammatory markers and renal functions. *Acta Paediatr.* 2005;94:1732-1737.

[177] Wang, Y; Chen, X; Klag, MJ; et al. Epidemic of childhood obesity: implications for kidney disease. *Adv. Chronic. Kidney Dis.* 2006;13:336-351.

[178] Tikkinen, KAO; Auvinen, A; Huhtala, H; et al. Nocturia and obesity: a population-based study in Finland. *Am. J. Epidemiol.* 2006;163:1003-1011.

[179] Nead, KG; Halterman, JS; Kaczorowski, JM; et al. Overweight children and adolescents: a risk group for iron deficiency. *Pediatrics* 2004;114:104-108.

[180] Pinhas-Hamiel, O; Newfield, RS; Koren, I; et al. Greater prevalence of iron deficiency in overweight and obese children and adolescents. *Int. J. Obes. Relat. Metab. Disord.* 2003;27:416-418.

[181] Theriot, JA; Sayat, J; Franco, S; et al. Childhood obesity: a risk factor for omental torsion. *Pediatrics* 2003;122:e460-e462.

[182] Harrington, JW; Leung, AK. Omental infarction. *Consultant Pediatrician* (in press).

[183] Calle, EE; Rodriguez, C; Walker-Thurmond, K; et al. Overweight, obesity, and mortality from cancer in a prospectively studied cohort of US adults. *N. Engl. J. Med.* 2003;348:1625-1638.

[184] Must, A; Jacques, PF; Dallal, GE; et al. Long-term morbidity and mortality of overweight adolescents. A follow-up of the Harvard Growth Study of 1922 to 1935. *N. Engl. J. Med.* 1992;327:1350-1355.

[185] American Dietetic Association. Position of the American Dietetic Association: individual-, family-, school-, and community-based intervention for pediatric overweight. *J. Am. Diet. Assoc.* 2006;106:925-945.

[186] Chen, W; Chen, P; Chen, SC; et al. Lack of association between obesity and dental caries in three-year-old children. *Acta Paed. Sin.* 1998;39:109-111.

[187] Willershausen, B; Haas, G; Krummenauer, F; et al. Relationship between high weight and caries frequency in German elementary school children. *Eur. J. Med. Res.* 2004;9:400-404.

[188] Moore, LL; Singer, MR; Bradlee, ML; et al. A prospective study of the risk of congenital defects associated with maternal obesity and diabetes mellitus. *Epidemiology* 2000;11:689-694.

[189] Shaw, GM; Nelson, V; Moore, CA. Prepregnancy body mass index and risk of multiple congenital anomalies. *Am. J. Med. Genet.* 2002;107:253-255.

[190] Waller, DK; Mills, JL; Simpson, JL; et al. Are obese women at higher risk for producing malformed offspring? *Am. J. Obstet. Gynecol.* 1994;170:541-548.

[191] Watkins, ML; Rasmussen, SA; Honein, MA; et al. Maternal obesity and risk for birth defects. *Pediatrics* 2003;111:1152-1158.

[192] Robson, WL; Leung, AK. Hypertension in young children. *Postgrad. Med.* 1991;90(3):191-200.

[193] Dietz, WH; Robinson, TN. Overweight children and adolescents. *N. Engl. J. Med.* 2005;352:2100-2109.

[194] American Diabetes Association. Type 2 diabetes in children and adolescents. *Diabetes Care* 2000;23:381-389.

[195] Lifshitz, F; Moses, N. Growth failure, a complication of dietary treatment of hypercholesterolemia. *Am. J. Dis. Child* 1989;143:537-542.

[196] Owens, S; Gutin, B; Allison, J; et al. Effect of physical training on total and visceral fat in obese children. *Med. Sci. Sports Exerc.* 1999;31:143-148.

[197] Epstein, LH; Wing, RR; Penner, BC; et al. Effect of diet and controlled exercise on weight loss in obese children. *J. Pediatr.* 1985;107:358-361.

[198] Watts, K; Beye, P; Siafarikas, A; et al. Effects of exercise training on vascular function in obese children. *J. Pediatr.* 2004;114:620-625.

[199] Woo, KS; Chook, P; Yu, CW; et al. Effects of diet and exercise on obesity-related vascular dysfunction in children. *Circulation* 2004;109:1981-1986.

[200] Centers for Disease Control and Prevention. Prevalence of physical activity, including lifestyle activities among adults - United States 2000-2001 MMWR Morb Mortal Wkl Rep 2003;52:764-769.

[201] Jakicic, JM. Exercise in the treatment of obesity. Endocrinol Metab Clin North Am 2003;32:967-980.

[202] American Academy of Pediatrics, Committee on Communications: children, adolescents, and television. *Pediatrics* 1995;96:786-787.

[203] Epstein, LH; Paluch, RA; Gordy, CC; et al. Decreasing sedentary behaviors in treating pediatric obesity. *Arch. Pediatr. Adolesc. Med.* 2000;154:220-226.

[204] Durant, N; Cox, J. Current treatment approaches to overweight in adolescents. *Curr. Opin. Pediatr.* 2005;17:454-459.

[205] Kennedy, E; Powell, R. Changing eating patterns of American children: a view from 1996. *J. Am. Coll .Nutr.* 1997;16:524-529.

[206] Krebs-Smith, SM; Cook, A; Subar, AF; et al. Fruit and vegetable intakes of children and adolescents in the United States. *Arch. Pediatr. Adolesc. Med.* 1996;159:81-99.

[207] Wrotniak, BH; Epstein, LH; Paluch, RA; et al. Parent weight changes as a predictor of child weight change in family-based behavioral obesity treatment. *Arch. Pediatr. Adolesc. Med.* 2004;158:342-347.

[208] Epstein, LH; Valoski A; Wing, RR; et al. Ten-year follow-up of behavioral, family-based treatment for obese children. *JAMA* 1990;264:2519-2523.

[209] Faith, MS; Berman, N; Heo, M; et al. Effects of contingent television on physical activity and television viewing in obese children. *Pediatrics* 2001;107:1043-1048.

[210] Godoy-Mates, A; Carraro, L; Vieira, A; et al. Treatment of obese adolescents with sibutramine: a randomized, double-blind, controlled study. *J. Clin. Endocrinol. Metab.* 2005;90:1460-1465.

[211] Chanoine, JP; Hampl, S; Jensen, C; et al. Effect of orlistat on weight and body composition in obese adolescents: a randomized controlled trial. *JAMA* 2005;293:2873-2883.

[212] Hundal, RS; Inzucchi, SE. Metformin: new understanding, new uses. *Drugs* 2003;63:1879-1894.

[213] Webb, E; Viner, R. Should metformin be prescribed to overweight adolescents in whom dietary/behavioural modifications have not helped? *Arch. Dis. Child* 2006;91:793-794.

[214] Kay, JP; Alemzadeh, R; Langley, G; et al. Beneficial effects of metformin in normoglycemic morbidly obese adolescents. *Metabolism* 2001; 50:1457-1461.

[215] Freemark, M; Bursey, D. The effects of metformin on body mass index and glucose tolerance in obese adolescents. *Metabolism* 2001;50:1457-1461.

[216] Inge, TH; Krebs, NF; Garcia, VF; et al. Bariatric surgery for severely overweight adolescents: concerns and recommendations. *Pediatrics* 2004;114:217-223.

[217] Dennison, BA; Boyer, PS. Risk evaluation in pediatric practise: aids in prevention of 2childhood overweight. *Pediatr. Ann.* 2004;33:25-30.

[218] American Academy of Pediatrics, Committee on Nutrition. Prevention of pediatric overweight and obesity. *Pediatrics* 2003;112:424-430.

[219] Hill, JO; Trowbridge, FL. Childhood obesity: future directions and research priorities. *Pediatrics* 1998;101:570-574.

[220] Centers for Disease Control and Prevention. Ten strategies for promoting physical activity, healthy eating, and a tobacco-free lifestyle through school health programs. June 2003. Available at: http://www.cdc.gov/HealthyYouth /publications /pdf/ten_strategies. pdf. Accessed April 1, 2007.

[221] Flodmark, CE; Marcus, C; Britton, M. Interventions to prevent obesity in children and adolescents: a systematic literature review. *Int. J. Obesity* 2006;30:579-589.

In: Nutrition Research at the Leading Edge
Editors: R. E. Cassady, E. I. Tidswell, pp. 95-132
ISBN: 978-1-60456-053-4
© 2008 Nova Science Publishers, Inc.

Chapter III

Cardiovascular Health

Brian Lockwood
School of Pharmacy and Pharmaceutical Sciences,
University of Manchester, Manchester, UK

Introduction

Cardiovascular diseases (CVD) which affect the heart and circulatory system are known to cause millions of deaths each year worldwide, comprising the largest contribution to mortality in Europe and North America [1]. According to prevalence data from the National Health and Nutrition Examination Survey Ш, 64.4 million Americans have one or more types of CVD, of whom 25.3 million are aged 65 years or older, and accounted for 38.5% of all deaths in the US. The cost implications of this, both direct and indirect, have been estimated to be $368.4 million [2]. Consequently much research has been aimed at developing new treatments and new methods of prevention of CVD [3].

Known high-risk factors include smoking, diabetes, hypertension and hypercholesterolaemia, eating a diet high in saturated fats accelerate this process.

Individuals with a predisposition and those with established CVD are increasingly given advice relating to their dietary habits, particularly relating to their fat and cholesterol intake and the risk of developing coronary heart disease (CHD), which has been linked by both epidemiological studies and clinical trials [4]. Further to this, the National Cholesterol Education Program in the US, has shown that for every 10% reduction in cholesterol levels, CHD mortality is reduced by 13% and total mortality by 10% [2].

In CHD, atherosclerotic plaques form on the inner surface of arteries, which narrow the lumen and consequently reduces the blood flow. Low density lipoprotein (LDL) then deposits at lesion sites in the artery wall, and is oxidised, which causes modifications in lipoproteins, stimulates inflammatory reactions, and causes monocytes and macrophages to accumulate, forming foam cells with high lipid levels and atherosclerotic plaques [5].

Studies of lipid metabolism have shown that it is not the high cholesterol levels that cause artherosclerosis and CHD but rather the oxidised low density lipoprotein (LDL). The use of antioxidants (AO)s would therefore be expected to reduce the incidence of CHD and this has been shown in epidemiological studies [6].

Lipids are transported as lipoproteins in the blood. These include very low density lipoprotein cholesterol (VLDL-C), low density lipoprotein cholesterol (LDL-C) and high density lipoprotein cholesterol (HDL-C). LDL-C is removed from the circulation by binding with both plasma membranes and HDL-C, and is a less concentrated form of cholesterol. An increased level of LDL-C can result from a deficiency in the binding mechanism and is known as type II hypercholesterolaemia. This can be due to a genetic defect (familial hypercholesterolaemia) or multifactorial due to genetics, diet and lifestyle. As well as primary hypercholesterolaemia, increased cholesterol levels may be secondary to diabetes mellitus, hypothyroidism, pregnancy, renal failure, obesity, a high alcohol intake, poor diet and various drugs, such as beta-blockers, diuretics and oral contraceptives. Hypercholesterolaemia is known to be an important risk factor in the development of artherosclerosis and CHD, and studies have shown that a 1% decrease in serum cholesterol can lead to a 2% reduction in mortality. The aims of treatment are to increase HDL-C and decrease total cholesterol and LDL-C [7,8].

Although diet can be used to lower cholesterol levels, in many cases this is insufficient and pharmacological intervention is required. Although generally safe and well tolerated, some lipid-lowering drugs cause side effects. The statins, for example pravastatin and lovastatin, which are widely prescribed, have been reported to (rarely) cause hepatotoxicity, reflected by increases in serum transaminases, as well as myopathy leading to renal failure, reflected by increases in creatine phosphokinase [9]. The importance of these side effects is augmented by the fact that statins are usually taken for long duration.

Myocardial infarctions (MI) occur in patients who have established CHD where there is severe and/or prolonged impaired supply of oxygenated blood to the cardiac tissue. There are a wide range of risk factors associated with the development of CHD, including family history, hypertension, raised serum cholesterol, diabetes, smoking, poor diet and lack of exercise [1] .

There is evidence that a number of nutraceuticals are beneficial in the prevention or symptom reduction of CHD, these include black and green tea and their flavonoids, soy protein and isoflavones, essential fatty acids, flax lignans, coenzyme Q10, lycopene, policosanol and pycogenol, melatonin, resveratrol, grape seed proanthocyanidin extract (GSPE), lutein, carnitine, and DHEA. The aim of this chapter is to determine what effects these nutraceuticals have on the cardiovascular system and what evidence there is to support their use, both experimentally and clinically. This topic has been the subject of a number of publications, and tea and soy constituents have been researched to a much greater extent than other nutraceuticals.

Black and Green Tea

Tea is probably the most popular drink in the world, second only to water in terms of average per capita consumption, and annual worldwide per capita consumption of tea has been estimated at 40L/year [10].

It is derived from the leaves of the *Camellia sinensis* plant, and is traditionally grown and consumed in many regions of the world. It is usually cultivated in areas of high humidity, fair temperature, and acidic soils, at a range of altitudes. Freshly collected leaves require processing in order to inactivate endogenous enzymatic oxidation when producing green tea, or to control oxidation during production of oolong and black tea [5] .In the production of green 'unfermented' tea, the leaves are rapidly steamed for 1 minute and then dried, to deactivate the naturally occurring polyphenol oxidase enzymes [11], thereby inhibiting degradation of the natural polyphenols, which results in a product with similar chemical composition to the fresh leaves, endowing it with characteristic flavour [12]. The major components present are a group of structurally related catechins, epicatechin, epicatechin gallate, epigallocatechin, and epigallocatechin gallate, and in total, these catechins are 90% of the total flavonoids and account for 30-50% of green tea solids [11].

In the production of black 'fermented' tea, the leaves are allowed to dry for 16-20 hours until their moisture content is reduced to approximately 55%, then the rolling and cutting process promotes the oxidation, and therefore fermentation, of the tea polyphenols [11]. During the fermentation process, simple catechin polyphenols are converted into more complex and condensed polyphenolic compounds including theaflavins and their gallates, and thearubigin polymers [12]. The chemical composition of most black teas varies slightly depending on the extent of fermentation undergone [13], but thearubigins account for 47% of the total flavonoids [11]. Solar withering of the leaves followed by partial fermentation following rolling of the plant leaves is stopped by firing, to produce oolong tea, which contains monomeric catechins, theaflavins and thearubigins [13]. Another interesting component of tea is the amino acid, theanine (see later in Chapter 19), which has been shown to significantly reduce blood pressure in hypertensive rats [14].

Epidemiological studies have been carried out in order to evaluate the effect of tea consumption on the incidence of CVD, but the findings are to some extent contradictory, with beneficial, adverse, or no effects being reported [11]. Initially most research was on green tea, but recently research has also included black and oolong teas.

The Ability of Tea To Lower Plasma Lipid

One proposed mechanism by which tea may protect from CVD, is via its effects on lipid and lipoprotein levels, and a number of epidemiological studies have studied the relationship between tea consumption and a possible cholesterol-lowering potential [15].

In a study on 1371 Japanese men, increased consumption of green tea, from 3 to 10 cups per day, was associated with decreased serum concentrations of total cholesterol and triglyceride and an increased proportion of high density lipoprotein cholesterol together with a decreased proportion of low and very low lipoprotein cholesterols. The group of subjects consuming the highest level of tea, 10 cups daily, showed a significant decrease in the ratio of LDL-C to HDL-C [16].

A further inverse relationship between green tea consumption and serum cholesterol and triglyceride levels has been identified in another epidemiological study, also conducted in Japan. Whilst ingestion of 10 cups of green tea per day (estimated to contain 360-540mg of

EGCG) did not lower total plasma cholesterol levels of postmenopausal women, male subjects were found to have decreased serum levels of both total cholesterol and triglycerides [17].

One study was conducted to determine the effects of black tea consumption on the blood lipid profiles of a group of mildly hypercholesterolaemic adults, and showed significant reduction in cholesterol levels. Ingestion of 5 servings of black tea per day during the 3 weeks of the trial, reduced total cholesterol 6.5%, LDL-C 11.1%, apolipoprotein B 5% and lipoprotein(a) 16.4%, compared with a caffeine-containing placebo, but less markedly compared with the placebo without caffeine [18].

In vivo studies with rats have shown that tea catechins reduced the solubility of cholesterol in micelles, which could be linked to reduced intestinal absorption of cholesterol [15]. Also in rats it has been shown that green tea catechins and black tea polyphenols may exert their hypocholesterolaemic activity via a number of mechanisms, including increased faecal excretion of fat and cholesterol, up-regulated LDL receptors in liver cells, and reduced hepatic cholesterol concentration [15]. However, it is unknown whether this also occurs in humans.

A randomised controlled trial carried out in China investigated the cholesterol-lowering effect of a theaflavin-enriched (375mg) green tea extract on adults with mild to moderate hypercholesterolaemia. Patients taking the extract showed an 11.3% reduction in serum total cholesterol, and a 16.4% reduction in LDL-C, compared to placebo [15].

A study carried out on US patients ingesting 900ml black tea daily over four weeks, found no significant alteration in total cholesterol, LDL-C or HDL-C [19].

Smoking is a major risk factor for atherosclerotic diseases, as it is known to trigger vascular injury by platelet aggregation. P-selectin is induced by platelet aggregation, and is involved in the adhesion of white blood cells to epithelial cells, also plasma concentrations are higher in smokers. A recent study investigated the effects of green tea consumption on atherosclerotic biological markers in smokers. Participants drank 600ml of green tea per day for 4 weeks, and there was a significant decrease in P-selectin plasma concentrations, of the order of 55%, and 15 % reduction in oxidised LDL [20].

Activity of Tea on Endothelial Function

As endothelial dysfunction is associated with a state of increased oxidative stress, it follows that ingestion of antioxidants could reverse the associated impaired vascular function [19]. In addition to its importance in the development and progression of atherosclerosis and thrombogenesis, impaired vascular function is associated with CVD, and antioxidant tea flavonoids may mediate improvements in vascular function [21].

Endothelial cells that line blood and lymphatic vessels and the heart have an integral role in vascular homeostasis, mediating their effects via the production and release of chemical agents such as nitric oxide (NO). NO is integral to normal endothelial function, hence vasomotor tone, platelet activity, leukocyte adhesion, and vascular smooth muscle cell proliferation [11].

If the normal functioning of endothelial cells is disrupted, a loss of NO is often observed, impairing vasodilator function in conduit arteries and resulting in an increased risk of developing CVD [22]. This situation occurs in atherosclerosis when the production of NO in the endothelium is reduced, therefore providing antioxidant treatment in response to endothelial dysfunction and atherosclerosis may be able to decrease oxidative stress and improve endothelial health [11].

Increased antioxidant defences in the body and decreased production of reactive oxygen species may contribute to reduced breakdown and/or enhanced synthesis and release of endothelial-derived NO, and hence improve vascular function. In studies looking at the beneficial effect of tea flavonoids on endothelial function, brachial artery flow-mediated dilation (FMD) has been used as a marker of vasodilator function, which in turn reflects endothelial function [21].

The effects of both two hour and four week black tea ingestion on endothelial dysfunction in patients with coronary artery disease (CAD). Plasma tea flavonoids increased after ingestion during both regimens, and also improved endothelium-dependent flow-mediated dilation of the brachial artery [19].

Acute consumption of black tea showed a 65% improvement in brachial artery FMD; regular ingestion of black tea over a four week period was found to improve FMD 56%, whilst a 77% acute improvement was reported in those subjects who ingested black tea chronically [19].

Five cups of black tea per day were taken by patients with mild elevations in serum cholesterol or triglyceride concentrations over four weeks. There were insignificant changes in total, LDL, and HDL cholesterol, but endothelium-dependent FMD improved by approximately 41% [21].

Effects of Tea on Atherogenesis

CHD results in the death of over 6.5 million people worldwide each year and atherosclerosis of the coronary arteries is the cause of most incidences [1]. Epidemiological studies have shown that consumption of approximately two cups of black tea per day correlates with a decreased risk of developing CHD, and it is thought that this may be mediated by reduced incidence and degree of progression of atherogenesis in tea-drinking individuals [23].

Black and green teas have been shown to be equally effective in increasing the total plasma antioxidant status after a single dose, however another study showed green tea to be more effective than black. Epidemiological studies relating tea consumption with lipid levels showed a negative correlation in black tea drinkers in Norway, and no correlation in Japanese green tea drinkers [10]. Animal work using experimentally induced atherosclerosis showed an inverse association between both green and black tea consumption and atherogenesis. Low dose teas, 0.0625%, caused a decrease in atherosclerosis by 26-46%, while the high dose, 1.25% (the "typical" human level of consumption), caused a decrease of 48-63%. In normal animals, both teas produced some improvement in LDL, LDL/HDL ratios and triglyceride levels [10]. It is thought that the oxidation of both LDL cholesterol and VLDL contributes to the development of atherosclerosis [10]. Consequently, by preventing their oxidation a corresponding reduction in atherogenesis should be seen.

Human trials with both black and green tea have shown a significant increase in plasma antioxidant capacity approximately one hour after consumption of 1-6 cups of tea daily [23]. It is thought that this can protect cells and tissues from oxidative damage caused by scavenging oxygen-free radicals, after they are absorbed from the gut after ingestion. Significant decrease in foam cell formation, the early form of atherosclerosis, has been reported in animals after consumption of both green and black teas [10]. This may explain how green and black teas have a protective effect against CHD. One recent review of the literature on green tea concluded that green tea possessed stronger cardioprotective activity than black tea, or oolong, simply due to the greater antioxidant capacity [24]. The apparent significance of the antioxidant and other biological activity of the flavonoids metabolites, as demonstrated by *in vivo* activity, shows the importance of investigation into the metabolites themselves.

Effects of Tea on Hypertension

Hypertension is the most common form of CVD, and approximately 20 per cent of the adult populations suffer from this. Hypertension is also one of the major risk factors for cardiovascular mortality, which accounts for 20-50% of all deaths. Some of the evidence has been reviewed in 2004 [14]. In Chinese individuals, an association has been suggested between tea drinking and a reduction in blood pressure, but hypertension has now been investigated in individuals with a history of long term tea drinking.

An epidemiological study carried out in Norway found that subjects experienced a fall in systolic blood pressure with increased consumption of black tea, whilst a further study conducted in Japan showed no relation between green tea intake and blood pressure [14]. Clinical trials carried out in both Australia and England failed to show a correlation between short-term consumption of high quantities of green or black tea and a decrease in blood pressure. Animal studies conducted in Japan concluded that a substantial hypotensive effect was observed in rats following short-term supplementation of their diet with green tea extracts.

These variable results have caused some confusion over the possible anti-hypertensive effect of green and black teas. Further epidemiological work was initiated in 1996, involving the participation of Chinese adult habitual tea drinkers in Taiwan [14]. The long-term effects of tea drinking and various lifestyle and dietary factors were evaluated for the risk of developing hypertension [14]. An inverse relationship was found between consumption of tea and mean blood pressure of individuals. Participants who had consumed at least 120ml of tea per day for one year had a 46% lower risk of being diagnosed with hypertension than non-habitual tea drinkers. Increased consumption of 600 ml or greater was shown to reduce the risk by 65%. It was suggested that the threshold level of tea consumption likely to reduce the risk of developing hypertension would be 120ml or more of either green or oolong tea per day, for at least one year, as nearly 40% of the 1507 subjects without a history of hypertension consumed tea at this level [14].

Increased peripheral vascular tone is a characteristic of hypertension, and this could be a result of endothelial dysfunction and a state of oxidative stress is also commonly observed. The presence of superoxide radicals could result in impaired nitric oxide synthesis, or even increased deactivation of NO, which could explain the increased peripheral vascular resistance observed [14].

Tea polyphenols are known to act as potent antioxidants acting as free-radical scavengers, and causing chelation of transition metals and inhibition of enzymes [13,25].

It is thought that green and oolong tea extracts demonstrate anti-hypertensive effects due to their ability to reverse the endothelial dysfunction associated with hypertension, both through their antioxidant activity, and also their capacity to relax vascular smooth muscle [14].

Effects of Tea on Myocardial Infarction

In addition to the cardiac activities discussed, tea polyphenols are believed to have anti-platelet, anti-thrombotic and anti-inflammatory properties, and animal studies suggest that they may also improve vascular function. This suggests that ingestion of tea could minimise the risk of developing CHD and of suffering a MI [26].

Tea consumption and MI has been the subject of a number of epidemiological studies. Both inverse and converse relationships have been found in studies ranging from Saudi to Japan. The Boston Area Health Study reported that consumption at least one cup of black tea per day conferred roughly half the risk of suffering a MI compared with habitual non tea-drinkers [13]. The Zutphen Elderly Study claimed an inverse association between age-adjusted tea polyphenol intake and ischaemic heart disease, but not with MI incidence [23]. Another study on Dutch populations, this time in Rotterdam, found that tea drinkers consuming more than 375ml per day had a lower relative risk of MI than non tea-drinkers [26].

A meta-analysis of 17 studies on tea consumption in relation to MI, based on ten cohort studies and seven case-control studies, reported that an increase in tea consumption of three cups per day was associated with an 11% decrease in the incidence rate of MI. However, the authors urged caution as preferential publication of smaller studies appeared to suggest protective effects [27]. A later study in the US, involving acute MI patients, concluded that post-MI mortality was lower amongst moderate to heavy tea drinkers, consuming more than 14 cups of tea per week for a year prior to MI, compared with non tea drinkers [28].

Unfortunately, not all studies showed that tea consumption reduced the incidence of MI. Two studies conducted within the UK actually identified a positive correlation between tea consumption and CHD risk [27]. Lifestyle factors could have had a profound effect on the findings, and therefore further research needs to be carried out into the effects of tea consumption.

Soy

In 1999, the Food and Drug Administration approved manufacturers of soy foods to state the health claim that consumption of at least 25g of soy protein per day may be beneficial to a reduced risk of developing CHD. It has been claimed that much of the support for this decision was obtained from a meta-analysis published in 1999 [29]. The results of this analysis showed that consumption of soy protein instead of animal protein reduced LDL cholesterol levels by 7-24% depending upon initial cholesterol levels. However, it was not clear whether the benefits reported were due to the soy protein or the constituent isoflavones [30]. This lack of specificity of composition of many of the soy products used in research since that date still cause problems in interpreting the active fraction/s of the soy tested.

Animal and clinical evidence relating to consumption of soy and soy protein has been published in a number of areas of cardiac health.

Effects of Soy Consumption on Plasma Lipids

Over the last 30 years, numerous animal and human studies have indicated that ingestion of isoflavone-rich soy protein is associated with decreased LDL and unchanged or increased HDL-C plasma concentrations [3], but the results from several clinical trials have been less conclusive [29]. In hypercholesteraemic men and women, the relationship is particularly evident, but in normocholesteraemic men and women there is less consistency in results [31].

One trial involving hypercholesterolaemic postmenopausal women showed increased HDL-C and reduced non HDL-C in subjects receiving 40g of soy protein per day for 6 months. The soy supplements contained either 2.39mg isoflavones/g protein, or 1.39mg isoflavones/g protein. Patients in the group taking the low concentration of isoflavones, had significantly improved blood lipid profiles before 24 weeks, while the other group did not show improvement until later in the study [32].

In two previous studies, mildly hypercholesterolaemic men consumed either 50g of soy protein daily, and experienced an 11-12% reduction in total and LDL-C concentrations, and in another study showed a 5-6% reduction in total cholesterol after consumption of 25g of soy protein per day [32].

Other studies have also compared the effects of isoflavone-rich soy protein and isoflavone-depleted soy protein on the plasma lipid profiles of subjects [31]. One study found that consumption of high isoflavone content soy protein significantly decreased total and LDL cholesterol levels in subjects with the highest baseline LDL-C concentrations [31]. A study of premenopausal women found that subjects taking high isoflavone soy protein had lower LDL-C concentrations and lower ratios of total to HDL-C and of LDL-C to HDL-C than those women taking the low isoflavone soy protein [31]. These studies support the view that the isoflavone content of soy protein is responsible for the cholesterol-lowering capacity of soy products [28].

In postmenopausal women oestrogen replacement therapy causes a decrease in their plasma cholesterol concentrations [32]. Consequently, the oestrogenic activity of isoflavones, particularly genistein and daidzein, could assist in the reduction of cholesterol levels observed in mildly hypercholesterolaemic [32].

A number of mechanisms implicated in the cholesterol-lowering activity of the isoflavones include altered thyroid status; enhanced bile acid excretion, leading to reduced rates of cholesterol absorption [28]; and upregulation of LDL receptors [33].

A number of trials have investigated the effects of soy isoflavones on plasma lipid profiles.

An eight-week study with healthy middle-aged subjects supplemented with 55mg of isoflavonoids, showed that the isoflavonoids had no significant influence on serum lipid or lipoprotein concentrations [32]. A trial using healthy individuals taking soy milk for 4 weeks, showed significant increases in plasma genistein and daidzein concentrations, but revealed no significant effect on plasm cholesterol or triglyceride levels [34].

A recent meta-analysis of 23 trials published between 1995 and 2002 of the effects of soy protein containing isoflavones on the lipid profile of subjects concluded that soy protein containing isoflavones significantly reduced serum total cholesterol, LDL-C, and triacylglycerol, and significantly increased HDL-C. However, these changes were related to the level and duration of intake, and the gender and initial serum lipid concentrations of the subjects [35]. Compared to the earlier meta-analysis, there was a LDL cholesterol reduction of 5.25%, whereas 7-24% had been found previously. The reductions in total and LDL-C were found to be larger in men than in women, and trials using intakes of >80mg showed better results. Interestingly, three trials reviewed, in which tablet formulations containing extracted soy isoflavones were investigated, showed no significant effects on total cholesterol reduction.

The metabolism of daidzein results in formation of equol in a wide range of animal species, but is not normally present in humans until soy is ingested. It is not produced by germ-free animals or infants, but is a product of intestinal bacterial metabolism. Adult populations are split into "equol producers" and "nonequol producers", the latter making up 50-70% of the population. The perceived benefits of being an "equol producer" are that equol has enhanced estrogenic activity *in vivo*, compared to daidzein, and has the greatest antioxidant activity of all the isoflavones when measured *in vitro*. This increased antioxidant activity may provide greater inhibition of lipid peroxidation, and consequently greater reduction in risk of cardiovascular disease [36].

In conclusion, further research is necessary to prove that replacement of animal protein in the diet with soy protein could reduce plasma lipid and lipoprotein concentrations, and also establish the relative effects of the protein and isoflavonoid components.

Effects of Soy Consumption on Vascular Function

It is possible that phytoestrogens may have a beneficial effect on vascular function by acting directly on vessel walls, perhaps via improved arterial compliance and enhanced FMD [37]. A number of studies have been carried out to investigate the improvement in vascular function after treatment with soy products and isoflavones.

One trial found that dietary soy protein supplementation over three months significantly improved distal pulse wave velocity in normotensive male and postmenopausal female subjects, following reduction in the extent of vasoconstriction in peripheral resistance vessels. Although the trial showed that soy supplementation improved blood pressure and lipid status, it did not improve vascular function, and produced a decline in endothelial function in male subjects [38].

Atherosclerotic female macaques were fed a diet rich in isoflavones, and administration of acetylcholine dilated their arteries, and constriction was reported in those fed a low isoflavone diet. Later intravenous administration of genistein to those animals receiving the low isoflavone diet proved to dilate previously constricted vessels [39].

Infusion of genistein into the brachial artery of participants in one trial resulted in an increase in blood flow within the microcirculation of subjects' forearms following [33]. Another trial reported on arterial compliance in perimenopausal women following administration of 45mg of genistein (80mg of total isoflavonoids) over five to ten week periods and systemic arterial compliance showed a 26% improvement [40].

Consumption of soy products containing isoflavones may improve vascular function via a variety of mechanisms. Due to their structural similarities to oestrogen, it is thought that they may cause an effect by binding to oestrogen receptor (ER)β receptors present in the vasculature, and protect against atherosclerosis [33].

Postmenopausal women have shown improved large artery function, enhanced brachial artery FMD, and restoration of normal vasomotion after oestrogen therapy [38,41]. Impaired brachial artery FMD is positively associated with coronary artery endothelial dysfunction and with cardiovascular risk factors [38]. Dietary soy could improve vascular function, hence reducing CVD risk, through oestrogenic mechanisms [38].

Although some studies show beneficial results, others show uncertainty concerning the effects of soy isoflavones on vascular function. The effects of genistein on vascular reactivity show that it may affect development of atherosclerosis, and have some effect on angina, however further trials are necessary to confirm these findings and their possible benefits [41].

Effects of Soy on Atherogenesis

One of the major contributing factors implicated in the pathogenesis of CHD is atherogenesis of the coronary arteries, and many experimental studies have shown that diets rich in soy protein may have beneficial effects in preventing the onset and development of atherosclerosis [41].

After a trial involving male and female macaque monkeys it was found that those fed a diet containing intact soy protein (143mg/day isoflavonoid human equivalent) had less atherosclerosis than those fed protein from casein-lactalbumin, and those who consumed low isoflavone soy protein isolates (16mg/day isoflavonoid human equivalent) [41]. It was concluded that consumption of soy containing high isoflavonoid content, could aid the prevention of atherosclerotic plaque development in monkeys [41].

A number of *in vitro* studies and human trials have been carried out in order to identify mechanisms involved in the activity of isoflavones in atherogenesis.

LDL oxidation has a major role in the pathogenesis of atherosclerosis, as it acts as the trigger for a cascade of events including accelerated platelet aggregation, injury to arterial endothelial cells, and stimulation of foam cell and fatty streak development. It has been suggested that prevention of this oxidation process could result in an improvement in atherosclerosis, and soy isoflavones are known to have antioxidant properties [42].

In vitro experiments have indicated that both genistein and daidzein cause inhibition of LDL oxidation in the vascular subendothelium [42]. It is thought that this antioxidative activity of the isoflavones can be attributed to their ability to scavenge free radicals, consequently decreasing oxidative stress [29].

These data substantiate a widely held view that soy isoflavones exert an anti-atherogenic effect in humans through inhibition of LDL oxidation, because of their antioxidant activity. Alternative mechanisms of activity include binding to oestrogen receptors; reduction in hyperlipidaemia; inhibition of the migration and proliferation of smooth muscle cells by genistein; and inhibition of tyrosine kinase by genistein [41].

Effects of Soy Products on Blood Pressure

Hypertension is the most common form of CVD, and has been the subject of several trials comparing the cardioprotective effects of ingestion of soy protein. As can be seen, conflicting evidence has been collated from these trials. Some of the data concerning the effects of soy on blood pressure in hypertension have recently been reviewed [43]. A trial involving normotensive men and women concluded that soy protein supplementation, involving 40g protein and 118mg isoflavonoids daily for three months, resulted in a significant reduction in the systolic, diastolic and mean blood pressures [38]. In one study, consumption of a soy-based diet was found to attenuate the development of hypertension in spontaneously hypertensive rats. Trials in perimenopausal women ingesting soy protein containing 34mg isoflavonoids per day showed that subjects' diastolic blood pressure was significantly reduced [43].

A trial involving male and females with mild-to-moderate hypertension was carried out in which patients received 500ml of either soy milk for a three-month period. At the end of the trial, consumers of soy milk were found to have significantly lower systolic, diastolic and mean blood pressures [43].

This trial also revealed an inverse relationship between the decreases in blood pressure and the daily urinary isoflavonoid excretions, which consisted mainly of genistein, but also of equol, a metabolite of daidzein. Urinary excretion of genistein was found to strongly correlate with reductions in diastolic blood pressure, whilst lower systolic blood pressures tended to be associated with increased levels of urinary excretion of equol [43].

The data from another clinical trial, in which patients with essential hypertension received 55mg of isoflavonoids from red clover per day for eight weeks, showed no significant hypotensive effect. Red clover contained similar isoflavonoids, genistein, daidzein, plus their methylated derivatives, so similar results may have been expected [43].

A recent review of 22 randomised trials of soy protein containing isoflavones concluded that soy products should be beneficial to cardiovascular health because of their high content of PUFAs, fibre, vitamins, minerals, and low content of saturated fat, because studies on the effects of the isoflavones alone were found to have negligible effects on average [44].

n-3 and n-6 Essential Fatty Acids

A large amount of research has been carried out into the effects of a mediterranian diet, centred mainly around the fatty acid composition of the diet. The concomitant consumption of a wide range of other constituents may however be part of the overall benefits.

A high dietary intake of saturated fat is thought to increase cholesterol levels and increase the risk of atherosclerosis. n-3 and n-6 polyunsaturated fatty acids (PUFA)s are believed to be beneficial in preventing or reversing high cholesterol levels [45]. Modern health advice is to reduce cholesterol, saturated fat and trans fatty acid intake for reduction of serum cholesterol levels [46].

However, recommendations to replace saturated fatty acids (FA)s with unsaturated FAs, in order to improve coronary health, have resulted in replacement by n-6 rather than n-3 PUFAs. This has led to the modern, western diet including far more n-6 FAs than n-3, in a ratio of approximately 20-30:1, although ideally the ratio should be almost equal. Moreover, fish consumption, which was a source of n-3 oils, has decreased in latter years. Also, due to modern food industry and agricultural methods, with an emphasis on production, the n-3 content of many foods, including meat, fish, eggs and vegetables is much lower than formerly. As a result many people are deficient in the n-3 essential FA, α-linolenic acid (ALA) [47].

Both n-6 and n-3 FAs are precursors of longer-chain eicosanoids, such as prostaglandins, thromboxanes and leukotrienes. Those derived from n-6 FAs have opposing properties to those derived from n-3 and therefore a balance is required. A diet rich in n-6 and lacking in n-3 tends to lead to thrombi, blood aggregation and cardiovascular disease, as well as allergies, inflammation and diabetes. Fish oils have long been recognised as a source of long chain n-3 PUFAs, and many researchers have studied these oils. However, flaxseed provides the richest plant source precursor, ALA, which is converted to these long-chain FAs, and provides a way to correct deficiency and prevent diseases associated with decreased n-3 FAs. Only recently have the benefits of flaxseed as a source of these essential FAs been realised.

One advantage of ALA over fish oils is that the problem of insufficient intake of vitamin E does not occur when plant sources are used [47]. Moreover, as well as being a precursor for longer-chain n-3 FAs, ALA has clinically relevant effects in its own right, which offers another benefit over n-3-containing fish-oils [48].

Levels of PUFA intake also need to be maintained to avoid clinical deficiency [49].

Linoleic acid (LA) is the major dietary n-6 PUFA, and it is found in vegetable oils including safflower, sunflower and corn oils. It is integrated into phospholipid membranes and lipoproteins and can be elongated and desaturated *in vivo* to form other fatty acids such as arachidonic acid [4].

Eicosapentaenoic acid (EPA), docosahexaenoic acid (DHA) and ALA are all n-3 fatty acids. EPA and DHA are found primarily in fish oils, ALA is found in vegetable oils, particularly flaxseed, but also soybean and canola oil. EPA and DHA can be synthesised from

ALA in the liver, but this supplies only a small proportion of the total levels. Eating one or two portions of oily fish per week is recommended to obtain the required dietary amount of n-3 PUFAs, as only relatively low doses of n-3 PUFAs of the order of 20mg/kg per day are required [50].

A large trial carried out in 1994 investigated the effect of an ALA-rich, Mediterranean diet in the survivors of a first myocardial infarction (MI). The MI survivors were randomly assigned to the experimental diet (n=302), or continued with their normal diets. The diet included a high intake of ALA, and more bread, root vegetables, green vegetables and fruit. Patients were also advised to eat more fish, less meat and replace butter and cream with margarine supplied by the study, which was canola-oil (rapeseed oil) based and provided about 5% ALA. A reduction of coronary events and cardiac deaths of close to 70% was seen in the experimental group over five years. There were significantly lower deaths in the group on the ALA-rich diet. In the experimental group there were only eight deaths, three from cardiac causes and none were sudden. The high intake of fruits and vegetables in the experimental group led to a significantly higher concentration of antioxidants in the plasma, measured over one year. Although these may well have increased the positive effects of the experimental diet, it was concluded that the increase in ALA in the diet also seemed to have significant consequences for coronary health. However, the number of dietary variables allowed in the diet make assessment of the affect of ALA difficult to judge.

Plant Provided PUFAs

Low saturated fatty acid diets are thought to be associated with a lower risk of cardiovascular disease mortality, however the majority of trials in this area have shown there to be no beneficial effects. The critical dietary factor appears to be dietary enrichment with PUFAs, which has been positively linked to a decreased risk of CHD mortality. [51].

LA is the major dietary fatty acid regulating LDL-C metabolism, by down-regulating LDL-C production and improving its hepatic receptor-dependent clearance. One major trial investigated the effect of inclusion of 11.7g/day LA in the diet, and revealed that this produced a 39% lower prevalence odds ratio for coronary artery disease [52]. Dietary intake must be above a certain critical threshold, of the order of 12.6g/day, in order to dictate the hyperlipidaemic effects of the other dietary fat components including cholesterol, for this action to take place. The corresponding levels of ALA and EPA+DHA are 1.7g/day and 0.5g/day respectively, and this level of dietary supplementation results in a n-6: n-3 FA ratio of approximately 6:1[45].

Data from a number of human trials suggest that ALA may protect against CHD. In one such study, The National Heart, Lung and Blood institute Family Heart Study, 1.1g/day, ALA correlated with a 40% reduction in mortality from coronary artery diseases [52]. The mechanism of action of dietary ALA may be related to cardiac function, rather than plasma lipids. ALA is not thought to be as effective as LA in modulating either LDL cholesterol production and clearance, or in increasing hepatic LDL receptor activity, but ALA has been found to reduce C-reactive protein, interleukin-6 (IL-6) and serum amyloid A, which are inflammatory markers associated with atherogenesis [45].

It is clear that there are benefits derived from substituting n-6 PUFAs for saturated fats, which leads to a reduction in cardiovascular deaths, via reduction in cholesterol levels. It is not known whether the benefits associated with consumption of ALA are independent, or are related to its biotransformation to EPA and DHA.

One study revealed a significant reduction in non-fatal myocardial infarction when adipose tissue contained high levels of ALA and low levels of *trans* fatty acids. This association was more marked for individuals with a low dietary fish and hence low EPA and DHA consumption [53].

Higher consumption of ALA has been found to result in lower prevalence of carotid artery plaques and a reduced intima-media thickness of the carotid arteries. It was thought that this could be caused by the conversion of ALA to EPA and DHA, both of which have been associated with cardioprotective effects [52]. This conversion has been monitored previously in subjects taking 40g flaxseed oil for 23 days, and the n-6:n-3 ratios in subjects dropped to 1:2, from a control value of 30:1 [54].

A possible relationship between high intake or blood levels of ALA and prostate cancer has been investigated, by carrying out a meta analysis of reports on the use of ALA in fatal coronary heart disease. Epidemiological studies have previously shown an increased risk of prostate cancer in men with high intakes of ALA. It was concluded that ALA consumption might be associated with an increased risk of prostate cancer. The dietary sources of the ALA, either from meat, or from vegetables, may be the cause of the increased risk, due to concomitant intake of many components which are prostate cancer risk factors, in high meat diets [55].

Obesity is one of the main risk factors for CHD. Another risk factor is aortic compliance, or elasticity, which is related to arterial function. A decrease in aortic compliance occurs in advancing age, hypertension, diabetes and artherosclerosis [56]. Middle-aged, obese subjects were supplemented with 20g of flaxseed oil daily over a four-week study, and improved aortic compliance with a resulting improvement in arterial function was reported. This finding may have significant effects in elderly, diabetic or obese patients, all of whom show a tendency of decreased aortic elasticity.

The studies involving ALA suggest it does impart important protection from cardiovascular disease, however, it is still not certain whether the benefits of ALA are due to its inherent activity, or through its conversion to EPA and DHA [45].

In a crossover study [57], flaxseed oil capsules were taken three times daily (20g oil per day, containing 12g ALA) and compared to 50g flaxseed flour per day, containing 12g ALA. In healthy women the bioavailability of ALA was similar in each case, resulting in lowered blood lipids. Also, there was no weight gain in the subjects, indicating that other energy sources had been displaced from the diet.

In another experiment [57], flaxseed flour sprinkled on foods was compared with bread made from the flour, both providing 50g/day of flaxseed for four weeks. Fatty acid profiles of the subjects did not differ significantly between the two groups, and no weight gain was reported. It therefore appears that the form in which flaxseed is consumed whether flour, oil or in baked goods, does not seem to affect the bioavailability of the ALA.

The optimum amount of ALA is about one or two teaspoons of the oil daily (2-9g) [58]. While still in the seed the oil can keep for years, but once extracted it should be carefully stored and shelf-dated, as it is sensitive to heat and light. Freezing is an alternative way of ensuring that the oil is in prime condition while being stored. Moreover, plant oils are often hydrogenated during processing, which destroys the ALA found in the pure oil. It is therefore important to ensure that flaxseed oil purchased for its therapeutic properties is not in this form [59].

PUFAs from Fish Sources

The main dietary source of EPA and DHA is fish, and fish consumption has been shown to decrease risk of sudden cardiac death. One investigation into the consumption of fish and heart rate, found lower heart rate in men who consumed fish. [60].

Another study found that supplementation with 3g each of EPA and DHA caused an increase in systemic arterial compliance, and a reduction in pulse pressure and total vascular resistance. Both fatty acids were also found to lower plasma total and VLDL triacylglycerol [61]. The effects of supplementation of 4g/day of purified EPA and DHA were studied in mildly hyperlipidaemic men over 6 weeks. Of the two, only DHA, but not EPA, was shown to reduce ambulatory blood pressure and heart rate. DHA supplementation led to a small increase in EPA levels, but EPA supplementation did not change DHA levels, thereby demonstrating the metabolic pathway [62].

There is growing evidence that EPA and DHA levels are responsible for a decreased risk of ischaemic heart disease mortality. One study revealed that increased plasma levels of combined DHA and EPA and possibly ALA lowered the risk of fatal ischemic heart disease, but not non-fatal heart attacks. A possible explanation for this was suggested that n-3 PUFAs have antiarrhythmic action [63]. A meta-analysis of randomised controlled trials on the effects of n-3 PUFAs in coronary heart disease suggested that both dietary and non-dietary supplementation with n-3 PUFAs may decrease mortality due to myocardial infarction, sudden death and overall mortality in patients with coronary heart disease [64].

EPA and DHA are antiarrhythmic agents due to their ability to prevent calcium overload in cardiac myocytes during periods of stress, where they have a membrane stabilising effect. The n-6 PUFAs, particularly LA are thought to be arrhythmogenic, due to their metabolism to arachidonic acid, prostaglandin and thromboxane [65].

The decreased blood pressure and vascular resistance are due to an increased arterial compliance. It has also been shown that EPA and DHA produce a dose-dependent reduction in tumour necrosis factor-α and IL-6 and hence have an anti-inflammatory effect, which may slow atherogenesis. In addition, EPA and DHA reduced atherosclerotic plaque development through the reduction of vascular adhesion molecules, such as vascular cell adhesion molecule-1 (VCAM-1). EPA and DHA are thought to reduce coronary heart disease mortality through a combination of these mechanisms [45].

In healthy individuals from three countries, 2.4g of both EPA and DHA were supplemented daily to their diets. An increase in LDL-C, but decrease in very low density lipoprotein (VLDL) was observed. Triacylglycerol levels were reduced via inhibition of hepatic triglyceride and VLDL apoB secretion. This suggests that other beneficial effects of n-3 PUFAs, rather than lipid metabolism, are responsible for the decreased risk of coronary mortality [66]. Activity of the n-6 fatty acids is thought to be the reverse of this situation.

In addition, EPA and DHA have an antithrombotic effect, cause a reduction in pro-aggregatory eicosanoids, such as thromboxane B2 which takes place as a result of EPA competing in the arachidonic acid cascade. Reduced platelet aggregation and reduced coagulation factors have been reported, which may reduce cardiovascular [45].

Comparison of Flaxseed and Fish Oils

Due to the health benefits of n-3 FAs compared to n-6 oils, research has been carried out to see if flaxseed has the same advantages as marine sources on lipoprotein metabolism. However, evaluation of many human studies [67], led to the conclusion that ALA was equivalent to n-6 fish oils and not as beneficial as n-3 fish oils in its effects on lowering serum cholesterol, unless ingested in very large quantities (60mL oil). This is because long chain n-3 FA production from ALA depends on the amount of n-6 FA already present. Fish oils provide long chain n-3 PUFAs, eicosapentaenoic acid (EPA, 20:5n-3) and docosahexaenoic acid (DHA, 22:6n-3), whereas flaxseed provides an n-3 precursor, which must be converted to these beneficial long chain n-3 PUFAs. Since most people have a vast excess of n-6 FAs, the n-6 pathways are preferred and long-chain ω6 FAs, are produced (18:2n-6 →20:4n-6). The conversion of the n-3 precursor to the long-chain FAs from ALA is therefore more significant over a long time period of time, or with very large intakes.

In a controlled, randomised, double-blind, crossover study [68], the effect of low dose flaxseed or fish oils on subjects consuming diets with a high or low polyunsaturated/saturated FA diet was investigated. All subjects took olive oil capsules (consisting mostly of oleic acid, 18:1n-9) for three months as a placebo. They were then randomly assigned to take flaxseed oil (35mg of ALA daily) or fish oil (35mg of EPA) in capsules for 3 months, before crossing over to the other supplement. Blood samples and diet records were taken every 3 months. Neither flaxseed oil nor fish oil capsules significantly altered plasma total, LDL-C and HDL-C. However, it was found that fish oil reduced plasma triacylglycerides in the low polyunsaturated/saturated group, but was not seen in the flaxseed oil subjects but this may have been due to the small dose used.

There is a large body of evidence to suggest that n-3 PUFAs contribute to reducing mortality from cardiac diseases via a range of pathways, thereby decreasing the risk factors of raised blood pressure and cholesterol, which are closely related to cardiovascular diseases. Eating fish regularly maintains a constant input of EPA and DHA, but in non-fish eaters it is obvious that taking these in supplement form could be beneficial [49]. However, for a person who consumes no fish in their diet it would presumably be advantageous to take a marine oil supplement.

Inexplicable conflicting evidence has been reported from some studies, such as the association of ALA with an increased risk of prostate cancer, but this link has not been investigated with fish oils, and it is possible that these may protect against prostate cancer [55]. Consequently, supplementation with purified EPA and DHA could be the best course of action.

One study making a direct comparison of the effects of tuna fish oil, evening primrose oil, soy oil and sunflower oil, concluded that the fish oil containing 6% EPA and 27% DHA may have significant beneficial effects on cardiovascular health, as it alone from the oils tested produced significant changes in vascular response [69].

In a number of studies into the effects of dietary FAs on cardiac indicators, FA intake is carefully controlled, however, this is not always the case, and personal dietary choices may have conflicted with the aims of the trials. Also, beneficial effects reported may have been caused by either the fatty acid itself or its metabolic products. As a high saturated fat intake is a specified risk factor for cardiovascular disease, substitution with alternative fatty acids such as PUFAs, may lower this risk. In all the trials the PUFAs have been well tolerated and no significant side-effects have been reported.

A range of structurally unrelated compounds have also been implicated in beneficial effects on CVD. These include the flax lignans, coenzyme Q10, lycopene, policosanol, pycnogenol, melatonin and resveratrol, GPSE, lutein and carnitine.

Flax Lignans

Flaxseed contains about 35-45% fixed oil, with ALA accounting for at least 50% of the total. Data concerning the ALA effects has been dealt with in the section "n-3 and n-6 Essential fatty acids. In addition to this, it contains the lignan, secoisolariciresinol diglucoside (SDG) at levels of 10-30mg/g of defatted flaxseed, and fibre [70].

Understanding of the cause of the beneficial cardiac effects of flax was aided greatly by Canadian researchers who compared the effects of high and low flaxseed diets in rabbits. They found that hypercholesterolaemic atherosclerosis was reduced by 46% in rabbits fed 7.5g/kg whole flaxseed. Later they showed that there was a 69% reduction in atherosclerosis in subjects fed flaxseed containing reduced ALA (3%), with a non- significant decrease in serum total cholesterol (TC) and LDL-C, and next they used 15mg/kg SDG supplementation and found 73% reduction in development of hypercholesterolaemic atherosclerosis. This result clearly shows the involvement of the lignan, SDG, in the outcome [70].

In a small human trial the effect of partially defatted flaxseed (low ALA) was investigated in hyperlipidemic men and women [71]. The subjects ate four control muffins (no flaxseed) or four test muffins (defatted flaxseed) daily, for two 3-week periods in a randomised, crossover design. There was a 2-week washout period between each test period. Serum samples were obtained and analysed for serum lipids. The defatted flaxseed reduced the serum concentrations of total cholesterol and LDL cholesterol in similar amounts to those given full-fat flaxseed in previous experiments, quoted by the authors. However, there was no effect on serum lipoprotein. As well as the lignan effects there are also beneficial effects from the seed coat gum of flaxseed, which may be responsible for the hypolididemic action. Additional trials are required in which all the components are isolated, to determine exactly which part of the flaxseed is contributing to these effects.

Recently the outcomes of clinical trials using flaxseed or oil in a range of subjects have been compared. Five trials out of six trials involved the use of flaxseed (38-50 g/day), and showed significant reduction in TC and LDL-C, and three out of four trials using flaxseed oil showed no reduction in cholesterol parameters. However, one trial using a very high dose, 60g/day of flaxseed oil for two weeks showed a decrease in triglyceride levels, and there were also reductions in TC and LDL-C levels in specific patient groups [72]. Research directed towards the specific involvement of SDG, has shown that there is an inverse relationship between serum enterolactone (major SDG metabolite) levels, and risk of acute cardiac events [73].

The coat of flaxseed contains viscous soluble and insoluble fibre, and the former is thought to be involved in cardiac protection. One meta-analysis has shown that 2-10 g/day, approximately 26-130 g of flaxseed, of viscous soluble fibre produces a small and significant decrease in TC and LDL-C [72].

Coenzyme Q10

Coenzyme Q10 (CoQ10) is a powerful antioxidant, and free radical scavenger, and is manufactured and used as a medicine in Japan [65]. It occurs naturally in the body and is mainly located in the mitochondria of myocardium, liver and kidney cells. It is an electron carrier in the mitochondrial synthesis of ATP, and has membrane stabilising effects [74]. It has been used for the treatment of cardiovascular diseases including heart failure, hypertension, angina and arrhythmias, but the evidence to support its use is contradictory. Significantly reduced levels of myocardium CoQ10, of the order of 50% normal levels, have been reported in heart failure in animals and humans [75]. Contradictory results have been reported in trials using CoQ10 supplementation in heart failure patients, but a meta-analysis of eight clinical trials supported its use [76]. However trials involving doses of less than 100mg/day produced negative results, and it has been suggested that doses of 150-200 mg/day should be used [75].

Clinical studies indicate that CoQ10 may be useful as a treatment for hypertension, as it causes a decrease in total peripheral resistance, and is thought to act as an antagonist of vascular superoxide [77]. A number of clinical trials have shown that supplementation causes a fall in blood pressure [77]. A trial involving 109 patients showed when the CoQ10 dose was adjusted to produce a blood concentration above 2μg/ml, a marked reduction in blood pressure occurred from 159/94 to 147/85 and 51% of patients were able to discontinue their previous anti-hypertensive medication [78]. CoQ10 may act by decreasing peripheral vascular resistance, or as a superoxide antagonist, or decrease cytoplasmic redox potential of the endothelium [77]. It is quite possible that CoQ10 may act via a variety of mechanisms.

Conflicting evidence exists for the benefits for cardiac patients. One observational non-randomised study claimed that administration of up to 50-150mg or 300mg/day CoQ10 could successfully treat refractory congestive heart failure. Administration of CoQ10 was found to improve the ejection fraction and functional status of the patient and it improved the patient's heart failure classification. In addition, clinical symptoms improved after 3 months, including arythmias in 63% of the patients. However, in another study using 200mg/day, CoQ10 did not affect ejection fraction, peak oxygen consumption, or exercise duration in patients with congestive heart [79].

The administration of 120mg/day of CoQ10 for 28 days have been reported to reduce angina, improve ventricular function and reduce total arrhythmias [80].

A trial using patients with hypertrophic cardiomyopathy supplemented with 200mg/day CoQ10 reported symptomatic relief of fatigue and dyspnoea, and improvements in measurements of left ventricular thickness and diastolic function. Successful outcomes required blood levels greater than 2μg/ml. This is thought to be due to an improvement in myocardial bioenergetics and ATP production [81].

It has been reported that CoQ10 supplementation at a level of 4mg/kg prior to stress, caused by surgery, improves the recovery of rats after cardiac operations. CoQ10 apparently improves the efficiency of mitochondrial energy production, therefore more energy is available for contractile function. Reduced troponin I release suggests that CoQ10 reduces myocardial damage. Supplementation in humans may result in increased cardiac recovery and hence reduced hospital stays [82].

Overall, evidence is available concerning the benefits of CoQ10 in many cardiovascular diseases, and it has been suggested that supplementation should be sufficient to raise serum blood levels to at least 2.5μg/ml [83].

Although CoQ10 is an endogenous compound, and no side-effects or tolerability problems have been reported, beta-blockers may reduce the efficacy of CoQ10, because they interfere with CoQ10 dependent enzymes [84] and statins have been reported to deplete CoQ10 [85]. It has been claimed that concomitant CoQ10 supplementation with statins could counteract this reduction in CoQ10 levels [85].

CoQ10 could possibility be used prior to cardiac surgery, to increase cardiac recovery, decrease myocardial damage, prevent arrhythmias, decrease angina, lower blood pressure and overall improve the clinical outlook of the patient. As CoQ10 may reduce hypertension, it may help to prevent more serious complications, such as myocardial infarction.

Lycopene

High levels of lycopene are present in tomato juice, sauce and oleoresin, plus a number of red fruits and vegetables, for example watermelons, pink grapefruit and pink guava [86]. It is closely related to beta-carotene and it is thought to reduce the risks of coronary heart disease. Lycopene is found in blood plasma and other body tissues, and low levels of lycopene are thought to be responsible for many chronic diseases. A recommended daily intake of 35mg has been suggested [87], but a review of the lycopene content of tomatoes and tomato products and their contribution to dietary lycopene, reported that most people do not obtain sufficient dietary amounts [88]. In lieu of sufficient dietary intake of lycopene, increased intake should be sought from foods or nutraceutical supplement.

The most widely studied carotenoid is β-carotene. A large, multi-centre study showed that a high level of β-carotene from a normal diet, based on adipose tissue concentrations, was associated with a reduced risk of myocardial infarction, particularly in smokers [89]. However further studies failed to show a reduction in CVS in smokers receiving β-carotene supplements and indeed suggested that supplements of β-carotene may be harmful in smokers, causing high mortality due to heart disease and lung cancer [90]. It was suggested that there might be other dietary contributions to the AO effect seen from a diet high in fruits and vegetables, besides the effect of β-carotene.

Lycopene is one micronutrient, often consumed with β-carotene in the diet, that may be responsible for the protective effects noticed. In a large study carried out in 10 different countries, the effects of α-carotene, β-carotene and lycopene were studied in a population of men (average age 54 years) from coronary care units, who had undergone a first acute myocardial infarction [91]. The carotenoid concentration was measured from subcutaneous adipose tissue, since the adipose tissue levels of carotenoids are derived mainly from the diet and provide a better indication of dietary status than serum levels. Lycopene showed the greatest protective effect of the three carotenoids measured, after the results had been corrected for age, obesity, smoking and other risk factors.

Another study was carried out to determine why Lithuanian men have four times higher mortality from coronary heart disease than Swedish men do [92]. 101 men aged 50 from Sweden, with no serious acute or chronic diseases were compared to a similar population of 109 men from Lithuania. There were only small differences between the two groups in traditional risk factors (hypertension, smoking, high cholesterol levels), but when comparing the resistance of LDL to oxidation, there was a lower resistance to oxidation in the men from Lithuania. There were also lower plasma concentrations of β-carotene, lycopene and γ-tocopherol in these men. These lower concentrations of AOs are due to the different diets of the two countries. It seems from this study that factors other than the usually cited risk factors are responsible for differences in mortality between Swedish and Lithuanian men. The AO status may well account for these differences and as already described lycopene is one of the best dietary AOs and may therefore help to prevent CVS.

Oxidation of LDL is also associated with the formation of artherosclerotic plaques leading to strokes. Diets containing fruits and vegetables rich in AOs could therefore also offer protection against strokes. In a study of 26,593 male smokers, aged 50 to 69, with no history of stroke in Finland, the subjects were asked to complete a detailed questionnaire about diet [93]. During a 6.1-year follow-up, 736 cerebral infarctions, 83 subarachnoid haemorrhages and 95 intracerebral haemorrhages occurred. The associations between these events and dietary intake were found to be significant only for β-carotene, but not for other nutrients, including flavonols, vitamin C, vitamin E, lutein and lycopene.

Although these reports suggest a beneficial effect of carotenoids and AOs on heart disease, and lycopene seems to be responsible for these outcomes, there is not yet conclusive evidence that lycopene itself contributes to the protective effects of fruit and vegetable consumption. A diet rich in fruits and vegetables where many micronutrients are available to act synergistically is therefore recommended at this stage, rather than individual supplements.

Initial research focussed on serum cholesterol levels, but more recently oxidative stress induced by ROS has been highlighted. Lycopene has been shown to significantly lower levels of oxidation of LDL, but it has also been shown to reduce the levels of breath pentane, another biomarker of oxidation [94]. However, other mechanisms of action, including modulation of intracellular gap junction communication; hormonal, immune system and metabolic pathways may also be involved [87].

Reactive oxygen species (ROS) and the oxidative damage they cause have been connected with the pathogenesis of atherogenesis and carcinogenesis [87]. Because of its antioxidant and free radical scavenging activity lycopene is thought to slow the progression of atherosclerosis, through the inhibition of the oxidative processes which convert circulating LDL carrying cholesterol, to oxidised LDL. The oxidation of LDL is thought to be a key step in the atherogenic process, oxidised LDL is taken up by macrophages inside the arterial wall which leads to the formation of foam cells and atherosclerotic plaques [94].

Other mechanisms of action have also been proposed, including inhibition of hydroxymethylglutaryl coenzyme A (HMG-CoA) reductase and thereby inhibition of cholesterol synthesis, LDL degradation, alterations in the size and composition of LDL particles, plaque ruptures and altered endothelial functions [94]. More research is needed to determine what exact mechanisms of action this compound has.

Population based evidence of the effects of lycopene have been collated from 10 European countries. It was found that lycopene levels were most protective against myocardial infarction when compared to other antioxidants [91]. Only limited research into the effects of lycopene in cardiovascular disease has been carried out. A clinical trial in Finland, which investigated the relationships between lycopene, atherosclerosis and coronary heart disease, concluded that middle aged men with low levels of serum lycopene had an increased intima-media thickness of the common carotid artery wall and an increased risk of acute coronary event or stroke, demonstrating that lycopene had a significant hypocholesterolemic effect in men [95]. Another study looking at lycopene and myocardial infarction risk concluded that low levels of adipose tissue lycopene are associated with an increased risk of heart attacks [92].

A recent study of the effects of supplementation with 250mg daily of tomato extract (containing 15mg of lycopene) demonstrated a reduction in blood pressure in patients with type-1 hypertension over the 8 week treatment period [96]. Work comparing the effects of lycopene with those of tomato juice in rats, showed both reduced the extent of lipid peroxidation, but only tomato juice improved post-ischaemic ventricular function, myocardial infarct size, and cardiomycete apoptosis, concluding that tomato juice, not lycopene is responsible for the cardioprotective effects [97].

Overall, lycopene appears to aid in the prevention of coronary heart disease, probably due to its antioxidant properties. More evidence is required before clinical use in the prevention of coronary heart disease.

Policosanol

Policosanol has been claimed to be as effective as the currently available lipid lowering drugs such as the statins for lowering lower plasma cholesterol [98]. Policosanol was developed in Cuba as a biproduct of the sugarcane industry, and used worldwide as a nutraceutical, and as a major cardiac medicine in the caribbean region [99].

Policosanol is a mixture of long chain fatty alcohols and other constituents obtained by solvent extraction and saponification of the wax from sugarcane, but may also be produced from beeswax and spinach wax, and an extract from wheatgerm oil has been used in a number of clinical trials [100]. The main components are octacosanol (62.9%), triacontanol (12.6%) and hexacosanol (6.2%) [99].

During motor endurance experiments on mice, it was noted that octacosanol caused altered hepatic and serum lipid concentrations. This led researchers to investigate the possible role of octacosanol and policosanol on serum lipids and its possible use as a cholesterol-lowering agent. A number of studies have been carried out in a number of animal species and policosanol was shown to reduce total cholesterol, LDL-C in a dose-deoendent way, whilst HDL-C was unchanged [101].

There have been in excess of 60 clinical trials published, mainly in Cuba, since 1992 concerning the effectiveness of policosanol as a lipid lowering agent. One double-blind clinical trial investigating the effect of in patients with type 2 hypercholesterolemia and additional coronary risk factors, showed policosanol 5 mg/day (and 10mg/day) after 12 weeks of treatment significantly reduced serum LDL-C by 18.2% (and 25.6%) and total cholesterol by 13.0% (17.4%). In addition there was a significant increase in HDL-C by 15.5% (and 28.4%), and triglycerides stayed constant up to 12 weeks, but significantly lowered later [98]. A range of other trials produced results with similar benefits. Studies demonstrated that the ability for lowering cholesterol were maintained over two years, but greatest reduction was seen after 6-8 weeks of treatment. Studies using higher doses above 20mg per day have not been undertaken, but may have greater effect. Importantly, no rebound effects have been recorded after stopping the treatment [99]. Details from a large number of clinical trials on patients with both primary and type II hypercholesteraemia appear to confirm that policosanol causes reduction in LDL-C, and total cholesterol, while HDL-C usually rises [101].

In non-insulin-dependent diabetes mellitus (NIDDM), hyperglycaemia may induce artherosclerosis leading to coronary heart disease, which is a main cause of death in these patients. It is therefore important to maintain low cholesterol levels in NIDDM patients by using glycaemic control, dietary measures and medication. Policosanol was used in a double-blind study, and patients with stable glycaemic control were given policosanol 5mg twice a day for twelve weeks [102]. Both total cholesterol and LDL-C were significantly reduced in the test group. Side effects were mild and at week 12, no side effects were reported in the policosanol group and the treatment did not affect glycaemic control.

Conflicting evidence has been published from a trial using 20mg daily of wheat germ policosanol in patients with normal to mildly elevated plasma cholesterol concentrations. Although the composition of this source of policosanol is very similar to that of sugarcane, no beneficial effects were seen [103].

A comparative study was carried out to compare 10mg/day policosanol and 20mg/day lovastatin in patients with hypercholesterolaemia and NIDDM [104]. Patients received either policosanol or lovastatin daily for twelve weeks. Both treatments were effective in lowering LDL-C and total cholesterol, without affecting glucose control. Policosanol was found to be safe and well tolerated, whereas lovastatin caused increased serum values of aspartate aminotransferase, creatine phosphokinase, and alkaline phosphatase as well as causing more frequent adverse effects (including five patients who withdrew from the study).

One animal study was carried out to determine the effect of oral pre-treatment with policosanol, two hours before isoprenaline-induced myocardial infarction. Policosanol reduced the size of the myocardial injury and also decreased the number of polymorphonuclear neutrophils (PMN) and mast cells in the damaged areas. The clinical value of these findings is unclear [105].

Policosanol is not thought to act like the statins which may cause inhibition of HMG-CoA reductase. It has been shown that policosanol inhibits cholesterol biosynthesis, probably at a stage prior to mevalonate formation, but direct inhibition of HMG-CoA reductase is thought to be unlikely [99]. Polycosanol is also possibly involved in increasing LDL cholesterol uptake in the liver by increasing numbers of LDL receptors, and is also thought to increase the rates of breakdown of serum LDL [98].

Further effects of policosanol, which may be indirectly beneficial to cardiac health have been reported. Both animal experiments and human studies have shown that it has an effect on platelets, brought about by lowering thromboxane B2 and elevating serum prostacyclin levels [98]. Anti-ischemic effects reported in animal studies may be responsible for this. It has been claimed that the antiplatelet effect of 20 mg is equal to that of 100 mg aspirin, but it acts by an alternative route, very few side-effects have been reported in clinical trials [98,99]. During long term use weight loss, polyuria and headaches have been described on rare occasions. Healthy volunteers reported no adverse effects after single doses of 1000mg, and 500mg/kg has been given orally to rats, with no reports of adverse effects. No drug interactions have been reported with other medicines in concomitant use during trials [99]. Policosanol has shown no adverse effects in non-insulin dependent diabetes mellitus patients with hypercholesteraemia [102], but it should not be used in pregnant or breast-feeding women, or in children until the possibility of adverse effects has been investigated [99].

Overall, policosanol may have a use in a number of cardiovascular diseases. The search for safe lipid lowering agents continues, and the low incidence of side effects makes it a promising choice. Safety needs further investigation and possible long term side-effects or serious drug interactions, for example with the statins, need evaluating. Standardised alkanol content of the product needs agreeing, thereby allowing precise comparison of published work. It has been claimed that most clinical trials have been carried out by only one group, in Cuba, and also that the origin of most policosanol on sale in the US is beeswax, not sugarcane, hence the possibility of unrepeatable effects [106].

Pycnogenol

Pine bark has been used historically for treating inflammatory diseases, which gives some credence to the use of pycnogenol. A range of cardiovascular effects have also been reported, including vasorelaxant effects, ability to inhibit angiotensin converting enzyme (ACE), and increase in the microcirculation by increasing capillary resistance [107].

One clinical trial using pycnogenol (150 mg/day for 6 weeks) increased the plasma polyphenol levels and antioxidant activity in subjects and also lowered LDL-C and increased HDL-C [108].

Pycogenol has been investigated for its activity in hypertensive patients and found to improve the endothelial function. A dose of 100mg daily for 12 weeks allowed reduction of the dose of nifedipine, a calcium channel antagonist, used for control of hypertension. This antihypertensive effect may be caused by a number of factors. Endothelin 1, which is a potent endogenous vasoconstrictor, levels decreased by 20% after dosing with pycnogenol. There was also a reduction in thromboxane B2 levels, and an increase in NO, which is an endothelial relaxing factor. There was no evidence to suggest that pycogenol acted as an ACE inhibitor [109], as had been claimed in an earlier publication [107].

Chronic venous insufficiency (CVI) results in swelling, and is particularly prominent in lower legs. It has a prevalence of 10-15% in men and 20-25% in women, and is usually treated with compression therapy. Although not life-threatening, if untreated it may progress to static oedema and ulcerations. One study investigated the effect of pycogenol at a dose of 360 mg/day over 4 weeks in CVI showed a significant reduction in the circumference of the lower limbs and improvement of subjective symptoms such as pain, cramps and feeling of heaviness. This activity of pycogenol is thought to be caused by stimulation of NO synthesis and acting as a free radical scavenger, leading to the relaxation of constricted blood vessels. Pycogenol is thought to counteract edema by sealing leaky capillaries, as a result of its high affinity for proteins,. In addition it significantly decreased cholesterol and LDL-C values in blood, and HDL levels remained unaffected [110].

Pycnogenol has recently been investigated for prophylaxis of deep vein thrombosis in long-haul flights of 8 hours 15 minutes average duration. 198 subjects were treated with 200mg pycnogenol 2-3 hours before the flight, followed by 200mg 6 hours later, and 100 mg the following day. In the control group there were 5 thrombotic events, one deep vein thrombosis (DVT) and 4 superficial thromboses, while the treatment group showed only symptoms of localised phlebitis [111]. Later work on oedema reduction during long haul flights reported significant reduction in oedema by passengers receiving the same dosage regimen [112]. A further trial by the same group investigated the effects on 18 patients with venous ulcers over 6 weeks. In this pilot study, combination of both oral and topical pycnogenol treatment, a faster reduction in the ulcerated area was observed, than that seen using oral treatment alone [113].

The possibility that pycogenol may be useful for inhibition of platelet aggregation induced by cigarette smoking has been investigated. The activity may be due to NO synthesis, thereby inhibiting thromboxane A2 production. The adverse effect on bleeding time produced by aspirin, is not shared by pycnogenol. It has noe been shown that 100mg pycnogenol has the same activity as 500mg aspirin [107].

It can be seen that pycogenol has a wide range of activities having beneficial effects on reducing many cardiovascular disease risk factors including DVT. As yet there is no clear evidence as to dosage levels, and safety data including drug interactions require studying.

Melatonin

In vivo research on animals has shown that melatonin overcomes cardiac injury after arterial occlusion followed by reperfusion. It appears that melatonin is more powerful than other antioxidants tested, in terms of ameliorating hypoxia and reoxygenation damage [114]. Intraperitoneal doses of 150 µg/kg were found to be most effective [115]. Humans dosed with 3mg oral melatonin showed dramatic increase in plasma melatonin concentrations, at 1830 ± 848 pg/ml, compared to 14 ± 11 pg/ml before ingestion showing maximal levels at 75 minutes after ingestion . This shows that in humans melatonin attenuates the reflex sympathetic increases that occur in response to orthostatic stress [116].

Resveratrol

There is evidence to suggest that resveratrol acts as an ontioxidant and inhibits both LDL oxidative susceptibility *in vivo,* by both chelating and free radical scavenging mechanisms. Cardioprotection is thought to result from its ability to inhibit platelet aggregation. At a physiological concentration of 1.2 µg/L, resveratrol was shown to reduce platelet aggregation by ~ 41% in healthy subjects, and this was raised to 78.5% by increasing the dose [117]. Cardioprotective effects of resveratrol may also be contributed to by inhibition of endogenous cholesterol biosynthesis, by inhibition of the rate limiting enzyme in cholesterol biosynthesis, squalene monooxygenase [118]. This may explain the protective effects on cardiovascular disease.

Grapeseed Proanthocyanidin Extract (GSPE)

GSPE is often considered alongside resveratrol as one of the main reasons for the apparent health of the French population who are both high wine and fat consumers, but have a low mortality from cardiac diseases. GSPE is a potent antioxidant, with activity levels above vitamins C and E [101].

Recent studies performed on isolated rat hearts given red wine extract before ischaemic arrest have provided evidence that grape proanthocyanidin extract (GSPE) from red wine are effective cardioprotective agents [119]. The red wine extract reduced myocardial infarct size as well as improving post-ischaemic ventricular functions. In another study by the same group [119], rats given oral GSPE for three weeks were resistant to subsequent ischaemic injury to the isolated hearts.

Other research has shown that as well as acting as a cardioprotective agent directly, GSPE also prevent artherosclerosis, which is a major risk factor for heart disease. It has been shown that *oxidation* of the polyunsaturated lipid components of LDL damages arteries and it is only this oxidised form of cholesterol that leads to artherosclerosis [58]. To determine whether the French paradox was due to the AO properties of red wine, an *in vitro* study was carried out [120]. Dealcoholised Californian red wine was used to prepare the proanthocyanidin extract, and LDL from the blood of normolipidaemic, non-smoking volunteers was used for the investigation. The extract caused an inhibition of 60% and 98% of the oxidation of LDL seen in the controls at concentrations of 3.8mmol/L and 10mmol/L respectively.

A similar experiment was carried out in humans using samples of dealcoholised red and white wine were tested for AO activity. The red wine samples were 20 times more active than the white wine samples [121].

However, not all red wines have the same protective effect. It has been shown from research on more than sixty different red wines from eleven different countries, that the GSPE content and therefore the AO properties vary greatly between different wines [122].

Red wines from Chile have a higher flavonol content than those from France, Italy, Australia and California. This could be explained by the climate in the grape-growing regions, the thickness of the grape skins, the time of grape harvesting and the actual winemaking process, which could all affect the flavonoid content.

It is interesting that many by-products of the wine industry are now being used in the nutraceutical industry. The industry produces the grape seeds and grape skins from winery waste and develops them as dietary supplements [123].

Although it has been presumed that the GSPE protect against CVD by their AO activity, most studies did not measure artherosclerosis directly. One *in vivo* study, however, did determine the effect of a GSPE extract from grape seeds directly on artherosclerosis [124]. In this study, an extract containing 73.4% GPE was obtained by freeze-drying an aqueous solution of grape seeds. The serum lipid profile did not change dramatically in the GSPE-fed rabbits, but serum LDL-C and the LDL/HDL ratio decreased at six weeks in the 1% GPE group and HDL-C decreased at eight weeks in the 0.1% GPE group. There was a lower amount of aortic plaque in the GPE group. The activity of the GSPE was thought to be related to prevention of LDL oxidation in the arterial cell wall.

Another use for GSPE that has been widespread in Europe is in the treatment of vascular disorders. These include varicose veins, venous insufficiency, and microvascular problems such as retinopathies. In France GPE are the active ingredients in a proprietary product used for microcirculatory disorders, called Endotelon. The AO properties of the GPE are largely responsible for their vascular properties [125].

A number of actions on the tissues of the arterial wall have been reported for GPSE, including inhibition of histidine decarboxylase involved in the atheromatous process, vascular relaxation, by increasing endothelial NO production, and inhibition of endothelin-1 formation [126]. Recent research using the atherosclerotic hamster model, found approximately 49 and 63% reduction in foam cells, which is a biomarker of the early stage of atherosclerosis, following administration of 50 and 100 mg/kg GSPE, respectively. In a human trial, GSPE supplementation of 100mg twice daily, significantly reduced oxidised LDL [127].

One human study using GPSE supplementation in conjunction with a novel niacin chromium, was shown to yield favourable effects on cholesterol and LDL. It was also shown to improve cardiac functional assessment including post-ischemic left ventricular function, reduced myocardial infarct size, reduced ventricular fibrillation and tachycardia, and reduced the levels of ROS [127].

Although research has shown that AOs are beneficial to most people to prevent many different diseases, some trials have not produced the expected results. Some AOs act as pro-oxidants depending on the timing of administration during oxidation processes and the individuals involved. It has been suggested that some individuals have higher rates of lipid peroxidation and are therefore at higher risk from diseases such as artherosclerosis and CVD, but in other individuals very high levels of AOs may actually cause pro-oxidation, worsening the damage. It may therefore be useful for populations to be screened to determine which people are at high risk and would benefit from AOs, rather than a general recommendation for everyone to increase in their AO intake [128]. However, the trials reviewed here indicate that in general AOs can be recommended, as such cases are rare.

Lutein

There is increasing scientific evidence that incidence of CHD is inversely related to consumption of fruits and vegetables. A comparative study of fruit and vegetable consumption and antioxidant status in Belfast, N. Ireland, (low fruit and vegetable consumption, high rate of heart disease) and Toulouse, France, (high fruit and vegetable consumption, low rate of heart disease), showed only one difference, namely the plasma concentrations of lutein and cryptoxanthin were twice as high in the Toulouse population [129]. Another epidemiological study reported that individuals with highest serum lutein plus zeaxanthin had a significantly reduced risk of CHD, and a further study showed a significant inverse relationship between lutein intake and the risk of stroke [130]. An *in vivo* study on middle aged men and women showed that in an *in vitro* artery cell wall system, lutein inhibited LDL-induced migration of monocytes to human artery cell walls, and further that this effect was more pronounced if the cells were pre-treated with lutein. There was also an inverse relationship between serum lutein levels and the progression of intima-media thickness (IMT) in the carotid arteries. Using an *in vivo* mouse model, progression of IMT was found to decline with increasing levels of plasma lutein [131].

Carnitine

Carnitine is found in high concentrations in heart muscle, where it has important functions, including preventing lactic acid formation, which is damaging to the myocardium. It has been shown that there is a reduction of up to 50% of both free and total carnitine in the failing heart [132].

During myocardial ischaemia, blood flow to the heart is reduced, and carnitine levels in myocardial muscle decrease by as much as 40% [133]. This results in an increase of free FAs and their metabolites within the cell cytoplasm, and a reduction of the oxidative processes necessary for energy production [134]. Supplementation with carnitine may be of use in patients with ischaemic heart disease.

In a study of patients suffering from exercise-induced stable angina with classical onset and improvement with rest or after the use of sub-lingual nitroglycerine [134]. The patients were treated with 2g/day carnitine orally for six months, added to their normal therapy. Medication being used by the patients included nitro-compounds, calcium channel blockers, β-blockers, antihypertensives, diuretics, cardiac glycosides, antiarrhythmics, anticoagulants and hypolipidaemics. Results showed significant and progressive improvements in cardiac function and quality of life. Although there were no differences in glycaemia or high-density lipoprotein HDL-C, there was a small but significant decrease in total cholesterol and triglycerides. There was also a significant reduction of cardioactive drug consumption as seen in table 1.

**Table 1. Percentage decreases in heart medication
seen in patients taking carnitine supplementation**

Medication	% decrease
Nitroglycerides	60
Other nitro-derivatives	40
Nifedipine	33
Diltiazem	47
β-blockers	36
Antihypertensives	44
Cardiac glycosides	35
Diuretics	34
Anticoagulants	44
Antiarrythmics	70
Hypolipidaemics	61

These results indicate that carnitine may be of importance in the control of exercised-induced stable angina, either alone or in combination with other heart medication.

In the year following myocardial infarction, patients are prone to cardiac complications, which often result in death. Patients who had suffered recent acute myocardial infarction received 2g carnitine twice daily, for one year, in addition to the standard cardioactive medication. Positive results were seen in terms of cardiac events and life expectancy with significant differences for nearly all the parameters studied. Particularly striking were the differences in mortality of 1.2% in the carnitine group compared to 12.5% in the control group receiving no carnitine. This study clearly showed that the addition of carnitine had benefits for the patients in the year following myocardial infarction [135].

In a similar study, patients with suspected acute myocardial infarction, were supplemented with 2g carnitine daily, in three divided doses. After 28 days of treatment, the mean infarct size was significantly reduced in the carnitine group, as were cardiac events, including angina pectoris, left ventricular failure and arrhythmias. No side effects were noted and the use of other heart medication was reduced [133].

Carnitine has also been used to shorten recovery time in children with heart failure who were given carnitine, at a dose of 50mg/kg/day for fifteen days. The children in the test group showed a marked improvement over the controls and decreased recovery time [136].

In conclusion, the role of carnitine in heart disease seems promising. The reduction in mortality in post myocardial infarction patients is very encouraging, as are the many other significant improvements to cardiac parameters seen with carnitine supplementation.

Some individuals may be genetically predisposed to carnitine deficiency, and this is associated with cardiomyopathy and skeletal muscle dysfunction, both of which can be treated with carnitine supplementation. Carnitine deficiency may also be acquired and can result in failing myocardium [132]. One clinical trial has shown a significant beneficial effect when treating MI patients with carnitine at a dose of 9g/day for 5 days, followed by 6g/day for the next 12 months [137]. Carnitine supplementation has also used in patients with a range of arythmias [65].

Short-term administration of creatine supplements to patients with CHD did not increase cardiac ejection fraction, but did increase skeletal muscle phosphocreatine and improvements in muscle strength, endurance and metabolism [132].

Dhea

Several epidemiological studies have found significant inverse relationships between serum dehydroepiandrosterone sulphate (DHEAS) and cardiovascular morbidity and mortality of men, suggesting that DHEA is a risk factor for CHD. However, DHEAS level does was not linked to cardiovascular risk in postmenopausal women, and DHEA supplementation in women caused decreased HDL-C levels [138]. Another study found that plasma levels of DHEAS were decreased in patients with congestive heart failure (CHF) in proportion to its severity, and that oxidative stress was associated with decreased levels of DHEAS [139].

Conclusion

The published data outlined from a wide variety studies and clinical trials suggest that dietary supplementation with certain nutraceuticals can improve cardiovascular health, both for healthy individuals and for those with cardiac problems. High quality evidence from studies involving soy protein supplementation of subjects' diets was sufficient for the Food and Drug Administration to give their approval to manufacturers of soy foods to use the health claim that "consumption of at least 25g of soy protein per day is related to a reduced risk of developing CHD" [30].

Meta-analyses of trials on a number of nutraceuticals used in this area have been carried out. Teas have been found to have produced conflicting results to date [27], while those for soy variably show decrease in total and LDLC, sometimes demonstrating significant decrease [30,35], sometimes no benefits [140]. Even analyses showing benefits suggest that the effects may be caused by other factors [141].Fish oil and EPA/DHA meta-analyses appear to confirm positive effects on blood pressure [142,143], and also beneficial effects on levels of cardiac morbidity [64,144]. CoQ10 appears well established as atreatment for congestive heart failure, and two analyses confirm this [76,145]. Policosanol appears to be more effective than plant sterols/stanols in reducing LDLC [146].

There are many green tea and soy nutraceutical products for consumers to purchase and now a number of formulated nutraceutical supplements have become available. In addition a number of other nutraceuticals are also available, with claims for improvement in cardiovascular health. A number of these entities are able to reduce various risk factors associated with cardiovascular diseases, such as cholesterol or hypertension, others are antiarrhythmic and therefore can reduce coronary heart disease mortality. However it is difficult to accurately define a recommended dosage, due to the fact that many of these nutraceuticals may be obtained as part of a healthy diet, resulting in some people having higher levels in their body compared to others. For effective cardiovascular protection, monitoring of plasma levels may be required before these products can be safely and effectively used to reduce cardiovascular disease [4].

References

[1] Walker R, Edwards C. *Clinical Pharmacy and Therapeutics.* Third Edition. London: Churchill and Livingstone; 2003.

[2] Juturu V, Gormley J J. Nutritional supplements modulating metabolic syndrome risk factors and the prevention of cardiovascular disease. *Curr. Nutr. Food Sci.* 2005; 1: 1-11.

[3] Merz-Demlow B E, Duncan A M, Wangen K E, *et al.* Soy isoflavones improve plasma lipids in normocholesterolemic, premenopausal women. *Am. J. Clin. Nutr.* 2000; 71: 1462-1469.

[4] Payne E, Potts L, Lockwood B. Nutraceuticals for cardiovascular protection. In Starks T P (Ed) *Focus on Nutrition Research* 2006, in press.

[5] Dufresne C J, Farnworth E R. A review of latest research findings on the health promotion properties of tea. *J. Nutr. Biochem.* 2001; 12: 404-421.

[6] Sanders T A B, Dean T S, Grainger D, Miller G J, Wiseman H. Moderate intakes of intact soy protein rich in isoflavones compared with ethanol-extracted soy protein increase HDL but do not influence transforming growth factor β_1 concentrations and hemostatic risk factors for coronary heart disease in healthy subjects. *Am. J. Clin. Nutr.* 2002; 76: 373-377.

[7] Castano G, Mas R, Fernandez L, *et al.* Effects of policosanol on postmenopausal women with type II hypercholesterolemia. *Gynecol. Endocrin.* 2000; 14 :187-195.

[8] Craig C R, Stitzel R E. *Modern Pharmacology.* 4th ed. USA: Little, Brown and company, 1994.

[9] Farnier M, Davignon J. Current and future traeatment of hyperlipidemia: the role of statins. *Am. J. Cardiol.* 1998; 82: 3J-10J.

[10] Vinson J A, Teufel K, Wu N. Green and black teas inhibit atherosclerosis by lipid, antioxidant, and fibrinolytic mechanisms. *J. Agric. Food Chem.* 2004; 52: 3661-3665.

[11] Kris-Etherton P M, Keen C L. Evidence that the antioxidant flavonoids in tea and cocoa are beneficial for cardiovascular health. *Curr. Opin. Lipidol.,* 2002; 13: 41-49.

[12] Mukhtar H, Ahmad N. Tea polyphenols: prevention of cancer and optimizing health. *Am J. Clin. Nutr.* 2000; 71: 1698S-1702S.

[13] Siddiqui I A, Afaq F, Adhami V M, Ahmad N, Mukhtar H. Antioxidants of the beverage tea in promotion of human health. *Antiox. Redox. Signal.* 2004; 6: 571-582.

[14] Yang Y C, Lu F H, Wu J S, Wu C H, Chang C J. The protective effect of habitual tea consumption on hypertension. *Arch. Int. Med.* 2004; 164: 1534-1540.

[15] Maron D J, Lu G P, Cai N S, *et al.* Cholesterol-lowering effect of a theaflavin-enriched green tea extract. A randomized controlled trial. *Arch. Int. Med.* 2003; 163: 1448-1453.

[16] Imai K, Nakachi K. Cross sectional study of effects of drinking green tea on cardiovascular and liver diseases. *BMJ* 1995; 310: 693-6.

[17] Nakachi K, Matsuyama S, Miyake S, Suganuma M, Imai K. Preventive effects of drinking green tea on cancer and cardiovascular disease: epidemiological evidence for multiple targeting prevention. *BioFactors* 2000; 13: 49-54.

[18] Davies M J, Judd J T, Baer D J, *et al.* Black tea consumption reduces total and LDL cholesterol in mildly hypercholesterolemic adults. *J Nutr* 2003; 133: 3298S-3302S.

[19] Duffy S J, Keaney J F Jr, Holbrook M, *et al.* Short- and long-term black tea consumption reverses endothelial dysfunction in patients with coronary artery disease. *Circulation* 2001; 104: 151-156.

[20] Lee W, Min W-K, Chun S, *et al.* Long - term effects of green tea ingestion on atherosclerotic biological markers in smokers. *Clin. Biochem,* 2005; 38; 84-7,

[21] Hodgson J M, Puddey I B, Burke V, Watts G F, Beilin LJ. Regular ingestion of black tea improves brachial artery vasodilator function. *Clin. Sci.* 2002, 102, 195-201.

[22] Vita, JA. Tea consumption and cardiovascular disease: effects on endothelial function. *J. Nutr.* 2003; 133: 3293S-3297S.

[23] Rietveld A, Wiseman S. Antioxidant effects of tea: evidence from human clinical trials. *J. Nutr.* 2003, 133, 3285S-3292S.

[24] Cheng T O. All teas are not created equal: the Chinese green tea and cardiovascular health. *Int. J. Cardiol.* 2006; 108: 301-8.

[25] Arts I C W, Hollman P C H, Feskens E J M, *et al.* Catechin intake might explain the inverse relation between tea consumption and ischemic heart disease: the Zutphen Elderly Study. *Am. J. Clin. Nutr.* 2001; 74: 227-232.

[26] Geleijnse J M, Launer L J, van der Kuip D A M, Hofman A, Witteman J C M. Inverse association of tea and flavonoid intakes with incident myocardial infarction: the Rotterdam study. *Am. J. Clin. Nutr.* 2002; 75: 880-886.

[27] Peters U, Poole C, Arab L. Does tea affect cardiovascular disease? A meta-analysis. *Am. J. Epidemiol.* 2001; 154: 495-503.

[28] Mukamal K J, Maclure M, Muller J E, Sherwood J B, Mittleman M A. Tea consumption and mortality after acute myocardial infarction. *Circulation* 2002, 105, 2476-2481.

[29] Lichtenstein, AH. Soy protein, isoflavones and cardiovascular disease risk. *J. Nutr.* 1998; 128: 1589-1592.

[30] Anderson J W, Johnstone B M, Cook-Newell M E. Meta-analysis of the effects of soy protein intake on serum lipids. *N E J. Med* .1995; 333: 276-82.

[31] Wangen K E, Duncan A M, Xu X, Kurzer M S. Soy isoflavones improve plasma lipids in normocholesterolemic and mildly hypercholesterolemic postmenopausal women. *Am. J. Clin. Nutr.* 2001; 73: 225-231.

[32] Potter S M, Baum J A, Teng H, *et al.* Soy protein and isoflavones: their effects on blood lipids and bone density in postmenopausal women. *Am. J. Clin. Nutr.* 1998; 68: 1375S-1379S.

[33] Nestel P. Role of soy protein in cholesterol-lowering. How good is it? *Arterioscl. Thromb. Vasc. Biol.* 2002; 22: 1743-1744.

[34] Mitchell J H, Collins A R. Effects of a soy milk supplement on plasma cholesterol levels and oxidative DNA damage in men – a pilot study. *Eur. J. Nutr.* 1999; 38: 143-148.

[35] Zhan S, Ho S C. Meta-analysis of the effects of soy protein containing isoflavones on the lipid profile. *Am. J. Clin. Nutr.* 2005; 81: 397-408.

[36] Setchell K D R, Brown N M, Lydeking-Olsen E. The clinical importance of the metabolite equol – a clue to the effectiveness of soy and its isoflavones. *J. Nutr.* 2002; 132: 3577-3584.

[37] Squadrito F, Altavilla D, Morabito N, *et al.* The effect of the phytoestrogen genistein on plasma nitric oxide concentrations, endothelin-1 levels and endothelium dependent vasodilation in postmenopausal women. *Atherosclerosis* 2002; 163: 339-47.

[38] Teede H J, Dalais F S, Kotsopoulos D, *et al.* Dietary soy has both beneficial and potentially adverse cardiovascular effects: a placebo-controlled study in men and postmenopausal women. *J. Clin. Endocrinol. Metab.* 2001; 86: 3053-3060.

[39] Honore E K, Williams J K, Anthony M S, Clarkson T B. Soy isoflavones enhance coronary vascular reactivity in atherosclerotic female macaques. *Fertil. Steril.* 1997; 67: 148-54.

[40] Nestel P J, Yamashita T, Sasahara T, *et al.* Soy isoflavones improve systemic arterial compliance but not plasma lipids in menopausal and perimenopausal women. *Arterioscl. Thromb. Vasc. Biol.* 1997; 17: 3392-8.

[41] Anthony M S, Clarkson T B, Williams JK. Effects of soy isoflavones on atherosclerosis: potential mechanisms. *Am. J. Clin. Nutr.* 1998 68: 1390S-1393S.

[42] Anderson J W, Smith B M, Washnock C S. Cardiovascular and renal benefits of dry bean and soybean intake. *Am. J. Clin. Nutr* .1999; 70: 464S-474S.

[43] Rivas M, Garay R P, Escanero J F, *et al.* Soy milk lowers blood pressure in men and women with mild to moderate essential hypertension. *J Nutr* .2002, 132, 1900-1902.

[44] Sacks F M, Lichtenstein A, Van Horn L, *et al.* Soy Protein , Isoflavones , and Cardiovascular Health: An American Heart Association Science Advisory for Professionals From the Nutrition Committee. *Circulation* 2006; 113: 1034-1044.

[45] Wijendran V, Hayes K. Dietary n-6 and n-3 fatty acid balance and cardiovascular health. *Ann. Rev. Nutr.* 2004; 24:597-615.

[46] Hoffman D R. Fatty acids and visual dysfunction. Food Science and Technology (New York) (2000), 96(*Fatty Acids in Foods and Their Health Implications* (2nd Edition)), 817-841.

[47] Simopoulos AP. Essential fatty acids in health and chronic disease. *Am. J. Clin. Nutr.* 1999; 70: 560S-569S.

[48] Cunnane S C, Zhen-Yu C, Yang J, *et al.* α-Linoleic acid in humans: direct functional role or dietary precursor? *Nutrition* 1991; 7: 437-439.

[49] Uauy R, Valenzuela A. Marine oils: Benefits of n-3 fatty acids. *Nutrition* 2000; 16: 680-684.

[50] Demaison L, Moreau D. Dietary n-3 polyunsaturated fatty acids and coronary heart disease-related mortality: a possible mechanism of action. *Cell. Mol. Life Sci.* 2002; 59:463-477.

[51] Bruckner G. Fatty acids and cardiovascular diseases. Food Science and Technology (2000), 96 (*Fatty Acids in Foods and Their Health Implications* (2nd Edition)), 843-863.

[52] Djoussé L, Folsom A, Province M, Hunt S, Ellison R. Dietary linolenic acid and carotid atherosclerosis: the National Heart, Lung and Blood Institute Family Heart Study. *Am. J.Clin. Nutr.* 2003; 77:819-825.

[53] Baylin A, Kabagambe E, Ascherio A, Spiegelman D, Campos H. Adipose tissue α-linolenic acid and non-fatal acute myocardial infarction in Costa Rica. *Circulation* 2003; 107:1586-1591.

[54] Allman MA, Pena NM, Pang D. Supplementation with flaxseed oil versus sunflower oil in healthy young men consuming a low fat diet: effects on platelet composition and function. *Eur. J. Clin. Nutr.* 1995; 49: 169-178.

[55] Brouwer I, Katan M, Zock L. Dietary α-linolenic acid is associated with a reduced risk of fatal coronary heart disease, but increased prostate cancer risk: a meta-analysis. *J. Nutr.* 2004; 134:919-922.

[56] Nestel P, Pomeroy SE, Sasahara T, *et al.* Arterial compliance in obese subjects is improved with dietary plant n-3 fatty acid from flaxseed oil despite increased LDL oxidizability. *Arterioscl. Thromb Vasc. Biol.* 1997; 17: 1163-1170.

[57] Cunnane S C, Ganguli S, Menard C, *et al.* High α linoleic acid flaxseed (*Linum usitatissimum*) : some nutritional properties in humans. *Br J Nutr* 1993; 69: 443-453.

[58] Erasmus U. *Fats that heal fats that kill: the complete guide to fats, oils and cholesterol.* 2nd edition. Burnaby BC, Canada: Alive Books, 1993.

[59] Cunnane S C. α-Linoleic acid in human nutrition and disease. *Nutrition* 1991; 7: 436.

[60] Dallongeville J, Yarnell J, Ducimetière P, *et al.* Fish consumption is associated with lower heart rates. *Circulation* 2003; 108:820-825.

[61] Nestel P, Shige H, Pomeroy S, Cehun M, Raederstorff D. The n-3 fatty acids eicosapentaenoic acid and docosahexaenoic acid increase systemic arterial compliance in humans. *Am. J. Clin. Nutr.* 2002; 76:326-330.

[62] Mori T, Bao D, Burke V, Puddey I, Beilin L. Docosahexaenoic acid but not eicosapentaenoic acid lowers ambulatory blood pressure and heart rate in humans. *Hypertension* 1999; 34:253-260.

[63] Lemaitre R, King I, Mozaffarian D, Kuller L, Tracy R, Siscovick D. n-3 polyunsaturated fatty acids, fatal ischemic heart disease and non-fatal myocardial infarction in older adults: the Cardiovascular Health Study. *Am. J. Clin. Nutr.* 2003; 77:319-325.

[64] Bucher H, Hengstler P, Schindler C and Meier G. N-3 polyunsaturated fatty acids in coronary heart disease: A meta-analysis of randomised controlled trials. *Am. J. Med.* 2002; 112:298-304.

[65] Chung M. Vitamins, Supplements, Herbal medicines, and Arrhythmias. *Cardiol. Rev.* 2004; 12:73-84.

[66] Rivellese A, Maffettone A, Vessby B, *et al.* Effects of dietary saturated, monounsaturated and n-3 fatty acids on fasting lipoproteins, LDL size and post-prandial lipid metabolism in healthy subjects. *Atherosclerosis* 2003; 167:149-158.

[67] Harris WS. n-3 Fatty acids and serum lipoproteins: human studies. *Am J Clin Nutr* 1997; 65(suppl): 1645S-1654S.

[68] Layne K S, Goh Y K, Jumpsen J A, *et al.* Normal subjects consuming physiological levels of 18:3(n-3) and 20:5(n-3) from flaxseed or fish oils have characteristic

differences in plasma lipid and lipoprotein fatty acid levels. *J. Nutr.* 1996; 126: 2130-2140.

[69] Khan F, Elherik K, Bolton-Smith C, *et al.* The effects of dietary fatty acid supplementation on endothelial function and vascular tone in healthy subjects. *Cardiovasc. Res.* 2003; 59: 955-962.

[70] Westcott N D, Muir A D. Flax seed lignan in disease prevention and health promotion. *Phytochem. Rev* .2004; 2: 401-417.

[71] Jenkins D J A, Kendall C W C, Vidgen E, *et al.* Health aspects of partially defatted flaxseed, including effects on serum lipids, oxidative measures, and ex vivo androgen and progestin activity: a controlled crossover trial. *Am. J. Clin. Nutr.* 1999; 69: 395-402.

[72] Stavro P M, Marchie A L, Kendall C W C, *et al.* Flaxseed, fiber, and coronary heart disease: clinical studies. *Flaxseed in Human Nutrition* (2nd Edition) 2003. 288-300.

[73] Bloedon L T, Szapary P O. Flaxseed and cardiovascular risk. *Nutr Rev* 2004; 62: 18-27.

[74] Witte K, Clark A, Cleland J. Chronic Heart Failure and Micronutrients. *J. Am. Coll. Cardiol.* 2001; 37:1765-1774.

[75] Sole M, Jeejeebhoy K N. Conditioned nutritional requirements and the pathogenesis and treatment of myocardial failure. *Curr. Opin. Clin. Nutr. Metab. Care* 2000; 3: 417-424.

[76] Soja A M, Mortensen S A. Treatment of congestive heart failure with coenzyme Q10 illuminated by meta-analyses of clinical trials. *Mol. Asp. Med.* 1997; 18: S159-68.

[77] McCarty M. Coenzyme Q versus Hypertension: does CoQ decrease endothelial superoxide generation? *Med. Hypoth.* 1999; 53:300-304.

[78] Langsjoen P, Langsjoen P, Willis R, Folkers K. Treatment of essential hypertension with coenzyme Q10. *Mol. Asp. Med.* 1994; 15: S265-S272.

[79] Khatta M, Alexander B, Krichten C, Fisher M, Freudenberger R, Robinson S, Gottlieb S. The effect of coenzyme Q10 in patients with congestive heart failure. *Ann. Int. Med.* 2000; 132:636-640.

[80] Singh R, Wander G, Rastogi A, *et al.* Randomised, double-blind placebo-controlled trial of coenzyme Q10 in patients with acute myocardial infarction. *Cardiovasc. Drug Ther.* 1998; 12:347-353.

[81] Langsjoen P, Langsjoen A, Willis R, Folkers K. Treatment of hypertropic cardiomyopathy with coenzyme Q10. *Mol. Asp. Med.* 1997; 18: S145-S151.

[82] Rosenfeldt F, Pepe S, Linnane A, *et al.* Coenzyme Q10 protects the aging heart against stress, studies in rats human tissues and patients. *Ann. N Y Acad. Sci.* 2002; 959:355-359.

[83] Langsjoen P, Folkers K, Lyson K, *et al.* Effective and safe therapy with coenzyme Q10 for cardiomyopathy. *Klinische Wochenschrift* 1988; 66:583-590.

[84] Kishi T, Kishi H, Folkers K. Inhibition of cardiac CoQ10-enzymes by clinically used drugs and possible prevention. In: Folkers K, Yamamura Y eds. *Biomedical and Clinical aspects of Coenzyme Q.* Vol 1. Amsterdam: Elsevier/ North Holland Biomedical Press; 1977:47-62.

[85] Preedy V, Mantle, D. Adverse effect on coenzyme Q10 levels. *Pharm J* 2004; 272:13.

[86] Rao A, Agarwal S. Role of lycopene as antioxidant carotenoid in the prevention of chronic diseases: A Review. *Nutr. Res.* 1999; 19:305-323.

[87] Rao A, Agarwal S. Role of antioxidant lyopene in cancer and heart disease. *J. Am. Coll. Nutr* .2000; 19:563-569.

[88] Rao A, Waseem Z, Agarwal S. Lycopene content of tomatoes and tomato products and their contribution to dietary lycopene. *Food Res. Int.* 1998; 31:737-741.

[89] Kardinaal A F, Kok F J, Ringstad J, *et al.* Antioxidants in adipose tissue and risk of myocardial infarction: the EURAMIC Study. *Lancet* 1993; 342: 1379-84. An

[90] Anonymous The effect of vitamin E and beta carotene on the incidence of lung cancer and other cancers in male smokers. The Alpha-Tocopherol, Beta Carotene Cancer Prevention Study Group. *N. Engl. J. Med.* 1994; 330: 1029-35.

[91] Kohlmeier L, Kark J D, Gomez-Gracia E, *et al.* Lycopene and myocardial infarction risk in the EURAMIC Study. *Am. J. Epidemiol.* 1997; 146: 618-26.

[92] Kristenson M, Zieden B, Kucinskiene Z, *et al.* Antioxidant state and mortality from coronary heart disease in Lithuanian and Swedish men : concomitant cross sectional study of men aged 50. *BMJ* 1997; 314: 629-33.

[93] Hirvonen T, Virtamo J, Korhonen P, Albanes D, Pietinen P. Intake of flavonoids , carotenoids, vitamins C and E, and risk of stroke in male smokers. *Stroke* 2000; 31: 2301-6.

[94] Rao A. Lycopene, tomatoes and the prevention of coronary heart disease. *Exp. Biol. Med.* 2002; 227:908-913.

[95] Rissanen T, Voutilainen S, Nyyssönen K and Salonen J. Lycopene, atherosclerosis and coronary heart disease. *Exp. Biol. Med.* 2002; 227:900-907.

[96] Engelhard Y N, Gazer B, Paran E. Natural antioxidants from tomato extract reduce blood pressure in patients with grade - 1 hypertension : a double-blind, placebo-controlled pilot study. *Am. Heart J.* 2006; 151: 100.e1-100.e6.

[97] Das S, Otani H, Maulik N, Das D K. Lycopene , tomatoes , and coronary heart disease. *Free Rad. Res.* 2005; 39: 449-455.

[98] Más R, Castaño G, Fernandez L, *et al.* Effects of policosanol in patients with type II hypercholesterolemia and additional coronary risk factors. *Clin. Pharmacol. Ther.* 1999; 65:439-447.

[99] Gouni-Berthold I and Berthold H. Policosanol: Clinical pharmacology and therapeutic significance of a new lipid lowering agent. *Am. Heart J.* 2002; 143:356-365.

[100] Hargrove J, Greenspan P, Hartle D. Nutritional significance and metabolism of very long chain fatty alcohols and acids from dietary waxes. *Exp. Biol. Med.* 2004; 229:215-226.

[101] Rapport L, Lockwood B 2001 *Nutraceuticals.* Pharmaceutical Press, London. 164pp.

[102] Torres O, Agramonte A, Illnait J, Mas Ferreiro F, Fernandez L, Fernandez J. Treatment of hypercholesterolemia in NIDDM with policosanol. *Diabetes Care* 1995; 18:393-397.

[103] Lin Y, Rudrum M, van der Wielen R P J, Trautwein E A, *et al.* Wheat germ policosanol failed to lower plasma cholesterol in subjects with normal to mildly elevated cholesterol concentrations. *Metab. Clin. Exp.* 2004; 53: 1309-1314.

[104] Crespo N, Illnait J, Mas R, *et al.* Comparative study of the efficacy and tolerability of policosanol and lovastatin in patients with hypercholesterolemia and noninsulin dependent diabetes mellitus. *Int. J. Clin. Pharmacol. Res.* 1999; 19: 117-127.

[105] Noa M, Herrera M, Magraner J, Mas R. Effect of Policosanol on Isoprenaline-induced Myocardial Necrosis in Rats. *J. Pharm. Pharmacol.* 1994; 46:282-285.

[106] Anon. A close look at coenzyme Q10 and policosanol. *Harvard Health Lett.* 2002; 13: 1-3.

[107] Packer L, Rimbach G, Virgili F. Antioxidant activity and biologic properties of a procyanidin-rich extract from pine (*Pinus maritima*) bark, pycnogenol. *Free Rad. Biol. Med* 1999; 27:704-724.

[108] Devaraj S, Vega-López S, Kaul N, *et al.* Supplementation with a pine bark extract rich in polyphenols increases plasma antioxidant capacity and alters the plasma lipoprotein profile. *Lipids* 2002; 37:931-934.

[109] Liu X, Wei J, Tan F, *et al.* Pycogenol, French maritime pine bark extract, improves endothelial function of hypertensive patients. *Life Sci.* 2004; 74:855-862.

[110] Koch R. Comparative study of venostasin and pycnogenol in chronic venous insufficiency. *Phytother. Res.* 2002; 16:S1-S5.

[111] Belcaro G; Cesarone M R, Rohdewald P, *et al.* Prevention of venous thrombosis and thrombophlebitis in long-haul flights with pycnogenol. *Clin. Appl. Thrombosis/hemostasis* 2004; 10: 373-7.

[112] Cesarone M R, Belcaro G, Rohdewald P, *et al.* Prevention of edema in long flights with pycnogenol. *Clin. Appl. Thrombosis/Hemostasis* 2005; 11: 289-294.

[113] Belcaro G, Cesarone M R, Errichi B M, *et al.* Venous ulcers : microcirculatory improvement and faster healing with local use of Pycnogenol. *Angiol.* 2005; 56: 699-705.

[114] Reiter R J, Tan D-X. Melatonin: a novel protective agent against oxidative injury of the ischemic/reperfused heart. *Cardiovasc. Res.* 2003; 58: 10-19.

[115] Chen Z, Chua C C, Gao J, Hamdy R C, Chua B H L. Protective effect of melatonin on myocardial infarction. *Am. J. Physiol.* 2003; 284: H1618-H1624.

[116] Ray C A. Melatonin attenuates the sympathetic nerve responses to orthostatic stress in humans. *J. Physiol.* 2003; 551: 1043-1048.

[117] Bhat K P L, Kosmeder J W II, Pezzuto J M. Biological effects of resveratrol. *Antiox. Redox. Signal* 2001; 3: 1041-1064.

[118] Laden B P, Porter T D. Resveratrol inhibits human squalene monooxygenase. *Nutr. Res.* 2001; 21: 747-753.

[119] Das DK, Sato M, Ray PS, *et al.* Cardioprotection of red wine: role of polyphenolic antioxidants. *Drugs Exp. Clin. Res.* 1999; 25: 115-120.

[120] Frankel EN, Kanner J, German JB, Parks E, Kinsella JE. Inhibition of oxidation of human low-density lipoprotein by phenolic substances in red wine. *Lancet* 1993; 341: 454-457.

[121] Serafini M, Maiani G, Ferro-Luzzi A. Alcohol-free red wine enhances plasma antioxidant capacity in humans. *J. Nutr.* 1998; 128: 1003-1007.

[122] Anon. Not all red wines are equal, new research suggests. *Pharm. J.*1999; 262: 213.

[123] Shrikhande AJ. Wine by-products with health benefits. *Food Res. Int.* 2000; 33: 469-474.

[124] Yamakoshi J, Kataoka S, Koga T, Ariga T. Proanthocyanidin-rich extract from grape seeds attenuates the development of aortic atherosclerosis in cholesterol-fed rabbits. *Atherosclerosis* 1999; 142: 139-149.

[125] Fine AM. Oligomeric proanthocyanidin complexes: history, structure, and phytopharmaceutical applications. *Alt. Med. Rev.* 2000; 5: 144-151.

[126] Lurton L. Grape polyphenols: The assets of diversity. *Nutracos* September 2003; 39-43.

[127] Bagchi D, Sen C K, Ray, *et al.* Molecular mechanisms of cardioprotection by a novel grape seed proanthocyanidin extract. *Mutat. Res.* 2003; 523-524: 87-97.

[128] Halliwell B. The antioxidant paradox. *Lancet* 2000; 355:1179-1180.

[129] McClean R, McCrum E, Scally G, *et al.* Dietary patterns in the Belfast MONICA Project. *Proc. Nutr. Soc.* 1990; 49: 297-305.

[130] Alves-Rodrigues A, Shao A. The science behind lutein. *Toxicol Lett* 2004: 150: 57-83.

[131] Dwyer J H, Navab M, Dwyer K M, *et al.* Oxygenated carotenoid lutein and progression of early atherosclerosis: the Los Angeles atherosclerosis study. *Circulation* 2001: 103: 2922-7.

[132] Sole M J, Jeejeebhoy K N. Conditioned nutritional requirements and the pathogenesis and treatment of myocardial failure. *Curr.Opin. Clin. Nutr. Metabol. Care.* 2000; 3: 417-424.

[133] Singh R B, Niaz M A, Agaewal P, *et al.* A randomised, double-blind, placebo-controlled trial of L-carnitine in suspected acute myocardial infarction. *Postgrad. Med. J.* 1996; 72: 45-50.

[134] Cacciatore L, Cerio R, Ciarimboli M, *et al.* The therapeutic effect of L-carnitine in patients with exercise-induced stable angina: a controlled study. *Drugs Exp. Clin. Res.* 1991; 17: 225-335.

[135] Davini P, Bigalli A, Lamanna F, Boem A. Controlled study on L-carnitine therapeutic efficacy in post-infarction. *Drugs Exp. Clin. Res.* 1992; 18: 355-365.

[136] Ergur A T, Tanzer F, Cetinkaya O. Serum- free carnitine levels in children with heart failure. *J. Tropical. Ped.* 1999; 45: 168-169.

[137] Iliceto S, Scrutinio D, Bruzzi P, *et al.* Effects of L- carnitine administration on left ventricular remodeling after acute anterior myocardial infarction: the L- Carnitine Ecocardiografia Digitalizzata Infarto Miocardico (CEDIM) Trial. *J. Am. Coll. Cardiol.* 1995; 26: 380-7.

[138] Buvat J. Androgen therapy with dehydroepiandrosterone. *World J. Urol.* 2003; 21: 346-355.

[139] Moriyama Y, Yasue H, Yoshimura M, *et al.* The plasma levels of dehydroepiandrosterone sulfate are decreased in patients with chronic heart failure in proportion to the severity. *J. Clin. Endocrinol. Metab.* 2000; 85: 1834-40.

[140] Yeung J, Yu T-f. Effects of isoflavones (soy phyto-estrogens) on serum lipids: a meta -analysis of randomized controlled trials. *Nutr. J.* (2003), 2: 15.

[141] Gardner C D, Newell K A, Cherin R, Haskell W L. The effect of soy protein with or without isoflavones relative to milk protein on plasma lipids in hypercholesterolemic postmenopausal women. *Am. J. Clin. Nutr.* 2001; 73: 728-735.

[142] Morris M C, Sacks F, Rosner B. Does fish oil lower blood pressure ? A meta-analysis of controlled trials. *Circulation* 1993; 88: 523-33.

[143] Appel L J, Miller E R 3rd, Seidler A J, Whelton P K. Does supplementation of diet with ' fish oil ' reduce blood pressure? A meta-analysis of controlled clinical trials. *Arch. Int. Med.* 1993; 153: 1429-38.

[144] Harper C R, Jacobson T A. Usefulness of Omega - 3 Fatty Acids and the Prevention of Coronary Heart Disease. *Am. J. Cardiol.* 2005; 96: 1521-1529

[145] Soja A M, Mortensen S A. Treatment of chronic cardiac insufficiency with coenzyme Q10 , results of meta - analysis in controlled clinical trials. *Ugeskrift Laeger* 1997; 159: 7302-8.

[146] Chen J T, Wesley R, Shamburek R D, Pucino F, Csako G. Meta-analysis of natural therapies for hyperlipidemia: plant sterols and stanols versus policosanol. *Pharmacother* 2005; 25: 171-183.

In: Nutrition Research at the Leading Edge
Editors: R. E. Cassady, E. I. Tidswell, pp. 133-155
ISBN: 978-1-60456-053-4
© 2008 Nova Science Publishers, Inc.

Chapter IV

Passive Smoking as a Conditioner of Food Habits and Nutritional Status: Repercussions on Health

Rosa M. Ortega, Ana M. López-Sobaler, Aranzazu Aparicio,
Laura M. Bermejo, Elena Rodríguez-Rodríguez and M. Carmen Mena

Departamento de Nutrición. Facultad de Farmacia.
Universidad Complutense. Ciudad Universitaria s/n. 28040- Madrid, Spain

Abstract

Many studies have associated passive smoking with an increased risk of developing certain diseases. Smoking during pregnancy increases the risk of the newborn having a low birth weight (at term or pre-term), and of suffering impaired respiratory function and ischaemic heart disease etc. In children and adolescents, environmental exposure to tobacco smoke has been associated with abnormal lipid profiles and an increased risk of atherosclerosis. Passive smoking can also be the cause of reduced female fertility in the general population. The food habits of both active and passive smokers may also be negatively affected.

The diets of smokers tend to be less adequate than those of non-smokers. Exposure to tobacco smoke modifies the sense of taste and smell, leading to changes in food preferences and food intake, and eventually to a more imbalanced diet. Matters are made worse in that smokers may have greater needs of certain nutrients such as antioxidants. Thus, even with a normal intake of these nutrients, the nutritional status of smokers can be inadequate.

As with active smokers, passive smokers may show slightly unhealthy food habits and more imbalanced diets than non-smokers – either as a consequence of living with smokers (and therefore sharing their food habits) or via the direct modification of their food choices. Passive smokers consume fewer fruits and vegetables and have lower intakes of a number of nutrients, which might be reflected at the serum level. For example, exposure to tobacco smoke is associated with reduced folate levels, via which some of the effects of active and passive smoking on health may be made manifest. Like active smokers, passive smokers may have a greater need of certain nutrients. For example, they show lower plasma concentrations of antioxidants than do non-smokers not exposed to smoke, independent of the differences in dietary antioxidant intake.

The diet of passive smokers may be an important factor in the relationship between tobacco smoke exposure and health problems. Although the cessation of smoking and the avoidance of passive smoking is the ideal goal, it cannot always be attained. Dietary intervention may therefore be a useful and indeed necessary strategy to prevent or delay smoking-related pathologies.

Introduction

Tobacco smoke is composed of mainstream smoke, which is directly inhaled by the smoker, and sidestream smoke, generated by the spontaneous combustion of the cigarette. Environmental tobacco smoke (ETS) consists of sidestream smoke and the smoke exhaled by the smoker, also known as second-hand smoke. "Passive smoking" is the involuntary inhalation by a non-smoker of smoke generated in his neighbourhood by one or more smokers (Romero-Palacios, 2004).

Tobacco smoke contains over 4000 chemicals in the form of particles and gases. The particulate phase includes tar (itself composed of many compounds), nicotine, benzene and benzo(a)pyrene. The gas phase includes carbon monoxide, ammonia, dimethylnitrosamine, formaldehyde, hydrogen cyanide and acrolein (Bermúdez et al., 1994; Eiserich et al., 1995). Some of these have markedly irritant properties and some 60 are known or suspected carcinogens (Romero-Palacios, 2004). Thus, tobacco smoke is an important source of oxidative stress, whether exposure is active of passive (Cross et al., 1999).

Currently, exposure to ETS, or passive smoking, affects between 20% and 80% of the population depending on the country, and is associated with long- and short-term health risks, especially ischaemic heart disease and lung cancer (Romero-Palacios, 2004). Smoking and exposure to ETS are the main causes of preventable morbidity and premature disease and death in developed countries (US Department of Health Education and Welfare, 1971).

Exposure to ETS may occur in the home, at the workplace, or in public places. The degree of exposure depends on several factors, e.g., the number of smokers in the vicinity, how much they smoke, the duration of exposure, and the characteristics of the exposure location (Romero-Palacios, 2004).

The exposure of children to ETS is a worldwide problem. In 1996, a national survey carried out in China found that 53.6% of non-smoker children and adults were exposed to ETS, with exposure defined as being in the presence of tobacco smoke for at least 15 minutes per day for more than 1 day per week (Yang et al., 1999). In 1998, nearly half of all US children under 5 years of age were reported to be exposed to ETS (Samet and Yang, 2001). In the UK, 42% of English children and 60% of Scottish children were reported exposed to ETS by parental smoking (Samet and Yang, 2001). According to a number of studies from Spain, between 48% and 69% of children and teenagers are exposed to smoke in their homes (Fuertes et al., 2001). A recent study in Granada on a sample of 504 children between the ages of 3 and 6 found that 57.6% lived in houses polluted with tobacco smoke by their parents and other relatives (Muñoz et al., 2003) Such data, however, is not available in most countries. According to the World Health Organization, some 1000 million adult smokers, and at least 700 million children, breath household ETS (WHO, 1999).

The determination of cotinine in serum, urine, and saliva is commonly used as a measure of exposure (active or passive) to tobacco smoke (Pirkle et al., 1996). Cotinine is the major metabolite of nicotine and has a half-life of about 16 - 20 hours (Jarvis et al., 1988; Benowitz et al., 1983). The serum cotinine level reflects exposure to nicotine largely from the previous 1 - 2 days. Both the children of smokers (Pirkle et al., 1996) and other adults who live with smokers (Kim et al., 2004) have higher concentrations of cotinine in their blood and saliva.

Relationship between Passive Smoking and Health Problems

For many years it was thought that passive smoking was ofohittle or no importance, causing only mild irritation of the conjunctiva and upper respiratory tract. However, the sanitary and social importance of passive smoking is becoming ever more evident, and its many repercussions affect all population groups.

The evidence regarding the health risks of passive smoking comes from epidemiological studies that have assessed the association between exposure to ETS and its negative effects on health, and from our growing knowledge regarding the components of ETS and their toxicities.

Health Problems in Expectant Mothers and their in Utero-Exposed Children

Some of the studies published over the last 15 years show that smoking, both active and passive, is related to reduced female fertility (Nizard, 2005). Others suggest that exposure during pregnancy can have negative effects on the child such as delayed intauterine development, low birth weight, and an increased risk of sudden death (Kalinka et al., 2005; Ortega et al., 2004; Tong et al., 2005). The children of mothers who are passively exposed to ETS during pregnancy are more likely to suffer asthma and are at greater risk of negative developmental outcomes (Barber et al., 1996). Such exposure also seems to be related to the cognitive capacity of child, who might experience difficulties in the comprehension of written texts and show learning difficulties (Rauh et al., 2004; Ortega et al., 2004; Yolton et al., 2005).

Health Problems in Child Passive Smokers

Passive smoking in children has been the subject of many studies. Exposure occurs basically at home and in play environments. As children grow up, exposure to maternal smoking decreases and the influence of smoke from other sources, such as ETS in public places, increases. Such exposure, particularly maternal smoking, undoubtedly influences the development of asthma in children (Heraud and Herbelin-Wagne, 2002; Gilliland et al., 2002).

ETS clearly has an effect on the respiratory system. In newborns and young infants, this may lead to an increased risk of suffering infections, including pneumonia and bronchitis (which can more be more severe than normal). Chronic respiratory problems such as childhood asthma may develop, and lung development may be slowed down (Mannino et al., 2001; Klerman., 2004).

Exposure to ETS has also been related to acute otitis in the first four years of life (the most common cause of deafness in children) (Klerman., 2004), and bacterial meningitis, the prevalence of which is greater among children exposed for longer periods (Iles et al., 2001).

Some authors report exposure to ETS to be associated with a greater risk of sudden death in babies (Tong et al., 2005), and with a greater probability of complications developing during surgery requiring general anaesthesia (Drongowski et al., 2003).

The results of other studies indicate ETS to have neurotoxic activity. Thus, constant exposure to ETS could have a negative influence on certain cognitive abilities in children and adolescents, e.g., greater difficulty in learning to read, greater difficulty in correctly solving mathematical problems, and perhaps even defects in the development of spatial vision (Yolton et al., 2005).

In adolescents, exposure is associated with an increased prevalence of headaches and eye irritation (Borzecki et al., 2005), and with the appearance of metabolic syndrome, perhaps including increased resistance to insulin (Weitzman et al., 2005).

Currently there is no clear scientific evidence of a direct relationship between exposure to ETS and an increased risk of childhood cancer (World Health Organization International Agency for Research on Cancer, 2002).

Health Problems in Adult Passive Smokers

Exposure to ETS has been causally related to lung cancer; this has been reported in many large epidemiological studies and by numerous groups of experts (National Research Council, 1986; US Environmental Protection Agency, 1992; Scientific Committee on Tobacco and Health, 1998; World Health Organisation, International Agency for Research on Cancer, 2002). Some studies also suggest that constant, prolonged exposure to ETS leads to other types of cancer such as leukaemia (Kasim et al., 2005).

Numerous observational and experimental studies have also causally related ETS exposure to coronary heart disease (California Environmental Protection Agency, 1997; Scientific Committee on Tobacco and Health, 1998; Samet., 2002); some studies also indicate that the risk of myocardial infarction is increased (Qureshi et al., 2005). Passive smokers (both children and adults) show increased total cholesterol, LDL-C and VLDL-C levels. Their total/HDL-C ratio is also increased and their HDL-C levels are lower (Holay et al., 2004; Azizi et al., 2002; Zhang, 1992; Neufeld et al., 1997; Whig et al., 1992; Feldman et al., 1991) – all of which increases the risk of developing atherosclerosis (Ambrose and Barua, 2004; Feldman et al., 1991).

Evidence also exists linking ETS to the worsening of asthma, reduced lung function, and other respiratory problems. However, these associations have not yet been declared causal (California Environmental Protection Agency, 1997; Scientific Committee on Tobacco and Health, 1998). Other studies show that people exposed to ETS are also at greater risk of periodontal problems (Arbes et al., 2001), and that they more commonly suffer allergies such as allergic rhinitis. This suggests ETS to be linked to a weakening of the immune system (Topp et al., 2005).

Recent studies associate ETS exposure to a reduction in bone mineral density, which may have a negative effect on development and the appearance of osteoporosis. Serum cotinine levels have been shown to be inversely correlated with bone mineral content in both males and females (Benson and Shulman, 2005).

Health Problems in Elderly Passive Smokers

In elderly people, exposure to tobacco smoke may have the same negative effects as in adults, but also appears to be directly related to the appearance and development of macular degeneration and even blindness (Khan et al., 2006). It has also been related to an increased incidence of cataracts (Ortega et al., 1994a).

Some studies have related prolonged and constant exposure to ETS to hearing losses, both in adults and the elderly (Nomura et al., 2005), although long-term longitudinal studies are need to confirm this.

It should be borne in mind that elderly people tend to remain indoors more often than younger people. If these places were smoke-polluted they would be in contact with ETS for longer, which might have a negative effect on their health (Simoni et al., 2003)

In summary, the disease load caused by smoking is huge, and its impact on public health around the world enormous – reason enough for programmes aimed at controlling smoking to be given high priority.

Changes in the Food Habits and Nutritional Status of Passive Smokers That May Increase Risks to Health

Reasons for Changes in Food Habits in Passive Smokers

Smokers' diets tend to be less adequate than those of non-smokers (Ortega et al., 1994b; Ortega, 2003; Ortega et al., 2004). Chronic cigarette smokers consume a smaller amount of phytonutrient-rich foods; this has been reported for smokers in the UK (Pollard et al., 2001), Canada (Palaniappan et al., 2001), the United States (Subar et al., 1990), and the Netherlands (Zondervan et al., 1996). The available evidence also indicates that the heaviest smokers invariably consume fewer fruits and vegetables than those who smoke fewer cigarettes per day (Ma et al., 2000; Birkett, 1999; Ortega et al., 1994b; Ortega et al., 2004). While the evidence is more limited, some epidemiological data suggest that male smokers are more likely than female smokers to consume fewer fruits and vegetables (Ma et al., 2000). Cigarette smokers appear to make up for the energy deficit created by consuming more dietary fats, especially saturated fats (Palaniappan et al., 2001; Ma et al., 2000; Birkett, 1999).

Non-smokers who live with smokers also have poorer dietary habits than those who live in non-smoking households. This relationship may be due to shared family lifestyle patterns. Some studies show that women married to smokers are significantly less likely to eat cooked or fresh vegetables more than once a day than women not exposed to ETS (Forastiere et al., 2000). In the study by Emmons et al., (1995), which involved 10,833 non-smokers, those exposed to ETS at home had significantly lower intakes of all the micronutrients studied compared to those free of household exposure. Exposure to ETS at the workplace was associated with lower intakes of vitamin C (but not the other micronutrients examined), fruits and vegetables. These authors indicate that home exposure to ETS was a stronger predictor of intake than workplace exposure (Table 1).

It should be remembered that parents have a decisive influence on the food habits and physical activity patterns of their children (Nicklas et al., 2004). Early childhood and the social environment in which the child takes his/her meals are widely assumed to be critical in the establishment of lifelong healthy eating habits. In their family life, the children of smokers are exposed to more imbalanced diets (Table 1).

Exposure to tobacco smoke modifies the sense of taste and smell, leading to changes in food preferences and food intake; the diets of passive smokers could therefore be more imbalanced. Active smokers certainly have a reduced sense of taste and smell (Reibel, 2003). Some studies indicate that smokers have a reduced capacity to recognise sweet, salty and sour tastes, and that the sensitivity of their tongue receptors to electric stimuli is slightly lower than that of non-smokers (Suliburska et al., 2004; Sato et al., 2002). The same can occur in passive smokers, and has been recorded in children. The children of smokers were found to be less able to identify certain smells than those who lived in generally smoke-free environments (Nageris et al., 2001).

It may also be the case that the lifestyles of passive smokers are more inadequate, perhaps because of the influence of the smokers with whom they live. In the U.K a study of 5036 non-smokers showed that those living with smokers ate more fried food, chips and butter, and less fruit and margarine than those living with other non-smokers (Thompson and Warburton, 1992). Koo et al., (1997), investigated the characteristics of non-smoking women from different countries (530 from Hong Kong, 13,047 from Japan, 87 from Sweden, and 144 from the U.S) who were married to either smokers or non-smokers. Independent of the country of residence, wives with smoking husbands generally ate less healthy diets, with a tendency to eat more fried food and less fruit than wives of non-smoking husbands. In addition, the women married to smokers scored worse in terms of behaviour regarded as healthy, e.g., avoiding obesity, controlling dietary cholesterol and alcohol, or taking vitamins and participating in preventive screening. These patterns suggest that wives who have never smoked but who have smoker husbands tend to share their less healthy dietary traits, and therefore to have dietary habits associated with an increased risk for lung cancer and heart disease.

Non-smoker women married to smokers also tend to be less well educated, to take fewer supplements, to drink alcohol more frequently, and to have lower vitamin A, C and calcium intakes, which may increase the risk of developing cancer (Matanoski et al., 1995). Passive smokers also have a lower consumption of vegetables and a lower folic acid intake than non-smoking women not exposed to EST (Ortega et al., 2004) (Tables 1 and 2).

Reasons for the Poorer Nutritional Status of Passive Smokers Even when their Intakes are Similar to those of Non-Smokers

Passive smokers may have higher requirements for some nutrients, such as antioxidants; thus, even with the same intake as non-smokers, they may have a poorer nutritional status.

Tobacco smoke contains a great variety of reactive oxygen species, reactive nitrogen species, free radicals, and many toxic compounds that together act as an important source of oxidative stress. Therefore, the antioxidant defences of both active and passive smokers can be placed under strain (Aycicek et al., 2005; Jacob, 2000). As seen in active smokers, passive smokers have lower levels of certain micronutrients, especially antioxidants. Exposure to even small quantities of tobacco smoke can affect the concentrations of antioxidant nutrients (Alberg, 2000), and thus lead to adverse effects. It should be remembered that the association between exposure and lower blood levels of nutrients might be underestimated if passive smokers classify themselves as non-smokers (Alberg, 2002) – something often seen.

Second hand smoke contains numerous oxidants and pro-oxidants that can produce free radicals and perhaps initiate lipid peroxidation (Church and Pryor, 1985). Free radicals are sequestered by antioxidants in the serum, thus providing greater protection against oxidation reactions. However, if this protection fails, peroxidation of LDL cholesterol may occur. This, plus the accumulation of cholesterol in macrophages, signals the start of atherosclerosis (Brown and Goldstein, 1983), and may be one of the reasons why cardiovascular diseases are more common among active smokers (Schectman et al., 1991). The circulating concentration of antioxidants in passive smokers is also lower than in non-smokers not exposed to EST (Valkonen and Kuusi, 1998).

Ascorbic acid levels can become reduced by two thirds within 90 minutes of being exposed to EST – something not seen with other antioxidants such as vitamin E, retinol, beta-carotene and uric acid (Valkonen and Kuusi, 1998). Acute exposure in non-smokers may therefore lead to deteriorated antioxidant defences in the serum, accelerate lipid peroxidation, and the accumulation of LDL cholesterol in the macrophages. It has even been suggested that the oxidative stress induced by second hand smoke may be worse in non-smokers than in active smokers, who are more accustomed to dealing with tobacco smoke (Glantz and Parmley, 1995)

Nutrient Intake and Nutritional Status: Changes in Passive Smokers

Differences in Energy Intake

Exposure to tobacco smoke leads to a reduction in appetite, which in turn leads to a reduction in the intake of food, and therefore of energy (Curtin et al., 1999) (Table 2). This loss of appetite has been associated with a reduction in neuropeptide Y in the hypothalamus in animals (Chen et al., 2005; Chen et al., 2006). In addition, nicotine can increase energy expenditure by 10 fold, leading to a reduction in body fat and body weight in active and passive smokers (Powledge, 2004; Pfeffer and Kaufer-Horwitz, 2001). One of the most representative examples of this is the often low birth weight of children borne to mothers who smoke (Ortega et al., 1998a; Steyn et al., 2006) - although it is also true that expectant mothers who smoke have a lower energy intake compared to their non-smoking counterparts (Ortega et al., 1998a).

Differences in the Intake of Macronutrients

Numerous studies have shown that the food habits of smokers are very different – and generally less healthy – than those of non-smokers (Dyer et al., 2003). Smokers consume fewer fruits, vegetables and wholemeal cereals than non-smokers (Ortega, 2003; Osler, 1998; Palaniappan et al., 2001), and thus their intake of carbohydrates, fibre, antioxidant vitamins and polyunsaturated fats is also lower (Reynolds et al., 2004; Schroder et al., 2002; Palaniappan et al., 2001; Dallongeville et al., 1998). In addition, they consume more meat, alcoholic drinks and coffee than non-smokers (Osler, 1998), which favours a higher intake of saturated fat and cholesterol (Palaniappan et al., 2001; Dallongeville et al., 1998) (Table 2). These habits are also taken up by those who live with smokers (Osler, 1998), and even though they are non-smokers their diets are also less healthy than those of other non-smokers (see Reynolds et al., 2004; Curtin et al., 1999; Crawley and While, 1996). It has been shown that people exposed to tobacco smoke have food habits similar to those of smokers, with a lower intake of water, fruits and vegetables (Alberg et al., 2000; Koo et al., 1997; Matanoski et al., 1995). This translates into a lower intake in fibre and vitamins than that seen in non-smokers (Hampl et al., 2001). They also have a higher consumption of alcohol and fried foods (Koo et al., 1997; Matanoski et al., 1995), and therefore greater intakes of ethanol and saturated fats and cholesterol than do non-smokers (Table 2).

Differences in Vitamin Intake and Vitamin Status

As mentioned above, passive smokers have less healthy food habits and tend to consume smaller quantities of fruits and vegetables. Therefore, their intake of vitamins and minerals also tends to be inferior. This, along with the direct effect of tobacco on antioxidant levels could lead to a lower concentrations of these vitamins in the blood (Alberg et al., 2000; Lewis et al., 2005) (Table 3).

Plasma concentrations of antioxidant vitamins are significantly lower in passive smoker infants and their mothers than in non-passive smoker infants and their mothers. In addition, lipid peroxidation and the oxidative stress index is remarkably higher in passive smoker infants and their mothers than in their non-passive counterparts. Significant correlations also exist between the oxidative and antioxidative parameters of passive smoker infants and their mothers (Aycicek et al., 2005).

As mentioned above, the compounds present in tobacco smoke are an important source of oxidative stress, and therefore the antioxidant capacity of active and smokers can be strongly challenged. Several studies report that active and passive smokers have lower levels of vitamin C, tocopherol, and carotenes (Alberg et al., 2000; Lykkesfeldt et al., 2000; Valkonen and Kuusi, 1998). This could be due to their greater use in the protection of cells from free radicals induced by tobacco smoke (Marangon et al., 1998), to a reduced intake of vitamin-rich foods (Ma et al., 2000), or both (Dallongeville et al., 1998).

Vitamin C is an effective free radical scavenger and is among the strongest determinants of plasma total antioxidant defence capability (Lykkesfeldt et al., 2000). The intake of vitamin C is lower in passive smokers than in non-smokers (Trobs et al., 2002). In addition, several studies that have quantified exposure to EST in passive smokers in terms of urine cotinine levels have shown that individuals with high cotinine levels take in smaller quantities of vitamin C (Wei et al., 2001). As with folates, the greater the duration of exposure to EST, the less vitamin C is consumed (Farchi et al., 2001) (Table 2). Numerous studies have shown that smoking, or being exposed to tobacco smoke, reduces the plasma concentration of this vitamin (Ayaori et al., 2000), even when exposure is minimal (Preston et al., 2003). In one study involving active, passive and non-smokers it was found that passive smokers had a plasma concentration of ascorbic acid intermediate between those of the others two groups, even when the intake of the vitamin was similar in all three groups (Tribble et al., 1993). In another study, a reduction in ascorbic acid levels was seen after exposure to EST (Valkonen and Kuusi, 1998). Even a short exposure led to a significant reduction, and therefore to an impairment of the antioxidant defence system (Valkonen and Kuusi, 1998) (Table 3).

During their intrauterine development, the children of smokers are effectively passive smokers, and thus suffer similar problems of low vitamin C levels. In addition, even though maternal blood levels of vitamin C may be similar to those of non-smokers, the milk of mothers who smoke contains less vitamin C than that of non-smokers. Thus, the breast-fed newborns of smoker mothers continue to have lower vitamin C levels after birth (Ortega et al., 1998b).

The length of time spent exposed to EST has an important effect on plasma vitamin C levels. One study involving passive smokers showed that women who spent 2 hours per day or less in the presence of EST had a higher plasma ascorbic acid level than those who were exposed for 2-8 hours per day (Mena, 2003).

Vitamin E is also a powerful antioxidant, and is the main lipophilic antioxidant in cell membranes. Protection against lipid peroxidation is achieved by its acting directly on a wide range of oxygen radicals (Jialal and Gruñid, 1993). However, the data coming from studies performed on vitamin E levels in smokers have been the centre of controversy.

The intake of vitamin E would appear to be lower in passive smokers than in non-smokers (Bruno and Traber, 2005). In addition, the concentration of this vitamin in the maternal milk of smokers is lower than that of non-smokers, even though dietary intake of the vitamin during pregnancy and maternal serum levels are similar to those of non-smoker mothers. Thus, children born to mothers who smoke (already intrauterine passive smokers) receive less vitamin E via their mothers' milk than do those born to non-smokers (Ortega et al., 1998a).

In vitro investigations have consistently demonstrated that cigarette smoke depletes plasma vitamin E as well as other antioxidants (Handelman et al., 1996). However, the plasma alpha- and gamma-tocopherol concentrations of smokers either do not differ (Leonard et al., 2003) or are lower (Bolton-Smith et al., 1991) than those that, compared to non-smokers, smokers and passive smokers have higher plasma concentrations of gamma-tocopherol, but not alpha-tocopherol (Dietrich et al., 2003b). Marangon et al., (1998) observed a plasma alpha-tocopherol level increase of 5% in smokers in comparison with non-smokers. Sobczak et al., (2004), however, indicate a statistically significant reduction in plasma alpha-tocopherol level in passive and active smokers compared to non-smokers, whereas smoking had virtually no influence on the gamma-tocopherol level.

It should be remembered that one of the reasons why lower tocopherol levels are not always seen in smokers is that, even though this vitamin suffers the oxidising effects of tobacco smoke it can be regenerated to its active form via the action of other antioxidants. This helps to maintain total tocopherol levels in plasma (Halliwell, 1996a).

The intake of beta-carotene is also lower in passive smokers compared to non-smokers, and is inversely related to the magnitude of exposure to ETS (Curtin et al., 1999; Dallongeville et al., 1998). In addition, people exposed to a greater degree show significantly lower serum beta-carotene levels (Farchi et al., 2001) (Table 3). This may be a reflection of the lower fruit and vegetable consumption of passive smokers since beta-carotene is the best biomarker of their recent intake (Ziegler et al., 1996).

In passive smokers, the duration of exposure to tobacco smoke seems to have an important influence on nutritional status. Mena (2003) found that women exposed to ETS for eight or more hours per day were more likely to show deficient serum beta-carotene levels (80%) than those exposed for 2-8 hours (20%) or those exposed for two hours or less (36.4%).

The fact that passive smokers have lower serum retinol concentrations than non-smokers may be due to the greater use of this antioxidant vitamin in the neutralisation of the free radicals in tobacco smoke, although they could also be a reflection of the effect of tobacco smoke on diet (Chelchowska et al., 2001) (Tables 2 and 3).

Both active and passive smoking are associated with a lower intake of folates (which is often low in the general population anyway) (Ortega et al., 2004), and with lower levels of serum and erythrocyte folic acid (Mannino et al., 2003). In addition, folate intake decreases with the duration of exposure (Ortega et al., 2004).

Exposure to tobacco smoke remains associated with lower serum and erythrocyte folate levels even after adjustment for folic acid intake (Mannino et al., 2003; Voutilainen et al.,

2001) (Table 3). These reduced folate levels may be one of the ways via which some of the health effects of active and passive smoking are eventually made manifest.

Differences in Mineral Intake and Status

Serum iron concentration can be higher in people most exposed to tobacco smoke since the carbon monoxide it contains provokes tissue hypoxia, to which the body reacts by increasing the synthesis of haemoglobin. This, of course, requires iron (Smith and Fischer, 2001) (Table 3). However, higher serum iron levels can be harmful since this mineral can contribute to increased oxidative stress (Whitfield et al., 2001).

The newborns of mothers who smoke (and who were therefore intra-uterine passive smokers) have lower levels of zinc, although an adequate maternal dietary intake of this mineral can resolve this problem (King, 2000). However, it is quite normal for such mothers – and indeed non-smoker mothers – not to take in sufficient zinc (Ortega et al., 1998a).

Table 1. Differences in food intake in active, passive and non-smokers

Food	Non smokers	Active smokers	Passive smokers	Reference
Animal Fat (servings/week)	8.2	9.4	8.3	Osler, 1998
Coffee (servings/week)	4.1	6.2	4.5	Osler, 1998
Cereals (g/day)	169		131	Curtin et al., 1999
(servings/week)	22.2	21.7	21.7	Osler, 1998
Eggs (servings/week)	1.8	1.8	1.7	Osler, 1998
Fish (servings/week)	1	0.7	0.8	Osler, 1998
Fruits (g/day)	235.5±142.4	203.5±187.5	197.0±160.0	Ortega et al., 2004
(servings/day)	1.3	0.7	1.2	Dietrich et al., 2003b
(servings/day)	0.96±0.03	0.52±0.04	0.86±0.06	Strauss, 2001
(servings/week)	5.8	4.2	5.6	Osler, 1998
Meat (g)	40.9		31.3	Curtin et al., 1999
(servings/week)	4.7	5.4	5.1	Osler, 1998
Vegetables (g/day)	272.1±124.1	235.8±122.0	231.1±108.4	Ortega et al., 2004
(g/day)	230		186	Curtin et al., 1999
(servings/day)	2.5	2.2	2.5	Dietrich et al., 2003b
(servings/week)	6.1	3.7	5.8	Osler, 1998
Alcoholic drinks (g/day)	34.8±82.0	71.6±111.3	31.7±66.8	Ortega et al., 2004

The dietary intake of calcium by passive smokers is often lower than that of non-smokers. The effects on health can be serious since tobacco also reduces the absorption of this mineral (Morabia et al., 2000) (Table 2).

In conclusion, passive smokers have less adequate food habits rendering them more susceptible to the serious health problems that can be provoked by tobacco. Active and passive smoking both lead to lower circulating concentrations of micronutrients, and consequently to a poorer nutritional status and increased health risks. The diet of passive smokers may be an important factor in the relationship between tobacco smoke exposure and health problems. Although the cessation of smoking and the avoidance of passive smoking is the ideal goal, it cannot always be attained. Dietary intervention may therefore be a useful and indeed necessary strategy to prevent or delay smoking-related pathologies.

Proposed Dietary Modifications for Passive Smokers

Dietary intervention could be helpful in preventing or delaying smoking-related disease.

With the aim of reducing the oxidative effects of tobacco smoke, several national and international bodies have indicated that the requirements of vitamin C in smokers (and by extension passive smokers) are greater than those of non-smokers (see Ortega, 2003; Cross et al., 1999). Taking a daily supplement of vitNªin C for two months reduces the level of F2-isoprostanes (an indicator of lipid peroxidation) in passive smokers (Dietrich et al., 2003a).

The Institute of Medicine (2000) estimates that smokers require 35 mg/day of vitamin C more than non-smokers since the metabolic turnover of this vitamin is double in these people (70 mg/day compared to 35.7 mg/day in non-smokers). Thus, the recommended vitamin C intake for smokers has been raised from 60 to 100 mg/day. However, it is not clear whether this is the most appropriate intake. Ortega et al., (2003) have calculated the intake of vitamin C necessary to bring the percentage of serum deficiencies in smokers down to that of non-smokers would require an intake of 150-200 mg/day. The same may be true for passive smokers.

Data available on vitamin E levels in smokers are controversial. Sobczak et al., (2004) indicate the plasma levels of alpha-tocopherol in passive and active smokers to be lower than those of non-smokers, whereas smoking had virtually no influence on the gamma-tocopherol level. Mena (2003) reports similar serum vitamin E levels in active and/or passive smokers, while Dietrich et al., (2003b) report smokers and passive smokers to have higher plasma concentrations of gamma-tocopherol but not alpha-tocopherol. Some studies have shown that certain indicators of oxidative stress can be improved with vitamin supplementation. For example, Jendryczko et al., (1993) found that despite their having similar plasma vitamin E concentrations, the erythrocytes of 25 children of smoker parents had an increased tendency (p<0.01) to peroxidise *in vitro* compared to those of 28 children of non-smoker parents. However, after supplementing both sets of children with 100 mg alpha-tocopherol acetate for 14 days, the susceptibility to erythrocyte peroxidation in the children of the smoker parents was partially improved.

Table 2. Differences in nutrient intake in active, passive and non-smokers

Nutrien	Non smokers	Active smokers	Passive smokers	Reference
Carbohydrates (%)	22.3		21.0	Curtin et al., 1999
Energy (Kcal)	1822		1636	Curtin et al., 1999
(MJ/day)	8.5±2.2	8.0±2.1	8.5±1.8	Ortega et al., 2004
Fiber (g/day)	15.0		13.0	Curtin et al., 1999
(g/day)	20.1±6.4	15.3±4.5	18.0±5.9	Tröbs et al., 2002
Alcohol (g/day)	2.5±5.4	5.2±8.4	2.6±5.1	Ortega et al., 2004
Linoleic Acid (g/day)	12.4±4.6	10.5±3.1	10.9±4.5	Tröbs et al., 2002
Beta-carotene (mg/day)	3.2±2.7	2.0±1.4	2.7±1.7	Trobs et al., 2002
(mg/day)	2,5	1,8	2,0	Dietrich et al., 2003b
(mg/day)	3,3		2,4	Curtin et al., 1999
(µg/day)	3429± 2044		-22.4±206.0 *	Farchi et al., 2001
Lycopene (µg/day)	4629	3197	3328	Dietrich et al., 2003b
Retinol (µg/day)	392	351	358	Dietrich et al., 2003b
(µg/day)	611.9±606.4		-37.1±63.4 *	Farchi et al., 2001
Vitamin E (alpha TE/day)	8.8	8.0	9.5	Dietrich et al., 2003b
(mg/day)	11.4±4.1	9.3±3.0	10.0±3.9	Tröbs et al., 2002
(mg/day)	9.0±3.8		0.01±0.38*	Farchi et al., 2001
Vitamin C (mg/day)	96.7±49.5	73.9±37.0	92.4±42.8	Tröbs et al., 2002
(mg/day)	86.5	66.4	89.1	Dietrich et al., 2003b
(mg/day)	94.2		83.8	Preston et al., 2003
(mg/day)	111.3±3.3	95.8±7.2	104.8±5.0	Strauss, 2001
(mg/day)	113	142	104	Tribble et al., 1993
(mg/day)	151.0±90.2		-5.2±7.7 *	Farchi et al., 2001
Cobalamin (µg/día)	5.4±3.5	5.3±2.5	4.9±2.8	Tröbs et al., 2002
Folate (µg/day)	181.7±72.4	159.1±65.7	165.2±66.6	Ortega et al., 2004
(µg/day)	318±173	252±110	276±173	Trobs et al., 2002
Iron (mg/day)	9.7		8.4	Curtin et al., 1999

* Difference with Non Smoker

Table 3. Differences in serum concentration/biochemical data in active, passive and non-smokers

Parameter	Non smokers	Active smokers	Passive smokers	Reference
Ascorbic acid (µmol/L)	42.6±12.9	41.8±14.7	43.4±12.4	Tröbs et al., 2002
(µmol/L)	60.8	40.3	59.1	Dietrich et al., 2003b
(µmol/L)	59±3.8		44±4.4	Valkonen y Kuusi, 1998
(µmol/L)	54.5	43.6	54.6	Dietrich et al., 2003b*
(µmol/L)	52.1		48.9	Preston et al., 2003
(µmol/L)	70	40	53	Tribble et al., 1993
(ng/mL)	0.94±0.30		-0.06±0.04 *	Farchi et al., 2001
(mg/dL)	0.94±0.36		-0.04±0.02*	Forastiere et al., 2000
Alpha tocopherol (µmol/L)	30.0	30.0	29.3	Dietrich et al., 2003b
(µmol/L)	22±1.4		21±1.4	Valkonen y Kuusi, 1998
(ng/mL)	10972±5023		-636.9±512.3 *	Farchi et al., 2001
(ng/mL)	10934±4902		-78.4±292*	Forastiere et al., 2000
(µmol/ mg cholesterol/L)	01.5±0.3	1.4±0.2	1.5±0.2	Tröbs et al., 2002
Gamma-tocopherol (µmol/L)	6.0	7.9	7.8	Dietrich et al., 2003b

Table 3. (Continued)

Parameter	Non smokers	Active smokers	Passive smokers	Reference
Alpha carotene (μmol/L)	0.064	0.036	0.039	Dietrich et al., 2003b
(ng/mL)	57.1± 70.0		-7.8±7.6 *	Farchi et al., 2001
(ng/mL)	57.0±69.4		-1.24±4.34*	Forastiere et al., 2000
Beta Carotene (μmol/L)	0.25	0.16	0.15	Dietrich et al., 2003b
(μmol/L)	1.06±0.75	0.73±0.43	0.97±0.56	Trobs et al., 2002
(ng/mL)	345.6±351.3		-32.0±32.9 *	Farchi et al., 2001
(ng/mL)	346.9±350.5		-21.9±19.1*	Forastiere et al., 2000
Total corotenoids (μmol/L)	1.84	1.51	1.52	Dietrich et al., 2003b
Plasma retinol (μmol/L)	2.21		1.86	Hozyasz and Chelchowska, 2004
(μmol/L)	2.17	2.33	2.06	Dietrich et al., 2003b
(ng/mL)	523.0±292.7		-13.4±29.5 *	Farchi et al., 2001
(ng/mL)	520.5±291.5		-10.6±17.0*	Forastiere et al., 2000
Cobalamin (pmol/L)	238±111	241±83	239±127	Tröbs et al., 2002
Folate (serum) (nmol/L)	18.7±6.1	17.1±6.6	18.8±6.3	Tröbs et al., 2002
(nmol/L)	18.4±6.7	16.5±5.5	16.7±6.5	Ortega et al., 2004
(log nmol/L)		-0.29*	-0.16 *	Mannino et al., 2003
Folate (Erythrocyte) (nmol/L)	889.3±421.5	879.6±393.1	828.9±385.0	Ortega et al., 2004
(nmol/L)		-86 *	-50 *	Mannino et al., 2003
Total Cholesterol (mg/dL)	227.3±49.7		-1.34±2.86*	Forastiere et al., 2000
HDL-Cholesterol (mg/dL)	43±11	38±10	42±11	Azizi et al., 2002
(mg/dL)	59±15	53±13	60±15	Tröbs et al., 2002
(mg/dL)	50.7±13.5		-0.80±0.79*	Forastiere et al., 2000
Trygicerides (mg/dL)	89.8±52.7		-0.12±3.0*	Forastiere et al., 2000
(mg/dL)	92±64	101±61	90±46	Tröbs et al., 2002
Homocystein (μmol/L)	11.9±4.9	12.4±4.0	11.1±3.4	Tröbs et al., 2002
(μmol/L)	8.8±2.4	9.4±2.9	8.27±1.99	Ortega et al., 2004
Lycopene (μmol/L)	0.73	0.71	0.67	Dietrich et al., 2003b
(ng/mL)	357.4±221.9		-32.7±30.0 *	Farchi et al., 2001
(ng/mL)	358.9±224.2		18.8±17.6*	Forastiere et al., 2000
(μmol/mmol cholesterol)	0.48		0.33	Hozyasz y Chelchowska, 2004

* Difference with Non Smoker

One of the reasons why lower serum vitamin E levels in active and/or passive smokers have not been generally found is the regeneration of the vitamin by other antioxidants (Halliwell, 1996b; Packer, 1992). Given this type of controversy it is currently questioned whether recommending smokers to increase their vitamin E intake via their diet or by supplements is a sound idea (Ortega, 2003).

Beta-carotene only has an antioxidant effect at certain doses and at certain concentrations of oxygen: at high concentrations and high partial pressures of oxygen it can, in fact, have pro-oxidant effects (Zhang and Omaye, 2000). More peroxidised radicals of beta-carotene are formed under such conditions, and there is a higher incidence of beta-carotene auto-oxidation (Palozza, 1998). There are some reports in the literature that supplementation with high doses of beta-carotene may be dangerous for smokers (Modnicki and Matlawska, 2005), even conditioning an increase in the incidence of lung cancer (Arora et al., 2001). It would therefore seem more appropriate to recommend smokers increase their intake of fruits and vegetables rather than take supplements (Modnicki and Matlawska, 2005; Ortega, 2003). In a study on ferrets administered a supplement with a physiological (low) or pharmacological (high) dose of beta-carotene (0.43 mg compared to 2.4 mg/kg body wt/day; equivalent to 6 and 30 mg/day respectively in humans) that were exposed to cigarette smoke for 6 months, it was seen that, in contrast with the pharmacological dose, the physiological dose had no potentially detrimental effects and may have afforded weak protection against the lung damage induced by cigarette smoke.

However, the use of antioxidant supplements by passive smokers may provide some protection against the increased oxidative stress they suffer. Taking a supplement of 3000 □g of beta-carotene, 60 mg of vitamin C, 30 I.U. of alpha-tocopherol, 40 mg of zinc, 40 □g of selenium, and 2 mg of copper for 60 days reduced the level of 8-hydroxy-2-deoxyguanosine, a marker of oxidative DNA damage (Howard et al., 1998). In addition, Moller et al., (2004) observed that long-term vitamin C supplementation at high doses (500 mg) together with vitamin E in moderate dose (182 mg) for four weeks reduced the steady-state level of oxidative DNA damage in the mononuclear blood cells of smokers.

Active and passive exposure to tobacco smoke has been associated with a lower intake of folate (Ortega et al., 2004) and lower serum and erythrocyte folate levels (Mannino et al., 2003). However, by tripling the recommended intake of folic acid (400 µg/day) serum levels similar to those of non-smokers can be attained (Ortega, 2003). Cafolla et al., (2002) indicate that following supplementation with 5 mg/day of folic acid, the serum and erythrocyte folate levels of smokers became similar to those of non-smokers. Therefore, active and passive smokers may be able to improve their health by increasing their intake of folates via fruits and vegetables or folate-fortified foods, or by taking folate supplements.

In summary, the question remains as to whether the recommended intakes of certain vitamins should be increased for smokers and passive smokers. More research is needed to determine the most appropriate levels of nutrients for these groups.

References

Alberg AJ, Chen JC, Zhao H, Hoffman SC, Comstock GW, Helzlsouer KJ. Household exposure to passive cigarette smoking and serum micronutrient concentrations. *Am. J. Clin. Nutr.* 2000; 72(6):1576-82.

Ambrose JA, Barua RS. The pathophysiology of cigarette smoking and cardiovascular disease: an update. *J. Am. Coll. Cardiol.* 2004;43(10):1731-7.

Arbes SJ Jr, Agustsdottir H, Slade GD. Environmental tobacco smoke and periodontal disease in the United Status. *Am. J. Public Health.* 2001;91(2):253-7.

Arora A, Willhite CA, Liebler DC. Interactions of beta-carotene and cigarette smoke in human bronchial epithelial cells. *Carcinogenesis.* 2001;22(8):1173-8.

Ayaori M, Hisada T, Suzukawa M, Yoshida H, Nishiwaki M, Ito T, Nakajima K,Higashi K, Yonemura A, Ohsuzu F, Ishikawa T, Nakamura H. Plasma levels and redox status of ascorbic acid and levels of lipid peroxidation products in active and passive smokers. *Environ Health Perspect.* 2000;108(2):105-8.

Aycicek A, Erel O, Kocyigit A. Decreased total antioxidant capacity and increased oxidative stress in passive smoker infants and their mothers. *Pediatr. Int.* 2005;47(6):635-9.

Azizi F, Raiszadeh F, Salehi P, Rahmani M, Emami H, Ghanbarian A, Hajipour R. Determinants of serum HDL-C level in a Tehran urban population: the Tehran Lipid and Glucose Study. *Nutr. Metab. Cardiovasc. Dis.* 2002;12(2):80-9.

Barber K, Mussin E, Taylor DK. Fetal exposure to involuntary maternal smoking and childhood respiratory disease. *Ann. Allergy Asthma Immunol.* 1996;76(5):427-30.

Benowitz NL, Kuyt F, Jacob P, Jones RT, Osman AL. Cotinine disposition and effects. *Clin. Pharmacol. Ther.* 1983;34:604-611

Benson BW, Shulman JD. Inclusion of tobacco exposure as a predictive factor for decreased bone mineral content. *Nicotine Tob. Res.* 2005;7(5):719-24.

Bermudez E, Stone K, Carter KM, Pryor WA. Environmental tobacco smoke is just as damaging to DNA as mainstream smoke. *Environ. Health Perspect.* 1994;102(10):870-4.

Birkett NJ. Intake of fruits and vegetables in smokers. *Public Health Nutr.* 1999;2:217-222.

Bolton-Smith, C., Casey, C. E., Gey, K. F., Smith, W. C. and Tunstall-Pedoe, H. Antioxidant vitamin intakes assessed using a food-frequency questionnaire: correlation with biochemical status in smokers and non-smokers. *Br. J. Nutr.* 1991; 65:337-346.

Borzecki A, Brzeski Z, Sodolski W, Wojcik A, Krakowska A, Pajak A. Tobacco smoking among adolescents-self-reported psycho-somatic health. *Przegl. Lek.* 2005;62(10):1099-101.

Brown MS, Goldstein JL. Lipoprotein metabolism in the macrophage: implications for cholesterol deposition in atherosclerosis. *Annu. Rev. Biochem.* 1983;52:223–261.

Bruno RS, Traber MG. Cigarette smoke alters human vitamin E requirements. *J. Nutr.* 2005;135(4):671-4.

Cafolla A, Dragoni F, Girelli G, Tosti ME, Costante A, De Luca AM, Funaro D, Scott CS. Effect of folic acid and vitamin C supplementation on folate status and homocysteine level: a randomised controlled trial in Italian smoker-blood donors. *Atherosclerosis.* 2002;163(1):105-11.

California Environmental Protection Agency. Health effects of exposureto environmental tobacco smoke. Sacramento, CA: Office of Environmental Health Hazard Assessment; 1997. Available at: *www.oehha.org/pdf/exec.pdf.*

Chelchowska M, Laskowska-Klita T, Szymborski J. Level of retinol and beta-carotene in plasma of smoking and non-smoking women. *Wiad. Lek.* 2001;54(5-6):248-54.

Chen H, Hansen MJ, Jones JE, Vlahos R, Bozinovski S, Anderson GP, Morris MJ. Cigarette Smoke Exposure Reprograms the Hypothalamic Neuropeptide Y Axis to Promote Weight Loss. *Am. J. Respir. Crit. Care Med.* 2006; [Epub ahead of print]

Chen H, Vlahos R, Bozinovski S, Jones J, Anderson GP, Morris MJ. Effect of short-term cigarette smoke exposure on body weight, appetite and brain neuropeptide Y in mice. *Neuropsychopharmacology.* 2005;30(4):713-9.

Church DF, Pryor WA. Free-radical chemistry of cigarette smoke and its toxicological implications. *Environ. Health Perspect.* 1985;64:111–126.

Crawley HF, While D. Parental smoking and the nutrient intake and food choice of British teenagers aged 16-17 years. *J. Epidemiol. Community Health.* 1996;50(3):306-12.

Cross CE, Traber M, Eiserich J, van der Vliet A. Micronutrient antioxidants and smoking. *Br. Med. Bull.* 1999;55(3):691-704.

Curtin F, Morabia A, Bernstein MS. Relation of environmental tobacco smoke to diet and health habits: variations according to the site of exposure. *J. Clin. Epidemiol.* 1999;52(11):1055-62.

Dallongeville J, Marecaux N, Fruchart JC, Amouyel P. Cigarette smoking is associated with unhealthy patterns of nutrient intake: a meta-analysis. *J. Nutr.* 1998;128(9):1450-7.

Dietrich M, Block G, Benowitz NL, Morrow JD, Hudes M, Jacob P 3rd, Norkus EP, Packer L. Vitamin C supplementation decreases oxidative stress biomarker f2-isoprostanes in plasma of nonsmokers exposed to environmental tobacco smoke. *Nutr. Cancer.* 2003a;45(2):176-84.

Dietrich M, Block G, Norkus EP, Hudes M, Traber MG, Cross CE, Packer L. Smoking and exposure to environmental tobacco smoke decrease some plasma antioxidants and increase gamma-tocopherol in vivo after adjustment for dietary antioxidant intakes. *Am. J. Clin. Nutr.* 2003b;77(1):160-6.

Drongowski RA, Lee D, Reynolds PI, Malviya S, Harmon CM, Geiger J, Lelli JL, Coran AG. Increased respiratory symptoms following surgery in children exposed to environmental tobacco smoke. *Paediatr. Anaesth.* 2003;13(4):304-10.

Dyer AR, Elliott P, Stamler J, Chan Q, Ueshima H, Zhou BF. Dietary intake in male and female smokers, ex-smokers, and never smokers: the INTERMAP study. *J. Hum. Hypertens.* 2003;17(9):641-54.

Eiserich JP, van der Vliet A, Handelman GJ, Halliwell B, Cross CE. Dietary antioxidants and cigarette smoke-induced biomolecular damage: a complex interaction. *Am. J. Clin. Nutr.* 1995;62(6 Suppl):1490S-1500S.

Emmons KM, Thompson B, Feng Z, Hebert JR, Heimendinger J, Linnan L. Dietary intake and exposure to environmental tobacco smoke in a worksite population. *Eur. J. Clin. Nutr.* 1995;49(5):336-45.

Farchi S, Forastiere F, Pistelli R, Baldacci S, Simoni M, Perucci CA, Viegi G; On behalf of the SEASD Group. Exposure to environmental tobacco smoke is associated with lower plasma beta-carotene levels among nonsmoking women married to a smoker. *Cancer Epidemiol. Biomarkers Prev.* 2001;10(8):907-9.

Feldman J, Shenker IR, Etzel RA, Spierto FW, Lilienfield DE, Nussbaum M, Jacobson MS. Passive smoking alters lipid profiles in adolescents. *Pediatrics.* 1991;88(2):259-64.

Forastiere F, Mallone S, Lo Presti E, Baldacci S, Pistelli F, Simoni M, Scalera A, Pedreschi M, Pistelli R, Corbo G, Rapiti E, Agabiti N, Farchi S, Basso S, Chiaffi L, Matteelli G, Di Pede F, Carrozzi L, Viegi G. Characteristics of nonsmoking women exposed to spouses who smoke: epidemiologic study on environment and health in women from four Italian areas. *Environ. Health Perspect.* 2000;108(12):1171-7.

Fuertes Fernández-Espinar J, Meriz Rubio J, Pardos Martínez C, López Cortés V, Ricarte Díez JI, González Pérez-Yarza E.. Prevalencia actual del asma, alergia e hiperrespuesta bronquial en niños de 6-8 años. *An. Esp. Pediatr.* 2001;54:18-26.

Gilliland FD, Li YF, Dubeau L, Berhane K, Avol E, McConnell R, et al.. Effects of glutation S-transferase M1, maternal smoking during pregnancy, and environmental tobacco smoke on asthma and wheezing in children. *Am. J. Respir. Crit. Care Med.* 2002; 166:457-63.

Glantz SA, Parmley WW. Passive smoking and heart disease: mechanisms and risk. *JAMA.* 1995;273:1047–1053.

Halliwell B. Antioxidants in human health and disease. *Annu. Rev. Nutr.* 1996b;16:33-50.

Halliwell B. Oxidative stress, nutrition and health. Experimental strategies for optimization of nutritional antioxidant intake in humans. *Free Radic. Res.* 1996a;25(1):57-74.

Hampl JS, Taylor CA, Booth CL. Differences in dietary patterns of nonsmoking adults married to smokers vs. nonsmokers. *Am. J. Health Promot.* 2001; 16(1):1-6.

Handelman GJ, Packer L, Cross CE. Destruction of tocopherols, carotenoids, and retinol in human plasma by cigarette smoke. *Am. J. Clin. Nutr.* 1996;63(4):559-65.

Heraud MC, Herbelin-Wagner ML. . Risk factors: environment, tobacco smoke. *Arch. Pediatr.* 2002;9(Suppl 3):377-83.

Holay MP, Paunikar NP, Joshi PP, Sahasrabhojney VS, Tankhiwale SR. Effect of passive smoking on endothelial function in: healthy adults. *J. Assoc. Physicians India.* 2004;52:114-7.

Howard DJ, Ota RB, Briggs LA, Hampton M, Pritsos CA. Oxidative stress induced by environmental tobacco smoke in the workplace is mitigated by antioxidant supplementation. *Cancer Epidemiol. Biomarkers Prev.* 1998;7(11):981-8.

Hozyasz KK, Chelchowska M. [Vitamin A levels among nonsmoking mothers of children with orofacial clefts married to a smoker]. *Przegl. Lek.* 2004;61(10):1083-5.

Iles K, Poplawski NK, Couper RT. Passive exposure to tobacco smoke and bacterial meningitis in children. *J. Paediatr. Child Health.* 2001;37(4):388-91.

Institute of Medicine, Food and Nutrition Borrad. Dietary references intakes for vitamin C, vitamin E, selenium and carotenoids, chapter 5: vitamin C. Washington DC: *National Academy Press*, 2000; 95:185.

Jacob RA. Passive smoking induces oxidant damage preventable by vitamin C. *Nutr. Rev.* 2000;58(8):239-41.

Jarvis MJ, Russell MAH, Benowitz NL, Feyerabend C. Elimination of cotinine from body fluids: implications for noninvasive measurement of tobacco smoke exposure. *Am. J. Public Health.* 1988; 78:696-698.

Jendryczko A, Szpyrka G, Gruszczynski J, Kozowicz M. Cigarette smoke exposure of school children: effect of passive smoking and vitamin E supplementation on blood antioxidant status. *Neoplasma.* 1993;40(3):199-203.

Jialal I, Grundy SM. Effect of combined supplementation with alpha-tocopherol, ascorbate, and beta carotene on low-density lipoprotein oxidation. *Circulation.* 1993;88(6):2780-6.

Kalinka J, Hanke W, Sobala W. Impact of prenatal tobacco smoke exposure, as measured by midgestation serum cotinine levels, on fetal biometry and umbilical flow velocity waveforms. *Am. J. Perinatol.* 2005;22(1):41-7.

Kasim K, Levallois P, Abdous B, Auger P, Johnson KC; Canadian Cancer Registries Epidemiology Research Group. Environmental tobacco smoke and risk of adult leukemia. *Epidemiology.* 2005;16(5):672-80.

Khan JC, Thurlby DA, Shahid H, Clayton DG, Yates JR, Bradley M, Moore AT, Bird AC; Genetic Factors in AMD Study. Smoking and age related macular degeneration: the number of pack years of cigarette smoking is a major determinant of risk for both geographic atrophy and choroidal neovascularisation. *Br. J. Ophthalmol.* 2006;90(1):75-80.

Kim H, Lim Y, Lee S, Park S, Kim C, Hong C, Shin D.Relationship between environmental tobacco smoke and urinary cotinine levels in passive smokers at their residence. *J. Expo. Anal. Environ. Epidemiol.* 2004;14 Suppl 1:S65-70.

King JC. Determinants of maternal zinc status during pregnancy. *Am. J. Clin. Nutr.* 2000;71(5 Suppl):1334S-43S.

Klerman L. Protecting children: reducing their environmental tobacco smoke exposure. *Nicotine Tob. Res.* 2004;6 Suppl 2:S239-53.

Koo LC, Kabat GC, Rylander R, Tominaga S, Kato I, Ho j H-C. Dietary and lifestyles correlates of passive smoking in Hong-Kong, Japan, Sweeden and the USA. *Soc. Sci. Med.* 1997; 45:159-69.

Leonard, S. W., Bruno, R. S., Paterson, E., Schock, B. C., Atkinson, J., Bray, T. M., Cross, C. E. and Traber, M. G. 5-Nitro--tocopherol increases in human plasma exposed to cigarette smoke in vitro and in vivo. *Free Radic. Biol. Med.* 2003;35:1560-1567.

Lewis SA, Antoniak M, Venn AJ, Davies L, Goodwin A, Salfield N, Britton J, Fogarty AW. Secondhand smoke, dietary fruit intake, road traffic exposures, and the prevalence of asthma: a cross-sectional study in young children. *Am. J. Epidemiol.* 2005;161(5):406-11.

Lykkesfeldt J, Christen S, Wallock LM, Chang HH, Jacob RA, Ames BN. Ascorbate is depleted by smoking and repleted by moderate supplementation: a study in male smokers and nonsmokers with matched dietary antioxidant intakes. *Am. J. Clin. Nutr.* 2000;71(2):530-6.

Ma A, Hampl JS, Betts NM. Antioxidants intakes and smoking status: data from the Continuing survey of Food Intakes by Individuals 1994-1996. *Am. J. Clin. Nutr.* 2000;71:774-80.

Mannino DM, Moorman JE, Kingsley B, Rose D, Repace J. Health effects related to environmental tobacco smoke exposure in children in the United States: data from the Third National Health and Nutrition Examination Survey. *Arch. Pediatr. Adolesc. Med.* 2001;155(1):36-41.

Mannino DM, Mulinare J, Ford ES, Schwartz J. Tobacco smoke exposure and decreased serum and red blood cell folate levels: data from the Third National Health and Nutrition Examination Survey. *Nicotine Tob. Res.* 2003;5(3):357-62.

Marangon K, Herbeth B, Lecomte E, Paul-Dauphin A, Grolier P, Chancerelle Y, Artur Y, Siest G. Diet, antioxidant status, and smoking habits in French men. *Am. J. Clin. Nutr.* 1998;67(2):231-9.

Matanoski G, Kanchanaraska S, Lantry D, Chang Y. Characteristics of nonsmoking women in NHANES I and NHANES I Epidemiologic Follow-up Study with exposure to spouses who smoke. *Am. J. Epidemiol.* 1995; 142:149-57.

Mena MC. El hábito de fumar como condicionante del estado nutricional en población femenina. *Tesis Doctoral Madrid.* 2003.

Modnicki D, Matlawska I. Carotenoids as components of dietary supplements recommended for smokers and persons passively exposed to cigarette smoke. *Przegl. Lek.* 2005;62(10):1188-9.

Moller P, Viscovich M, Lykkesfeldt J, Loft S, Jensen A, Poulsen HE.Vitamin C supplementation decreases oxidative DNA damage in mononuclear blood cells of smokers. *Eur. J. Nutr.* 2004;43(5):267-74

Morabia A, Bernstein MS, Antonini S. Smoking, dietary calcium and vitamin D deficiency in women: a population-based study. *Eur. J. Clin. Nutr.* 2000;54(9):684-9.

Muñoz C, Jurado D, Luna JD.. Exposición al humo de tabaco ambiental en niños en el medio familiar: creencias, actitudes y prácticas de los padres. *Prev. Tab.* 2003;5:11-8.

Nageris B, Braverman I, Hadar T, Hansen MC, Frenkiel S. Effects of passive smoking on odour identification in children. *J. Otolaryngol.* 2001;30(5):263-5.

National Research Council. *Environmental Tobacco Smoke: Measuring Exposures and Assessing Health Effects.* Washington, DC: Committee on Passive Smoking, Board on Environmental Studies and Toxicology, National Research Council; 1986.

Neufeld EJ, Mietus-Snyder M, Beiser AS, Baker AL, Newburger JW. Passive cigarette smoking and reduced HDL cholesterol levels in children with high-risk lipid profiles. Passive cigarette smoking and reduced HDL cholesterol levels in children with high-risk lipid profiles. *Circulation.* 1997;96(5):1403-7.

Nicklas T, Johnson R; American Dietetic Association. Position of the American Dietetic Association: Dietary guidance for healthy children ages 2 to 11 years. *J. Am. Diet. Assoc.* 2004;104(4):660-77.

Nizard J. What are the epidemiological data on maternal and paternal smoking?. *J. Gynecol. Obstet. Biol. Reprod* (Paris). 2005;34 Spec No 1:3S347-52.

Nomura K, Nakao M, Morimoto T. Effect of smoking on hearing loss: quality assessment and meta-analysis. *Prev. Med.* 2005;40(2):138-44.

Ortega RM, Andres P, Zamora MJ, Ortega A. The nutritional problems of the smoker. The role of diet in the appearance and progress of cataracts. *Rev. Clin. Esp.* 1994a;194(11):982-4.

Ortega RM, Lopez-Sobaler AM, Gonzalez-Gross MM, Redondo RM, Marzana I, Zamora MJ, Andres P. Influence of smoking on folate intake and blood folate concentrations in a group of elderly Spanish men. *J. Am. Coll. Nutr.* 1994b;13(1):68-72.

Ortega RM, Lopez-Sobaler AM, Martinez RM, Andres P, Quintas ME. Influence of smoking on vitamin E status during the third trimester of pregnancy and on breast-milk tocopherol concentrations in Spanish women. *Am. J. Clin. Nutr.* 1998a;68(3):662-7.

Ortega RM, Lopez-Sobaler AM, Quintas ME, Martinez RM, Andres P. The influence of smoking on vitamin C status during the third trimester of pregnancy and on vitamin C levels in maternal milk. *J. Am. Coll. Nutr.* 1998;17(4):379-84.

Ortega RM, Requejo AM, Lopez-Sobaler AM, Navia B, Mena MC, Basabe B, Andres P. Smoking and passive smoking as conditioners of folate status in young women. *J. Am. Coll. Nutr.* 2004;23(4):365-71.

Ortega RM. Nutrición del fumador. En: Requejo AM y Ortega RM, eds. Nutriguía. Manual de nutrición clínica en atención primaria. Ed. Complutense. *Madrid.* 2003. p. 324-331.

Osler M. The food intake of smokers and nonsmokers: the role of partner's smoking behavior. *Prev. Med.* 1998;27(3):438-43.

Packer L. Interactions among antioxidants in health and disease: vitamin E and its redox cycle. *Proc. Soc. Exp. Biol. Med.* 1992;200(2):271-6.

Palaniappan U, Jacobs Starkey L, O'Loughlin J, Gray-Donald K. Fruit and vegetable consumption is lower and saturated fat intake is higher among Canadians reporting smoking. *J. Nutr.* 2001;131:1952-1958.

Palozza P. Prooxidant actions of carotenoids in biologic systems. *Nutr. Rev.* 1998;56(9):257-65.

Pfeffer F, Kaufer-Horwitz M. *Nutrición en el adulto.* En: Casanueva E, Kaufer-Horwitz M, Pérez-Lizaur AB, Arroyo P. Nutriología Médica 2ª ed. 2001. Editorial Médica Panamericana. México. 104-119.

Pirkle JL, Flegal KM, Bernert JT, Brody DJ, Etzel RA, Maurer KR.. Exposure of the US population to environmental tobacco smoke: the Third National Health and Nutrition Examination Survey, 1988-91. *JAMA* 1996;275:1233-40.

Pollard J, Greenwood D, Kirk S, Cade J. Lifestyle factors affecting fruit and vegetable consumption in the UK Women's Cohort Study. *Appetite* 2001;37:71-79.

Powledge TM. Nicotine as therapy. PLoS. Biol. 2004;2(11):e404. *Epub* 2004 Nov 16.

Preston AM, Rodriguez C, Rivera CE, Sahai H. Influence of environmental tobacco smoke on vitamin C status in children. *Am. J. Clin. Nutr.* 2003;77(1):167-72.

Qureshi AI, Suri MF, Kirmani JF, Divani AA. Cigarette smoking among spouses: another risk factor for stroke in women. *Stroke.* 2005;36(9):e74-6. *Epub* 2005 Aug 4.

Rauh VA, Whyatt RM, Garfinkel R, Andrews H, Hoepner L, Reyes A, Diaz D, Camann D, Perera FP. Developmental effects of exposure to environmental tobacco smoke and material hardship among inner-city children. Neurotoxicol. *Teratol.* 2004;26(3):373-85.

Reibel J. Tobacco and oral diseases. Update on the evidence, with recommendations. *Med. Princ. Pract.* 2003;12 Suppl 1:22-32.

Reynolds P, Hurley SE, Hoggatt K, Anton-Culver H, Bernstein L, Deapen D, Peel D, Pinder R, Ross RK, West D, Wright W, Ziogas A, Horn-Ross PL. Correlates of active and passive smoking in the California Teachers Study cohort. *J. Womens Health* (Larchmt). 2004;13(7):778-90.

Romero-Palacios PJ. Asthma and tobacco smoke. *Arch. Bronconeumol.* 2004;40(9):414-8.

Samet JM, Yang G.. Passive smoking women and children. In: Samet JM, Yoon SY, editors. Women and the tobacco epidemic. Challenges for the 21st century. The World Health Organization in collaboration with the Institute for Global Tobacco Control and the Johns Hopkins School of Public Health. *Geneva: World Health Organization,* 2001.

Samet JM. Risks of active and passive smoking. *Salud. Publica. Mex.* 2002;44 Suppl. 1:S144-60.

Sato K, Endo S, Tomita H. Sensitivity of three loci on the tongue and soft palate to four basic tastes in smokers and non-smokers. *Acta Otolaryngol. Suppl.* 2002;(546):74-82.

Schectman G, Byrd JC, Hoffman R. Ascorbic acid requirements for smokers: analysis of a population survey. *Am. J. Clin. Nutr.* 1991;53: 1466–1470

Schroder H, Marrugat J, Elosua R, Covas MI. Tobacco and alcohol consumption: impact on other cardiovascular and cancer risk factors in a southern European Mediterranean population. *Br. J. Nutr.* 2002; 88(3):273-81.

Scientific Committee on Tobacco and Health, HSMO. *Report of the Scientific Committee on Tobacco and Health.* The Stationari Office.1998. 011322124x.

Simoni M, Jaakkola MS, Carrozzi L, Baldacci S, Di Pede F, Viegi G. Indoor air pollution and respiratory health in the elderly. *Eur. Respir. J. Suppl.* 2003;40:15s-20s.

Smith CJ, Fischer TH. Particulate and vapor phase constituents of cigarette mainstream smoke and risk of myocardial infarction. *Atherosclerosis.* 2001;158(2):257-67.

Sobczak A, Golka D, Szoltysek-Boldys I. The effects of tobacco smoke on plasma alpha- and gamma-tocopherol levels in passive and active cigarette smokers. *Toxicol. Lett.* 2004;151(3):429-37.

Steyn K, de Wet T, Saloojee Y, Nel H, Yach D. The influence of maternal cigarette smoking, snuff use and passive smoking on pregnancy outcomes: the Birth To Ten Study. *Paediatr. Perinat. Epidemiol.* 2006;20(2):90-9.

Strauss RS. Environmental tobacco smoke and serum vitamin C levels in children. *Pediatrics.* 2001;107(3):540-2.

Subar AF, Harlan LC, Mattson ME. Food and nutrient intake differences between smokers and non-smokers in the US. *Am. J. Public Health.* 1990;80:1323-1329.

Suliburska J, Duda G, Pupek-Musialik D. Effect of tobacco smoking on taste sensitivity in adults. *Przegl. Lek.* 2004;61(10):1174-6.

Thompson, D. H. and Warburton, D. M. (1992) Lifestyle differences between smokers, ex-smokers and non-smokers, and their implications for their health. *Psychology and Health* 1992;7: 311-321.

Tong EK, England L, Glantz SA. Changing conclusions on secondhand smoke in a sudden infant death syndrome review funded by the tobacco industry. *Pediatrics.* 2005;115(3):e356-66.

Topp R, Thefeld W, Wichmann HE, Heinrich J. The effect of environmental tobacco smoke exposure on allergic sensitization and allergic rhinitis in adults. *Indoor Air.* 2005;15(4):222-7.

Tribble DL, Giuliano LJ, Fortmann SP. Reduced plasma ascorbic acid concentrations in nonsmokers regularly exposed to environmental tobacco smoke. *Am. J. Clin. Nutr.* 1993;58(6):886-90.

Trobs M, Renner T, Scherer G, Heller WD, Geiss HC, Wolfram G, Haas GM, Schwandt P. Nutrition, antioxidants, and risk factor profile of nonsmokers, passive smokers and smokers of the Prevention Education Program (PEP) in Nuremberg, Germany. *Prev. Med.* 2002;34(6):600-7.

US Department of Health Education and Welfare. *The health consequences of smoking.* A report of the Surgeon General (DHEW Publication No. HSM 73-8704). Washington, DC: US Government Printing Office, 1971.

US Environmental Protection Agency. *Respiratory health effects of passive smoking: lung cancers and other disorders.* Washington, DC: Office of Research and Development, Office of Health and Environmental Assessment; 1992. US EPA Publication No. EPA/600/6-90/006F. Available at: *http://cfpub.epa.gov/ncea/cfm/recordisplay.cfm? deid_2835*

Valkonen M, Kuusi T. Passive smoking induces atherogenic changes in low-density lipoprotein. *Circulation.* 1998;97(20):2012-6.

Voutilainen S, Rissanen TH, Virtanen J, Lakka TA, Salonen JT; Kuopio Ischemic Heart Disease Risk Factor Study. Low dietary folate intake is associated with an excess incidence of acute coronary events: The Kuopio Ischemic Heart Disease Risk Factor Study. *Circulation.* 2001;103(22):2674-80.

Wei W, Kim Y, Boudreau N. Association of smoking with serum and dietary levels of antioxidants in adults: NHANES III, 1988-1994. *Am. J. Public Health.* 2001;91(2):258-64.

Weitzman M, Cook S, Auinger P, Florin TA, Daniels S, Nguyen M, Winickoff JP. Tobacco smoke exposure is associated with the metabolic syndrome in adolescents. *Circulation.* 2005;112(6):862-9

Whig J, Singh CB, Soni GL, Bansal AK. Serum lipids and lipoprotein profiles of cigarette smokers and passive smokers. *Indian J. Med. Res.* 1992;96:282-7.

Whitfield JB, Zhu G, Heath AC, Powell And LW, Martin NG. Effects of alcohol consumption on indices of iron stores and of iron stores on alcohol intake markers. Alcohol. *Clin. Exp. Res.* 2001;25(7):1037-45.

World Health Organization Division of Noncommunicable Disease Tobacco Free Initiative.. International consultation on environmental tobacco smoke (ETS) and child health consultation report. *Geneva: WHO,* 1999. Available from *http://www.who.int./toh*

World Health Organization International Agency for Research on Cancer IARC. Monographs on the Evaluation of Carcinogenic Risks to Humans. Volume 83 Tobacco Smoke and Involuntary Smoking Summary of Data Reported and Evaluation Tobacco smoking and tobacco smoke Involuntary smoking. 2002. Available at: *http://monographs.iarc.fr/ENG/ Monographs/vol83/volume83.pdf*

Yang G, Fant L, Tan J, et al.. Smoking in China. Findings of the 1996 National Prevalence Survey. *JAMA* 1999;2892:1247-53.

Yolton K, Dietrich K, Auinger P, Lanphear BP, Hornung R. Exposure to environmental tobacco smoke and cognitive abilities among U.S. children and adolescents. *Environ. Health Perspect.* 2005;113(1):98-103.

Zhang P, Omaye ST. Beta-carotene and protein oxidation: effects of ascorbic acid and alpha-tocopherol. *Toxicology.* 2000;146(1):37-47.

Zhang Y. Influence of smoking on cholesterol concentrations in serum lipo-protein of healthy subjects. *Zhonghua Liu Xing Bing Xue Za Zhi.* 1992 Apr;13(2):97-100.

Ziegler RG, Mayne ST, Swanson CA. Nutrition and lung cancer. *Cancer Causes Control.* 1996;7(1):157-77. Review.

Zondervan KT, Ocke MC, Smit HA, Seidell JC. Do dietary and supplementary intakes of antioxidants differ with smoking status? *Int. J. Epidemiol.* 1996;25:70-79.

In: Nutrition Research at the Leading Edge   ISBN: 978-1-60456-053-4
Editors: R. E. Cassady, E. I. Tidswell, pp. 157-174   © 2008 Nova Science Publishers, Inc.

Chapter V

Effectiveness of School-Based Environmental vs Individual Approaches to Diet, Physical Activity, and Sedentary Behavior Change Among Youth

D. Thompson[1], T. Baranowski, I. Zakeri,
R. Jago, J. Davis and K. Cullen
Children's Nutrition Research Center, Baylor College of Medicine
Houston, TX, USA

Abstract

Background. Schools offer unique channels for youth obesity prevention. School based programs can be categorized as having an individual, environmental, or a combined (individual + environmental) focus.

Purpose. This chapter reviews the literature on school based interventions focusing on diet, physical activity, and/or sedentary behavior reporting body composition as an outcome measure, and then characterizes these programs as having an individual, environmental, or combined focus. These categories are then examined in an attempt to determine which approach appears to be more effective at promoting change in body composition within the school setting.

Method. Primary inclusionary criteria were: school based interventions; a focus on diet, physical activity, and/or sedentary behavior; reporting body composition as an outcome measure; and emphasizing prevention rather than treatment. Secondary

[1] Corresponding Author: Debbe Thompson, PhD USDA/ARS Scientist/Nutritionist; Assistant Professor; Children's Nutrition Research Center, Baylor College of Medicine 1100 Bates Street, Houston, TX 77030; 713-798-7076 phone, 713-798-7098 fax, dit@bcm.tmc.edu , www.bcm.tmc.edu/cnrc I am currently a scientist with USDA/ARS, with a faculty appointment at the Children's Nutrition Research Center, Baylor College of Medicine

inclusionary criteria (to enhance confidence in the inferences drawn) included having an experimental design, with school as the unit of randomization; using appropriate statistical analysis methods to account for clustering within schools; inclusion in a peer-reviewed journal; and reporting results in English

Results. Eleven interventions met all inclusionary criteria. Three of the 11 achieved significant change in body composition (27% of total). Significant group differences in body composition were reported by two of the individual focus (29%), one (50%) of the environmental focus, and none (0%) of the combined focus interventions. No consistent differences in procedures, methods, or intervention components were found among the interventions that did or did not achieve change in body composition.

Conclusion. Both individual and environmental interventions promote change in diet, physical activity, and/or sedentary behavior and have demonstrated success in impacting body composition in a school setting. More research is needed to identify the approach, procedures, and methods that are most effective at promoting body composition change in a school setting.

KeyWords: Obesity prevention, youth, school-based, curriculum, environment.

Introduction

Youth obesity has risen dramatically over the past several decades [1, 2], and indications are that it is continuing to increase [2]. Obese youth are at greater risk of becoming obese adults [3], with increased risk of developing chronic diseases [4]. Elevated glucose, lipids, and blood pressure, risk factors for the most common chronic diseases, have been observed among obese youth [4]. Further, obese youth are more likely to suffer from social isolation [4], discrimination [4], stigmatization [5], depression [6], low self esteem [7] and body dissatisfaction [4], which likely impair their quality of life [8]. Thus, obesity impacts both physical and psychological health.

Obesity prevention may be easier than treatment, since it is generally accepted that once gained, excess weight is difficult to lose and keep off [9]. Focusing on obesity prevention among youth offers a unique opportunity to establish healthy behaviors early in life. Youth behavior may be more susceptible to modification because health habits are likely not as firmly established as those of adults [9]. Therefore, effective methods for preventing obesity among youth should be identified and implemented before habits become firmly entrenched and thus more resistant to change.

Diet [10-14] and/or physical activity [15-18] have been associated with obesity risk, and are therefore, common targets for obesity prevention interventions. Obesity risk has been negatively related to consumption of fruit [10], vegetables [11], and carbohydrates [13], while a positive relationship has been observed with dietary fat [12, 13], added sugar [12], and soft drink [14] consumption. Similar to diet, physical activity and obesity risk have been shown to have a negative relationship [16], while sedentary behaviors (i.e., physically inactive behaviors), such as television viewing, had a positive relationship with body composition measures [17, 18]. These relationships are of concern because youth diet and physical activity behaviors often fall below national recommendations and guidelines, as outlined below.

Youth dietary habits are less than desirable [14, 19-21] and likely track into adulthood [22-25]. Fewer than 20% of youth in the United States [19] met the national guideline of at least five servings of fruit and vegetables a day [26]. Although recent national data suggested the percentage of kcal from fat consumed by 2-17 year old youth decreased between 1989 and 1995, actual fat intakes did not decrease [20]. Instead, total kcal intake increased, thereby lowering the percentage of kcal from fat [20]. Alternatively, increasing fruit, juice, and vegetable consumption has been shown to help lower total fat intake [27-30]. Data from the USDA Continuing Surveys of Food Intakes by Individuals from 1977 and 1995 indicated the proportion of adolescent boys and girls consuming soft drinks, the biggest source of refined sugar in the diet, increased by 74% and 65%, respectively [21]. Energy intake and soft drink consumption were positively related among children and adolescents [21]. Although a positive relationship has been observed between adolescent soft drink consumption and weight gain over a 2-year period [14], the association between soft drink consumption and diet quality is controversial [21, 31].

Youth physical activity is also less than desirable. National organizations have issued guidelines or statements regarding the importance of physical activity in childhood [32]. Even so, many youth do not engage in enough physical activity to benefit from an active lifestyle. A third of high school youth reported not engaging in any vigorous activity; approximately three-fourths reported not engaging in moderate physical activity; and approximately 70% reported not attending daily physical education classes [33]. Declines in physical activity have been observed throughout childhood and adolescence [34]. Further, gender differences in physical activity have also been observed. Females were less active than males at all ages [35], with greater decreases in activity during adolescence [34]. Males were approximately 15-25% more active than females during the school-age years, and activity levels decreased 2.7% per year for males and 7.4% per year for females [35]. In a nationally representative sample of American high school students, the least active were more likely to be nonwhite females between the ages of 16 and 18 years [36]. Thus, it is apparent that youth do not meet the physical activity guidelines recommended for a healthy lifestyle.

Relationships among obesity, diet, physical activity, and sedentary behavior are complex. Interactions among youth diet and physical activity behaviors have been observed [6, 37-39], complicating the independent effects of diet and physical activity on body composition. For example, in young African American girls, physical activity was negatively associated with % kcal from fat [37, 38], but positively associated with % kcal from carbohydrate [37, 38]. Age may further complicate the relationship. A review article reported that consuming a healthy diet was a correlate of physical activity among children, but not adolescents [6], suggesting that other factors may affect the relationship as youth become older. Associations between sedentary behavior and diet have also been observed. For example, viewing two or more hours of television a day was associated with inadequate fruit, juice, and vegetable intake among White high school students, but not among African American or Hispanic students [39]. These findings suggest ethnicity may also impact the relationships between diet, physical activity, and sedentary behavior, thus adding an additional layer of complexity.

While more research is needed to identify and clarify these complex relationships, it is fairly well established that changes in diet, physical activity, and sedentary behavior are needed to help combat the youth obesity epidemic. Therefore, it is imperative that effective channels within which to promote youth obesity prevention behaviors be identified.

Schools offer a unique environment within which to promote obesity prevention behaviors. Over 90% of children in the United States are enrolled in schools [40], making this a potentially effective channel for reaching large numbers of youth. Schools have responsibility for the effective implementation of the physical education curriculum and for serving school meals [40], thereby providing incentives to partner with innovative programs promoting physical activity and/or healthy nutrition. Established social networks (e.g., teachers, administrative staff, peers, team sports, band, after-school programs, intramural sports, etc), classes (e.g., health, physical education, math, science), programs/services (e.g., Parent Teacher Organization, school health services), and communication channels (e.g., newsletters, closed-circuit television programs, automatic telephone call services, assemblies, etc) are in place in the school environment and can be tapped as a source of information dissemination, support, reinforcement, and modeling [41, 42]. The challenge for school based programs is to identify and capitalize on methods for utilizing these resources in an efficient and effective manner to promote behavior change.

School based interventions focusing on nutrition, physical activity, and/or sedentary behavior change can be categorized as having an *individual, environmental, or combined* (individual + environmental) focus. Interventions classified as having an *individual focus* typically take a curricular approach and emphasize change at the individual level. *Environmental focus* interventions attempt to provide a supportive environment within which to promote and support behavior change and maintenance within the school setting. Environmental focus programs typically target behaviors within the school environment (e.g., foods offered within the school cafeteria or in vending machines). *Combined focus* interventions (i.e., individual focus + environmental focus) integrate selected features of both approaches (e.g., classroom curriculum and healthy foods in the cafeteria). The purpose of this chapter is to review the available evidence on school based programs targeting diet, physical activity, and/or sedentary behavior that report body composition as an outcome measure, in an effort to identify which of these approaches is most likely to be successful at promoting change in body composition and to then elucidate program features commonly associated with success.

Method

Systematic searches of electronic databases (PubMed, Medline, PsychInfo) were conducted, using the following terms alone and/or in combination: body mass index (BMI), body composition, school, obesity prevention, diet, physical activity, environmental, behavioral, and individual. Manual searches of known relevant publications (such as Journal of School Health, Journal of Nutrition Education, etc) were also conducted. Once located, all manuscripts were evaluated against strict inclusionary/exclusionary criteria prior to inclusion in the review.

Inclusionary/Exclusionary Criteria

Inclusionary/exclusionary criteria were carefully developed with the intention of including only those studies that met strict research design and statistical analyses standards. Meeting these standards increased the likelihood that proper inferences could be drawn about program effectiveness.

Two types of inclusionary criteria were utilized in this review: content and method. Inclusionary criteria related to content were: school based interventions; emphasizing diet, physical activity, and/or sedentary behavior; reporting body composition as an outcome measure; and emphasizing prevention rather than treatment. Inclusionary criteria related to method included: research design issues, such as having an experimental design with school as the unit of randomization; using appropriate hierarchical or cluster-based statistical analysis methods to account for the group effect; and inclusion in a peer-reviewed journal. There were no limitations regarding geographic region or country, although the results needed to be reported in English.

Definitions

"School-based intervention" was defined as an intervention that was implemented during usual school hours. Therefore, interventions offered before or after school or during the summer were excluded. "Individual focused programs" was defined as those that offered a curricular approach to behavior change. "Environmental focused programs" was defined as those that attempted to change the school environment. "Combined focus programs" was defined as programs that offered features of both individual and environmental focused programs. "Diet" was defined as having a focus on selected nutrients (e.g., sodium, fat), kcal (e.g., total kcal, % kcal from fat), food groups (e.g., fruit, vegetables, carbohydrates), or healthy eating practices (e.g., general healthy food choices, heart healthy foods). "Physical activity" was defined as lifestyle, moderate, vigorous, and/or moderate-to-vigorous physical activity. "Sedentary behavior" was defined as physically inactive behaviors, such as video or computer games, television viewing, talking on the telephone, and/or computer use outside the school environment. "Body composition" measures were defined as BMI, ponderosity, skinfold, bioelectrical impedence, DEXA, hydrostatic weighing, waist circumference, waist:hip ratio, and/or a combination of these measures. "Prevention" was defined as an attempt to instill healthy diet and/or physical activity behaviors in an effort to decrease risk of developing obesity or other health problems, as opposed to having a focus on treating an existing obesity, weight, or health problem. "Experimental design" was defined as inclusion of more than one group, random assignment, with school as the unit of randomization. "Appropriate statistical analysis" was defined as analysis that adjusted for group effect (e.g., mixed model analysis, hierarchical modeling, scores averaged within schools).

Results

Systematic searches located 46 school based interventions published in peer-reviewed journals that focused on diet, physical activity, and/or sedentary behavior during the usual school day/year and reported body composition as an outcome measure. Of these, 35 were excluded because they did not focus on prevention, did not have an appropriate research design, and/or did not utilize appropriate statistical analysis procedures.

Eleven school based interventions met all the criteria [43-53]. Of these, seven (64%) had an individual focus [43-49], two (18%) had an environmental focus [50, 51], and two (18%) had a combined (individual + environmental) focus [52, 53]. Two of the seven interventions with an individual focus (29%) reported significant group differences in body composition [43, 48] while one of the two environmental-focus interventions (50%) reported significant group differences in body composition [51]. Neither of the combined focus interventions (0%) reported significant effects on body composition [52, 53].

Results of the interventions meeting all the criteria are presented in Table 1. Descriptive information (intervention type, focus, audience, and body composition measure), factors likely to impact the outcome (theoretical framework, intervention components, duration, implementor, and parent involvement), and effect on body composition (significant, non-significant) are presented in the table. Characteristics of the three interventions achieving change in body composition are presented below.

Programs Achieving Change in Body Composition

Overview

Three of the 11 (27%) school based interventions that met both content and method inclusionary criteria achieved a statistically significant change in body composition [43, 48, 51]. Features of the three interventions are presented in Table 1 and discussed below.

Type

Two of the three interventions achieving change in body composition (67%) had an individual focus [43, 48], while one had an environmental focus (33%) [51]. None of the successful interventions had a combined focus.

Intervention Focus

No common intervention foci (diet, physical activity, sedentary behavior) were found among the three interventions. One of the interventions focused on diet and physical activity [51], one focused on diet, physical activity, and sedentary behavior [43], and one focused on sedentary behavior alone [48].

Audience

No common audience was found among the three successful interventions. Two were implemented in middle schools [43, 51] and one in elementary schools [48].

Table 1. Program Characteristics

Author	Type	Focus	Audience	B/Comp Measure	Theory	Intervention Components	Duration	Who	Parent Focus	B/Comp Effect
Gortmaker et al [43] PLANET HEALTH	I	Diet PA SB	MS; 10 schools; 1295 students	Obesity (BMI + TSF)	Behavioral Choice SCT	TX=Classroom curriculum + enhanced PE class + fitness funds + teacher/staff wellness sessions CT=usual health and PE	2 years	TX = Teachers Trained	None mentioned	Sig effect in females, but not males
Harrell et al [44] CHIC	I	Diet PA	ES; 12 schools; 1274 students	BMI; Skinfolds (TSF, SSSF)	Bruhn and Parcel Model	TX=Classroom curriculum + enhanced PE class CT=usual health and PE	8 weeks	TX = Teachers Trained	Written report (child results)	NS
Harrell et al [45] CHIC-Risk	I	Diet PA	ES; 18 schools; 422 students	BMI; Skinfolds (TSF, SSSF)	Bruhn and Parcel Model	TX1=Classroom curriculum + enhanced PE class Tx2=small groups (high risk children only) - PE and/or diet CT=usual health and PE	8 weeks	TX1 = Teachers Tx2 = Teachers + RN Trained	Written report (child results)	NS
Neumark-Sztainer et al [46] NEW MOVES	I	Diet PA	HS; 6 schools; 201 girls (girls only)	BMI	SCT	TX=New Moves program = PA, nutrition, social support (replaced coed PE class) CT=minimal intervention – printed materials	1 semester + 8 week maintenance program	School faculty/staff + research team; school faculty/ staff trained	Postcards (TX only)	NS
Resnicow et al [47] TEACH-WELL	I	Diet	ES; 32 schools; 966 students (cohort)	Skinfolds (TSF, SSSF); Waist/hip	SCT	TX=GIMME-5 curriculum (children) + wellness program (teachers) CT=GIMME-5 curriculum only	2 years	Child TX/CT = Teachers Trained Teacher TX= wellness counselors	None mentioned	NS

Table 1. (Continued)

Author	Type	Focus	Audience	B/Comp Measure	Theory	Intervention Components	Duration	Who	Parent Focus	B/Comp Effect
Robinson [48, 72]	I	SB	ES: 2 schools; 192 students	BMI; Skinfolds (TSF); Waist/hip; Waist circm.	SCT	TX=Classroom curriculum CT=no treatment	6 months	TX=Teachers Trained	Home TV monitors; TV budget; newsletters (TX only)	SIG effect all b/comp measures
Sallis et al [49] SPARK	I	PA	ES: 7 schools; 955 students	Skinfold (TSF; CSF)	None	TX1 and 2=SPARK PE curriculum + PE equipment CT=usual PE + PE equipment	2 years	Tx1=certified PE specialist trained Tx2=PE teacher trained Tx3=PE teacher trained	Homework; weekly newsletters (TX only)	NS
Sahota et al [50, 73] APPLES	E	Diet PA	ES: 10 schools; 634 students	BMI	Health Promoting Schools Philosophy	TX=School action plans to promote diet and PA + changes to school meals + resources CT=usual health curriculum	1 year	TX=Teachers trained	Helped create action plans (TX only)	NS
Sallis et al [51] M-SPAN	E	Diet PA	MS: 24 schools; 1109 students	BMI	Cohen's Structural Ecological Model	TX=enhanced PE curriculum; enhanced opportunities for PA during leisure periods; changes to foods offered at all school sources; policy changes; student health committee; parent education; school incentives; social marketing CT: Not described	2 years	TX=School community, facilitated by research team; teachers and FS staff trained	Parent education; partic. in health policy mtgs. (TX only)	Sig effect for boys, but not girls

Table 1. (Continued)

Author	Type	Focus	Audience	B/Comp Measure	Theory	Intervention Components	Duration	Who	Parent Focus	B/Comp Effect
Caballero et al [53, 74, 75] PATH-WAYS	C	Diet PA	ES; 41 schools; 1704 students	% body fat BMI Skinfolds (TSF, SSSF)	SLT Principles of Am. Ind. Culture and practice Indigenious learning modes	TX=Classroom curriculum + FS modifications + new PE curriculum + family involvement CT=not described	3 years	Teachers and FS staff Annual training	Family action packs; family events at school	NS
Leupker et al [52] CATCH [76, 77]	C	Diet PA	ES; 96 schools; 5106 students	BMI Skinfolds (TSF, SSSF)	SCT Org. Change Model	TX1=classroom curriculum + enhanced PE + FS changes TX2=Tx1 + home curriculum CT=usual health, PE, FS programs	3 years	Teachers + PE specialist Trained	Tx2 only = home activity packets; family fun nights.	NS

Notes: B/comp=body composition; I=individual focus intervention; E=environmental focus intervention; C=combined focus intervention; PA=physical activity; SB=sedentary behavior; ES=elementary school; MS=middle school; HS=high school; BMI=body mass index; TSF=tricep skinfold; SSSF=subscapular skinfold; CSF=calf skinfold; circum=circumference; SCT=Social Cognitive Theory; SLT=Social Learning Theory; Am. Ind.=American Indian; Org=Organizational; TX=treatment; CT=control; PE=physical education; FS=food service; SIG=statistically significant effect; NS=nonstatistically significant effect

Theory

All of the successful interventions were based on a theoretical framework, but the frameworks differed [43, 48, 51]. The two individual focus interventions both utilized Social Cognitive Theory [54] alone [48] or in combination with another theory [43]. The environmental focus intervention [51] was based on Cohen's Structural Ecological Model [55].

Intervention Components

The two individual focus interventions followed a structured curriculum [43, 48]. The environmental focus intervention attempted to change the school culture, by emphasizing structural changes that facilitated healthy diet and physical activity behaviors [51]. For example, the intervention restructured the environment to provide more opportunities and incentives to engage in organized activity during the school day, and it provided health food alternatives within the school environment. Two of the interventions [43, 51] provided funds to help the schools achieve desired changes. One of the interventions [43] also included wellness sessions for classroom teachers and school staff.

Duration

All of the interventions achieving change in body composition had a duration of at least six months [43, 48, 51]. Two of the three interventions had a duration of two academic years [43, 51].

Implementor

The two individual focus interventions were implemented by classroom and/or physical education teachers [43, 48], while the environmental focus intervention was a collaborative effort that included school faculty and staff, students, parents, and members of the research team [51]. All of the successful interventions trained the implementation team [43, 48, 51].

Parent Involvement

Two of the successful interventions involved the parents [48, 51]. In the individual focus program, family members received a "TV budget" along with the child in an effort to reduce sedentary behavior [48]. In the environmental focus intervention [51], parents participated in school health policy meetings and received newsletters providing information on how to support youth diet and physical activity change. Although the remaining individual focus intervention did not mention parents [43], it is likely they were included because the intervention focused on reduction of home television viewing.

Synthesis

No intervention features were identified that separated successful and unsuccessful interventions. Insufficient studies were available to draw a strong conclusion regarding the relative effectiveness of individual vs environmental approaches.

Recommendation

Because of difficulties encountered in identifying interventions evaluated with sufficient methodological rigor to include in this review, it is clear that greater methodological rigor is greatly needed. Therefore, future interventions should adhere to strict research design and statistical analysis methods. Authors of future manuscripts reporting intervention outcomes should follow the reporting guidelines outlined in the CONSORT (for randomized controlled trials) [56] or TREND (for nonrandomized designs) [57] statement. Doing so will help ensure consistency in reporting practices, thereby enabling studies to be more easily compared, and enhancing the ability to identify features of successful interventions.

Conclusion

Individual [43, 48] and environmental [51] focus interventions have demonstrated success at changing body composition in a school setting. However, the lack of consistency in research design, statistical analyses, and reporting practices made it difficult to compare and evaluate the results. Standardized reporting procedures should be implemented to enhance the ease with which intervention studies can be compared and evaluated.

Future Directions

To advance the field and increase the potential effectiveness of school based obesity prevention programs, research needs to occur in several dimensions. These include: the identification and elucidation of effective intervention components; refinement of measurement tools, approaches, and techniques; and a critical examination of our approach to research. Each of these ideas is briefly presented below.

Elucidate Effective Intervention Components

Evidence suggests that in addition to broad based research in which several theories and multiple intervention components are integrated to create a comprehensive intervention, a parallel line of single theory research needs to be established. This single theory research is needed to help identify theoretical frameworks, mechanisms, and intervention components most likely to lead to successful behavior change. This research, in turn, could inform broader-based, more comprehensive interventions. Both of these approaches, single theory and broad based interventions research, are needed to help combat the obesity epidemic.

Mediators are intermediate variables in the pathway between independent and dependent variables and represent the mechanism(s) through which the independent variable exerts its effect on the dependent variable [58-60]. Focusing behavioral research on identifying and understanding how to best influence mediators should enhance the effectiveness of methods to achieve change in the desired direction [58, 61]. Mediation analysis is not common in behavioral research, including research related to school based youth obesity prevention interventions [59, 61]. Designing interventions to effect change in mediators would likely result in targeted, and thereby more effective, interventions.

Refine Measurement Approach, Methods, and Tools

The obesity prevention literature has not demonstrated widespread success in the identification of pathways of effect from intervention to change in body composition [40]. Part of the lack of success may be due to limitations in measurement [62]. The interventions may achieve change in mediators or behaviors, but measurement tools with low reliability and/or validity may mask the changes and lead to inappropriate conclusions regarding intervention effects on body composition, behavior, and mediating variables [62]. Only measurement tools with demonstrated acceptable reliability and validity coefficients for the intended population should be utilized in intervention research [62] and psychometric characteristics of measurement tools should be reported in intervention outcome results [62]. To increase the ease of comparison of intervention effects across diverse interventions, some common measures should be designated that all (or most) school based interventions utilize. A national collaborative body may be necessary to specify such measures. Consideration should also be given to establishment of a clearinghouse of measurement tools with acceptable reliability and validity coefficients, from which researchers could select, as well as the establishment of item pools from which tools specific to populations could be created [63]. Computer adaptive testing offers an innovative method for collecting highly valid and reliable data, while reducing participant burden [64, 65]. Item response theory can be used to create item pools that are valid measures of underlying constructs [63, 66].

Critically Examine Approach to Research

Much of the variance in diet, physical activity, and sedentary behavior is unexplained by current theories and models [40]. Therefore, current theories and conceptual models guiding behavioral research need to be critically examined [67]. Obesity is a multi-faceted problem, affected by a multitude of factors [68]. It is likely that effective solutions will need to take a broad-based approach and draw from a number of different disciplines and fields. Therefore, theories and conceptual models from other fields, such as developmental psychology, communication, marketing, parenting, and informatics, need to be examined and incorporated into multidisciplinary theoretical frameworks with which to approach the underlying issues and create innovative, more likely to be effective, interventions.

Greater effort also needs to be placed on the translation of behavioral research from the laboratory setting to applied settings that have the potential for a broad public health impact, such as in the school setting. For example, laboratory research may identify effective methods for helping youth become successful problem solvers. Incorporating this knowledge into school based obesity prevention programs is the logical application of this research, particularly since it is well-recognized that youth perceive problems when attempting to engage in healthy behaviors, such as being physically active [69, 70] or eating healthy [71]. Also, because so much attention is currently being focused on the youth obesity epidemic and extensive research in this area is currently being conducted, it is critical that non-significant, as well as significant, outcomes be published in an effort to eliminate duplication of effort, spur the generation of new ideas, and enhance the potential for collaboration among researchers.

Significance

Based on the current literature, there appears to be no relative advantage to individual, environmental, or combined focus programs in the school environment. Although few conclusions could be drawn, this review highlights the paucity of effective studies and emphasizes the need for consistency in reporting practices, as well as a critical examination of the methods guiding current research practices. Halting the youth obesity epidemic sweeping the nation is a daunting task. It is only with the willingness to take a critical look at the field and the manner in which school based research is designed, implemented, and reported will a solution to the problem be identified. This chapter outlines a plan for achieving this goal. It is clear that more research is necessary to provide insight into factors needed to develop effective school based obesity prevention interventions.

Acknowledgement

This research was largely funded in by a grant from the National Institutes of Health (NIH 5 R21 CA102470). This work is a publication of the United States Department of Agriculture (USDA/ARS) Children's Nutrition Research Center, Department of Pediatrics, Baylor College of Medicine, Houston, Texas and was funded in part by federal funds from the USDA/ARS under Cooperative Agreement No. 58-6250-6001. The contents of this publication do not necessarily reflect the views or policies of the USDA, nor does mention of trade names, commercial products, or organizations imply endorsement from the US government.

References

[1]   Troiano, R.P., et al., Overweight prevalence and trends for children and adolescents. *Archives of Pediatric Adolescent Medicine*, 1995. 149: p. 1085-1091.

[2]   Centers for Disease Control and Prevention. NCHS - Health E Stats - Prevalence of Overweight Among Children and Adolescents: United States, 1999-2000. Available: *http://www.cdc.gov/nchs/products/pubs/pubd/hestats/overwght99.htm.* Downloaded 8/16/01.

[3]   Serdula, M.K., et al., Do obese children become obese adults? a review of the literature. *Preventive Medicine,* 1993. 22: p. 167-177.

[4] Dietz, W.H., Health consequences of obesity in youth: childhood predictors of adult disease. *Pediatrics*, 1998. 101: p. 518-525.

[5] Kraig, K.A. and P.K. Keel, Weight-based stigmatization in children. *International Journal of Obesity*, 2001. 25: p. 1661-1666.

[6] Sallis, J.F., J.J. Prochaska, and W.C. Taylor, A review of correlates of physical activity of children and adolescents. *Medicine and Science in Sports and Exercise*, 2000. 32: p. 963-975.

[7] Kaplan, K.M. and T.A. Wadden, Childhood obesity and self-esteem. *Journal of Pediatrics*, 1986. 109: p. 367-370.

[8] Rippe, J.M., et al., Improved psychological well-being, quality of life, and health practices in moderately overweight women participating in a 12-week structured weight loss program. *Obesity Research,* 1998. 6: p. 208-218.

[9] Epstein, L.H., et al., Treatment of Pediatric Obesity. Pediatrics, 1998. 101: p. 554-570.

[10] Lloyd, T., et al., Fruit consumption, fitness, and cardiovascular health in female adolescents: the Penn State Young Women's Health Study. *American Journal of Clinical Nutrition*, 1998. 67: p. 624-630.

[11] Cullen, K., et al., Anthropometric, parental, and psychosocial correlates of dietary intake of African American girls. *Obesity Research*, 2004. 12(supplement): p. 20S-31S.

[12] Miller, W., et al., Dietary fat, sugar, and fiber predict body fat content. *Journal of the American Dietetic Association*, 1994. 94: p. 612-615.

[13] Tucker, L., G. Seljaas, and R. Hager, Body fat percentage of children varies according to their diet composition. *Journal of the American Dietetic Association*, 1997. 97: p. 981-986.

[14] Ludwig, D., K. Peterson, and S. Gortmaker, Relation between consumption of sugar-sweetened drinks and childhood obesity: a prospective, observational analysis. *Lancet*, 2001. 357: p. 505-508.

[15] Davies, P., J. Gregory, and A. White, Physical activity and body fatness in pre-school children. *International journal of Obesity Related Metabolic Disorders*, 1995. 19: p. 6-10.

[16] Berkowitz, R., et al., Physical activity and adiposity: a longitudinal study from birth to childhood. *Journal of Pediatrics,* 1985. 106: p. 734-738.

[17] Gortmaker, S., W. Dietz, and L. Cheung, Inactivity, diet and the fattening of America. *Journal of the American Dietetic Association*, 1990. 90: p. 1247-1252, 1255.

[18] Kronenberg, F., et al., Influence of leisure time physical activity and television watching on atherosclerosis risk factors in the NHLBI Family Heart Study. *Atherosclerosis*, 2000. 153: p. 433-43.

[19] Krebs-Smith, S., A. Cook, and A. Subar, Fruit and vegetable intakes of children and adolescents in the United States. *Archives of Pediatric Adolescent Medicine*, 1996. 150: p. 81-6.

[20] Morton, J. and J. Guthrie, Changes in children's total fat intakes and their food group sources of fat, 1989-1991 versus 1994-1995: implications for diet quality. *Family Economics and Nutrition Review*, 1998. 11(3): p. 44-57.

[21] Harnack, L., J. Stang, and M. Story, Soft drink consumption among US children and adolescents: Nutritional consequences. *Journal of the American Dietetic Association,* 1999. 99: p. 436-441.

[22] Stein, A., et al., Variability and tracking of nutrient intakes of preschool children based on multible administrations of the 24-hour dietary recall. *American Journal of Epidemiology,* 1991. 134: p. 1427-37.

[23] Singer, M., et al., The tracking of nutrient intake in young children: the Framingham Children's Study. *American Journal of Public Health,* 1995. 85: p. 1673-7.

[24] Resnicow, K., et al., 2-year tracking of children's fruit and vegetable intake. *Journal of the American Dietetic Association,* 1998. 98: p. 785-9.

[25] Kelder, S., et al., Longitudinal tracking of adolescent smoking, physical activity, and food choice behaviors. *American Journal of Public Health,* 1994. 84: p. 1121-6.

[26] United States Department of Health and Human Services. Healthy People 2000: national health promotion and disease prevention objectives. *DHHS Publication No. (PHS) 91-50212.* Washington, DC. Government Printing Office, 2000.

[27] Raynor, H., L. Epstein, and C. Gordy, Effects of increased fruits and vegetables and decreasing high-fat and/or high sugar during obesity treatment. *Annals of Behavioral Medicine,* 1999. 21(Supplement): p. S-019.

[28] Subar, A., et al., The 1987 National Health Interview Survey. *Amerian Journal of Public Health,* 1994. 84: p. 359-366.

[29] Keenan, D., et al., Use of qualitative and quantitative methods to define behavioral fat reduction strategies and their relationship to dietary fat reduction in the patterns of dietary change study. *Journal of the American Dietetic Association,* 1996. 96(1245-1250).

[30] Kristal, A., A. Shattuck, and H. Henry, Patterns of dietary behavior associated with selecting diets low in fat: reliability and validity of a behavioral approach to dietary assessment. *Journal of the American Dietetic Association,* 1990. 90: p. 214-20.

[31] Forshee, R. and M. Storey, Associations of adequate intake of calcium with diet, beverage consumption, and demographic characteristics among children and adolescents. *Journal of American College of Nutrition,* 2004. 23: p. 18-33.

[32] Sallis, J.F. and K. Patrick, Physical activity guidelines for adolescents: consensus statement. *Pediatric Exercise Science,* 1994. 6: p. 302-314.

[33] Centers for Disease Control and Prevention. CDC Surveillance Summaries. Youth Risk Behavior Surveillance - United States, 1999; *MMWR,* 49(SS-5), June 9, 2000.

[34] Pate, R.R., B.J. Long, and G. Heath, Descriptive epidemiology of physical activity in adolescents. *Pediatric Exercise Science,* 1994. 6: p. 434-447.

[35] Sallis, J.F., Epidemiology of physical activity and fitness in children and adolescents. *Critical Reviews in Food Science and Nutrition,* 1993. 33: p. 403-408.

[36] Pate, R.R., et al., Associations between physical activity and other health behaviors in a representative sample of US adolescents. *American Journal of Public Health,* 1996. 86(11): p. 1577-1581.

[37] Jago, R., et al., Relationship between physical activity and diet among African-American girls. *Obesity Research,* 2004. 12 Supplement: p. 55S-63S.

[38] Taylor, W., et al., Healthy Growth: project description and baseline findings. *Ethnicity and Disease*, 2002. 12: p. 567-77.

[39] Lowry, R., et al., Television viewing and its associations with overweight, sedentary lifestyle, and insufficient consumption of fruits and vegetables among US high school students: differences by race, ethnicity, and gender. *Journal of School Health*, 2002. 72(10): p. 413-421.

[40] Baranowski, T., et al., School-based obesity prevention: a blueprint for taming the epidemic. *American Journal of Health Behavior*, 2002. 26: p. 486-93.

[41] Resnicow, K. and T. Robinson, School-Based Cardiovascular Disease Prevention Studies: Review and Synthesis. *Annals of Epidemiology*, 1997. S7: p. S14-S31.

[42] Hooks, P., et al., Social networking as a recruitment strategy for Mexican American families in community health research. *Hispanic Journal of Behavioral Sciences*, 1986. 8: p. 345-55.

[43] Gortmaker, S., et al., Reducing obesity via a school-based interdisciplinary intervention among youth: Planet Health. *Archives of Pediatric Adolescent Medicine*, 1999. 153(4): p. 409-418.

[44] Harrell, J., et al., Effects of a school-based intervention to reduce cardiovascular disease risk factors in elementary-school children: The Cardiovascular Health in Children (CHIC) Study. *Journal of Pediatrics*, 1996. 128: p. 797-805.

[45] Harrell, J., et al., School-based interventions improve heart health in children with multiple cardiovascular disease risk factors. *Pediatrics*, 1998. 102: p. 371-380.

[46] Neumark-Sztainer, D., et al., New Moves: a school-based obesity prevention program for adolescent girls. *Preventive Medicine*, 2003. 37: p. 41-51.

[47] Resnicow, K., et al., Results of the TeachWell Worksite Wellness Program. *American Journal of Public Health*, 1998. 88: p. 250-257.

[48] Robinson, T., Reducing children's television viewing to prevent obesity. *Journal of the American Medical Association*, 1999. 282: p. 1561-67.

[49] Sallis, J.F., et al., The effects of a 2-year physical education program (SPARK) on physical activity and fitness in elementary school students. *American Journal of Public Health*, 1997. 87(8): p. 1328-1334.

[50] Sahota, P., et al., Randomized controlled trial of primary school based intervention to reduce risk factors for obesity. *British Medical Journal*, 2001. 323: p. 1-5.

[51] Sallis, J., et al., Environmental interventions for eating and physical activity: a randomized controlled trial in middle schools. *American Journal of Preventive Medicine*, 2003. 24: p. 209-217.

[52] Leupker, R., et al., Outcomes of a field trial to improve children's dietary patterns and physical activity: The Child and Adolescent Trial for Cardiovascular Health (CATCH). *Journal of the American Medical Association*, 1996. 275: p. 768-776.

[53] Caballero, B., et al., Pathways: a school-based, randomized controlled trial for the prevention of obesity in American Indian schoolchildren. *American Journal of Clinical Nutrition*, 2003. 78: p. 1030-8.

[54] Bandura, A., *Social Foundations of Thought and Action: A Social Cognitive Theory.* 1986, Englewood Cliffs, NJ: Prentice Hall.

[55] Cohen, D., R. Scribner, and T. Farley, A structural model of health behavior: a pragmatic approach to explain and influence health behaviors at the population level. *Preventive Medicine*, 2000. 30: p. 146-54.

[56] Begg, C., et al., Improving the quality of reporting of randomized controlled trials. The CONSORT statement. *Journal of the American Medical Association*, 1996. 276: p. 637-9.

[57] Des Jarlais, D., et al., Improving the reporting quality of nonrandomized evaluations of behavioral and public health interventions: the TREND statement. *American Journal of Public Health*, 2004. 94: p. 361-6.

[58] Baranowski, T., et al., Theory as mediating variables: why aren't community interventions working as desired? *Annals of Epidemiology*, 1997. S7: p. S89-S95.

[59] Bauman, A.E., et al., Toward a better understanding of the influences on physical activity: the role of determinants, correlates, causal variables, mediators, moderators, and confounders. *American Journal of Preventive Medicine*, 2002. 23(2S): p. 5-14.

[60] Baron, R.M. and D.A. Kenny, The moderator-mediator variable distinction in social psychological research: conceptual, strategic, and statistical consideration. *Journal of Personality and Social Psychology*, 1986. 51(6): p. 1173-1182.

[61] Baranowski, T., C. Anderson, and C. Carmack, Mediating variable framework in physical activity interventions: How are we doing? How might we do better? *American Journal of Preventive Medicine*, 1998. 15(4): p. 266-297.

[62] Baranowski, T., et al., Measurement of outcomes, mediators, and moderators in behavioral obesity prevention research. *Preventive Medicine*, 2004. 38: p. S1-13.

[63] Hays, R., L. Morales, and S. Reise, Item response theory and health outcomes measurement in the 21st century. *Medical Care*, 2000. 38(9 supplement): p. I128-42.

[64] Ware, J., et al., Applications of computerized adaptive testing (CAT) to the assessment of headache impact. *Quality of Life Research*, 2003. 12: p. 935-52.

[65] Gardner, W., et al., Computerized adaptive measurement of depression: a simulation study. *BMC Psychiatry*, 2004. 4: p. 13.

[66] Bjorner, J., M. Kosinski, and J. Ware, Calibration of an item pool for assessing the burden of headaches: an application of item response theory to the headache impact test (HIT). *Quality of Life Research*, 2003. 12: p. 913-33.

[67] Baranowski, T., et al., Are current health behavioral change models helpful in guiding prevention of weight gain efforts? *Obesity Research*, 2003. Supplement: p. 23S-43S.

[68] Goran, M.I. and M.S. Treuth, Energy expenditure, physical activity, and obesity in children. *Pediatric Clinics of North America*, 2001. 48(4): p. 931-953.

[69] Tappe, M.K., J.L. Duda, and P.M. Ehrnwald, Perceived barriers to exercise among adolescents. *Journal of School Health*, 1989. 59(4): p. 153-155.

[70] Allison, K.R., J.J.M. Dwyer, and S. Makin, Perceived barriers to physical activity among high school students. *Preventive Medicine*, 1999. 28: p. 608-615.

[71] Lytle, L., et al., Predicting adolescents' intake of fruit and vegetables. *Journal of Nutrition Education and Behavior*, 2003. 35: p. 170-5.

[72] Robinson, T., Can a school-based intervention to reduce television use decrease adiposity in children in grades 3 and 4? *Western Journal of Medicine*, 2000. 173: p. 40.

[73] Sahota, P., et al., Evaluation of implementation and effect of primary school based intervention to reduce risk factors for obesity. *British Medical Journal,* 2001. 323: p. 1-4.

[74] Davis, C., et al., Design and statistical analysis for the Pathways study. *American Journal of Clinical Nutrition,* 1999. 69(supplement): p. 760S-3S.

[75] Lohman, T., et al., Indices of changes in adiposity in American Indian children. *Preventive Medicine,* 2003. 37: p. S91-96.

[76] Lytle, L., et al., Changes in nutrient intakes of elementary school children following a school-based intervention: results of the CATCH study. *Preventive Medicine,* 1996. 25: p. 465-477.

[77] McKenzie, T., et al., Effects of the CATCH physical education intervention: teacher type and lesson location. *American Journal of Preventive Medicine,* 2001. 21: p. 101-09.

In: Nutrition Research at the Leading Edge
Editors: R. E. Cassady, E. I. Tidswell, pp. 175-189

ISBN: 978-1-60456-053-4
© 2008 Nova Science Publishers, Inc.

Chapter VI

Defining the Role of Saturated Fat in Carbohydrate Restricted Diets

James H. Hays[1],* Angela DiSabatmo[1], and K.M. Mohamed Shakir[2]
[1] Cardiovascular Research, Christiana Care Health System, Newark,
Delaware 19718; USA
[2] Endocrinology and Metabolism Department, National Naval Medical Center, Bethesda,
Maryland 20889-5600. USA

Abstract

Studies have shown elevated LDL cholesterol and other adverse responses with the addition of saturated fat to an otherwise balanced diet. Epidemiological studies have suggested that these adverse markers correlate with real adverse outcomes. There are, however, few studies documenting the effect of saturated fat intake in the face of carbohydrate restriction on markers of cardiovascular disease and, of course, there are no outcome studies. We will review the available data, including our own, and provide historic, epidemiological and physiologic reasons why the continuous intake of saturated fat may be needed to maximize the health benefits of a carbohydrate restricted diet.

The present epidemic of obesity could be related to the availability of excess food and the ability or need to decrease exercise. Humans appear to be better suited to avoid starvation than to avoid obesity when food is plentiful. Certainly some, and perhaps most, humans are programmed to overeat if possible. Clearly some escape obesity, however, and there are powerful physiologic controls on caloric balance suggesting that it should be possible to select a diet from abundance that will result in satiety or at least satisfaction, and result in healthy body weight. If this diet also improved survival from chronic illnesses like cancer, Type 2 diabetes mellitus and atherosclerotic cardiovascular disease, it could be considered an

---

* Correspondence concerning this article should be addressed to Dr. James H. Hays, M.D., FACP FACE, Cardiovascular Research, Christiana Health System, Newark, DE 19718, USA.

optimal diet. It would be the answer to the question; if we can eat anything, what should we eat? Surprisingly, the answer to this question may include a lot of saturated fat.

Over the last ten years, the principal author has prescribed a diet that advocates progressively increasing amounts of saturated fat primarily from red meat coupled with progressively more rigorous carbohydrate restriction. The primary motivation for this was to improve glycemic control in Type 2 diabetics and decrease insulin requirements in patients with Type 1 diabetes mellitus. When patients who adhered to the diet lost weight, it generated much excitement in those patients and certainly in the prescriber.

But would this prescription result in long-term deterioration of markers of glycemic control and cardiovascular disease? Because the patients could be closely followed and because of the availability of conventional therapy, particularly statins, that might be expected to minimize adverse effects, we observed patients with Type 2 diabetes mellitus for one year of follow-up after diet prescription [1]. Weight loss did not appear to be associated with deterioration in either glycemic control or serum markers of cardiovascular disease. A small prospective study seemed to confirm these observations [2] but we hasten to add that the lipid response to the diet appears to be complex [3]. It will not take long to review the preliminary data we have collected. It will also not take long to note other studies which show results of other carbohydrate restricted diets. No studies have long-term follow-up or hard endpoints like mortality or myocardial infarction. The data alone is suggestive but not convincing. We will therefore begin with a brief historical, epidemiological and physiological perspective to help the reader to understand why we are investigating a diet that has been said to defy "common sense" [4].

Comparison of gene sequences from diverse human populations suggests that we have descended from a group that left Africa as late as 50,000 years ago [5]. As we spread throughout the planet over the next 40,000 years, there was a remarkable decline in populations of mega fauna and archiological data supports the concept that this decline could be attributed to the efficiency of human hunters [6]. There seems to be widespread agreement that prehistoric humans ate predominantly meat but it should also be noted that zoological evaluation of modern humans clearly classifies us as predators [7]. The rise of agriculture over the last 10,000 years has changed our diets but not our physiology. It has been suggested that our conversion from hunter-gatherers to agrarians was one of necessity and was actually associated with a decline in longevity [8]. The progression of this process, however, has brought industrialized populations to a point where agriculture and animal husbandry make many foods available in abundance. Indigenous peoples across a broad range of cultures who have continued their hunter-gatherer or subsistence farming lifestyles longer than other humans may be particularly adept at avoiding starvation and equally adept at becoming obese when the food supply increases [9]. Our recent common genetic heritage, coupled with the overwhelming nature of the obesity epidemic, suggest that if changes in diet composition could be shown beneficial, then those recommendations could be made broadly.

Cardiovascular disease has long been the number one cause of death in most populations [10]. Epidemiological evidence that the extent of saturated fat intake in geographically diverse populations predicted an increased rate of cardiovascular disease convinced many that dietary intake of saturated fat should be restricted [11]. Studies linking serum risk factors, particularly LDL cholesterol levels, to morbidity and mortality [12,13] coupled with data showing adding dietary saturated fat increased serum LDL levels [14,15] put the nail in the coffin for most. The recognition that diabetic patients prescribed a carbohydrate restricted high fat diet were still dying of cardiovascular disease at an alarming rate led to recommendation of saturated fat restriction in this ever growing group also [16]. There are problems with these conclusions, however.

First, clear epidemiological evidence of increasing obesity when endogenous populations adopt a western diet could be blamed on increased intake of non-nutritive carbohydrate rather than saturated fat alone [17]. Other epidemiological observations suggest a high saturated fat diet may be amazingly cardioprotective. Indigenous people of Greenland appear to have little cardiovascular disease and almost no atheroscherosis. They have a uniquely favorable lipid profile and an antithrombogenic state [18].

These people were consuming an extremely high fat diet and the fact that chewed whale skin could provide vitamin C in their diets speaks to the avidity of their carbohydrate restriction [19] High intake of omega-3 fatty acids has been credited with these effects [20]. Interestingly, as this indigenous people is over run with abundance, maintaining intake of seal meat was the dietary factor most closely related to maintaining their beneficial cardiovascular profile [21] Dietary omega-3 fatty acids appear to be provided by consumption of marine mammals rather then deep water fish. Could it be possible that the saturated fat itself has an independent benefit?

The evidence that serum low density lipoprotein levels relate to the incidence of cardiovascular disease is clear. There remain other risk factors, however. LDL levels are similar in matched populations that do and do not have cardiovascular disease [22]. Diabetics [23], pre-diabetics, those with dysmetabolic syndrome [24],appear to have risk beyond that predicted by their LDL levels alone. The recent re-evaluation of the Whitehall data which correlated increased cardiovascular rates of events with increased levels of hemoglobin A1C that were well within the "normal range" [25] indicate that perhaps glucose levels are a more sensitive marker of cardiovascular disease than LDL levels. When we wonder, "how low should we go?" perhaps we should be thinking of glucose rather than LDL.

Finally, although adding saturated fat to a high carbohydrate diet will raise serum LDL levels, no study has linked total fat or saturated fat intake with adverse cardiovascular outcome [26]. Most importantly, there are very few observations of serum risk factors, let alone outcome studies, in which fat intake is increased in the face of carbohydrate restriction. One intriguing metabolic ward study done with liquid diets showed lowest LDL levels were observed when stearic acid was substituted for carbohydrate [27].

Several studies reported improvement in glycemic control and serum risk factors in patients with Type 2 diabetes mellitus when monounsaturated fat replaced carbohydrate in their diets [28-35]. It was difficult to implement these recommendations in clinical practice, however. The sources of monounsaturated fat are limited and it was difficult for patients to approach the level of 30% of total calories from these foods that seemed needed to achieve the results reported in the studies. We began suggesting the lay publication The Zone [36] to patients for practical guidance about a high monounsaturated starch restricted diet. We were still not satisfied. In 1995, as we gradually added saturated fat and eliminated starch from diets of patients, we saw weight loss without obvious deterioration in glycemic control or serum risk factors for cardiovascular disease (Table 1) [1]. Statistical analysis showed much of the weight loss could be attributed to changes in glycemic therapy but neither these changes nor changes in lipid lowering therapy appeared to exclude beneficial effects of the diet per se on weight loss as well as on serum total cholesterol levels. We were able to complete a six week prospective study in patients with dysmetabolic syndrome and documented atherosclerotic cardiovascular disease whose low density lipoprotein levels had been treated to 100 mg/dL or less with statins prior to entry in the study [2]. Several changes suggested an improved cardiovascular risk profile in the patients (Table 2). Why did adding saturated fat reduce weight yet fail to worsen serum markers of cardiovascular disease? Unfortunately, we can only speculate why these changes were observed.

Table 1. Showing Effect of High Saturated Fat-Starch Avoidance Diet in Patients with Type 2 Diabetes Mellitus

	Diet			
	The Zone (n=132)		High Saturated Fat Starch Avoidance (n = 151)	
Months	0	12	0	12
Weight (Kg)	91.8±24	94.0±25	91.7±49	86.9±23*
HgA1C (%)	8.79±1.8	7.86±1.7	9.34±2.3	6.95±1.5*
Triglycerides (mg/dL)	203±144	207±160	229±169	183±194
Cholesterol (mg/dL)	226±67	215±47	231±12.3	190±6.0*
HDL Cholesterol (mg/dL)	44±25	42±12	43±14	47±15
LDL Cholesterol (mg/dL)	139±45	131±37	133±42	105±38

All mean ± standard deviation. Data analyzed by multiple regression with difference from baselines regressed against elapsed time and amount of time on drugs with dummy variable representing diet groups [1]. *$p<0.05$ vs groups for effect of diet not related to changes in hypoglycemic or lipid lowering therapy. n = number of patients studied.

It has been our observation that the primary mechanism promoting weight loss is satiety [1]. The prospective study also suggested this mechanism [2]. With the emergence of the obesity epidemic, the concept of carbohydrate restriction has become a hot topic and the diet prescription of Dr. R.C. Atkins has finally been put to the test [37-40] after 40 years of casual and often vitriolic dismissal [41] The results show modest sustained weight loss and improvements in some risk factors for cardiovascular disease (Tables 3A and 3B). We have included in this analysis what we consider other versions of Dr. Atkins' diet as outlined in the popular books *Protein Power* [42] and *The South Beach Diet* [43]. All of these diet prescriptions share carbohydrate restriction and come to relatively similar recommendations about what carbohydrates to eat or avoid. Dr. Atkins' prescription was the one which openly advocated high saturated fat but this was only a temporary induction technique designed to induce ketosis and weight loss [44]. It was not intended to be maintained and ultimately patients were to consume a relatively low saturated fat diet. This position has recently been reiterated by the Atkins Institute [45]. Recent observations indicate Dr. Atkins' diet may also result in weight loss via a reduction in caloric intake [46].

Table 2. Showing the Effect of High Saturated Fat-Starch Avoidance Fat on Weight, Serum Glucose, Insulin and Lipids

	n=23		
	0 Weeks	6 Weeks	(p)
Weight (Kg)	113±19.5	107.5±18.9	<0.001
Waist (Inches)	48.4±5.1	46.2±4.7	<0.001
Body Fat (%)	37.3±5.9	36.6±6.3	0.02
Glucose (mg/dL)	106.1±17.7	98.3±9.3	0.04
Insulin (μIU/ml)	21.3±13.2	14.8±5.7	0.006
Triglycerides (mg/dL)	146.2±82.6	87.8±41.4	<0.001
Cholesterol (mg/dL)	167.9±84.9	161.1±41.4	0.48
HDL (mg/dL)	44.1±11.8	42.8±12.8	0.31
LDL (mg/dL)	100.5±27.3	103.6±38.9	0.64

Results of six week prospective study of patients with documented atherosclerotic coronary artery disease prescribed a high saturated fat starch avoidance diet. (p) comparison of baseline versus final observation [2]. n = number of patients studied.

Table 3A. Effect of Other Carbohydrate Restricted Diets on Weight

Study	Westman E.C. [51]	Foster G.D., et al [52]	Samoha F.F., et al [53]	Brehm B.J., et al [54]
Diet	Atkins	Atkins	Protein Power	Atkins
Duration	6 Months	12 Months	6 Months	6 Months
Control	None	Low Fat Diet	Low Fat Diet	Low Fat Diet
Weight Loss (Kg)	-9.0±5.3*	-4.4±6.7	-5.8±8.6**	8.5±1.0**
n (Completed Study)	51(41)	63(49)	132(79)	53(42)

There is reason to postulate that saturated fat intake could produce satiety. Saturated fat is known to delay gastric emptying. This effect may be mediated in part by gastrointestinal hormones like gastric inhibitory polypeptides and cholecystokinin [47]. Stearic acid, the primary saturated fatty acid in red meat, has a unique ability to stimulate insulin secretion [48]. There may even be a synergistic effect of cosecretion of cholecystokinin and insulin on brain satiety centers [49]. To maximize these potential effects, our patients are advised to always consume saturated fat as the first part of the meal. Unlike Dr. Atkins, we have insisted on an ongoing intake of limited portions of certain fresh fruits and non starchy vegetables. Ketonuria is carefully avoided in diabetic patients and is discouraged in non-diabetic subjects. We do not believe ketosis has played a significant role in weight loss associated with a high saturated fat starch avoidance diet although it is difficult to exclude increases in ketone levels below our level of detection. The study of Lewis et al suggests that ketosis adds little or nothing to weight loss versus calorie restriction alone [50]. At present, we postulate no "metabolic advantage" of this diet but attribute weight loss to satiety alone.

Table 3B. Effect of Other Carbohydrate Restricted Diets on Serum Lipids

	Westman E.C. [51]		Foster G.D., et al [52]		Samoha F.F., et al [53]		Brehm B.J., et al [54]	
	Baseline	Final	Baseline	Final[+]	Baseline	Final	Baseline	Final
Triglycerides (mg/dL)	130±62	74±33*	131.1±113.8	-17.0±13**	88±176	150±171**	148.7±13.4	113.9±15.3
Cholesterol (mg/dL)	214±35	203±42*	200.5±33.5	+0.1±9	181±52	184±48	296.3±6.6	205.5±6.8
LDL (mg/dL)	136±32	126±34*	129.5±30.0	+0.31±16.6	114±29	118±40	124.9±5.4	124.0±5.8
HDL (mg/dL)	52±14	62±15*	46.8±11.2	+11.0±19.4**	41±11	41±10	51.8±2.9	58.7±2.6

All values are means ± standard deviation except for final values in study of Foster et al [+]. These authors reported only changes (shown as mean ± SD) but did not report absolute values [37-40, 40A].

* = p <0.05 versus baseline. **= p <0.05 versus control group.

The lipid changes seen with the high saturated fat starch avoidance diet seem to parallel those reported in the studies with the Atkins diet [37-40]. If the decreases in serum triglyceride, glucose and insulin levels can be sustained, benefits might be expected. Our observations of improved glycemic control in patients with Type 2 diabetes mellitus and a suggestion of improved insulin sensitivity in non-diabetics has now been reported with the Atkins diet [46]. However, prior concerns of the effects of dietary saturated fat on serum cholesterol levels [51,52] require us to pay special attention to them. Why didn't low density lipoprotein levels rise?

Lipids are transported in aqueous serum as lipoproteins, a complex arrangement of triglycerides, cholesterol and proteins. Different lipoproteins have different functions and very different relationships to the incidence of cardiovascular disease. The gastrointestinal tract absorbs fat and cholesterol and packages it in chylomicrons whose characteristic apo protein is Apo B 47. Except in rare genetic syndromes or severe insulin deficiency, chylomicrons remain in the circulation only briefly after a meal. The post-prandial rise in triglycerides may have implications for cardiovascular risk [53] and may be associated with alterations in vascular endothelial function [54] that also could contribute to additional risk but no study has linked cardiovascular outcome with serum chylomicrons or Apo B 47 levels. Rather, the large convincing outcome studies have used fasting serum low density lipoprotein levels where 95% of the level does not reflect lipids directly absorbed from the diet but rather reflects the lipids "repackaged" by the liver associated with the lipoprotein Apo B 100. The liver produces Apo B 100 in response to free fatty acids and possibly to excess glucose to form triglycerides and releases these into the circulation as VLDL. The rate limiting factor in this production is activity of the hepatic enzyme Acetyl-CoA carboxylase [55]. The more fatty acids and glucose provided, the more VLDL is released into the circulation. It is only after intravascular processing that VLDL is transformed into denser, and more atherogenic, LDL. Thus it is not surprising that most carbohydrate restricted diet reports decreases in serum triglycerides. An accompanied increase in HDL cholesterol could be expected [56], and might especially add to an antiatherogenic effect, but it should be remembered that triglyceride levels alone are predictive of cardiovascular outcome if low enough limits are applied [57].

Although reducing VLDL production, and thus circulating Apo B 100 levels, might be expected to have beneficial effects, it must also be noted that some subtypes of VLDL and LDL have been suggested to be more atherogenic than others. In particular, small dense LDL and smaller HDL particles are suggested to be associated with atherogenesis [58,59]. If dietary manipulation had improved total VLDL and total LDL levels but also increased the concentrations of more atherogenic subtypes of these particles, there would be cause for concern. Our prospective study did not reveal adverse effects in patients who were with statins prior to dietary change [2] (Table 4).

We hasten to caution that one of the 23 patients in our study had a marked increase in LDL levels of 173 mg/dL to 291 mg/dL. We could detect no difference in dietary intake or statin compliance in this patient. We considered him a "hyperabsorber" and instructed him to stop the diet. Interestingly, Yancy et al [60] recently reported exclusion of two of 35 patients following the Atkin's diet because of adverse effects on serum lipids. We currently believe that approximately one in 20 or more may hyperabsorb cholesterol despite carbohydrate restriction and suggest close monitoring of serum lipids in patients on the diet.

Table 4. Showing Effect of High Saturated Fat-Starch Avoidance Diet on Serum Lipids

	0 Weeks	6 Weeks	(p)
LDL			
Number	1156±340.9	1122.9±368.2	0.68
Size (nm)	20.6±0.9	21.0±0.7	0.02
Medium (mg/dL)	37.9±26.4	26.6±27.9	0.31
Small (mg/dL)	35.4±39.5	26.6±27.9	0.31
VLDL			
Triglyceride (mg/dL)	113.5±81.2	57.4±43.9	< .001
Size (nm)	54.6±6.6	45.6±7.3	< .001
Large (mg/dL)	51.2±45.5	13.6±20.5	< .001
Medium (mg/dL)	40.2±38.6	15.4±13.3	< .001
Small (mg/dL)	17.6±11.0	15.4±13.3	0.54
HDL			
Size (nm)	8.61±0.39	8.77±0.42	0.01
Large (mg/dL)	19.9±12.2	19.5±12.0	0.76
Small (mg/dL)	23.5±4.4	22.6±38	0.26

Nuclear magnetic resonance spectroscopic analysis of serum lipids before and after high saturated fat starch avoidance diet. Despite pretreatment with statins to LDL levels less than 100, 10 of 23 patients had a metabolic syndrome profile before the diet. Eight of these 10 changed to a low risk profile. One low risk profile changed to high risk (see text) [2].

The recent availability of the drug ezetimibe has allowed us to make further observations. Because ezetimibe inhibits gastrointestinal cholesterol absorption it has an additive effect in patients on statins, which increase hepatic clearance of LDL. It appears to achieve an approximate 10% or more decrease in total LDL levels when added to statin therapy [61]. We prefer statins as first line therapy in patients with cardiovascular risk. They have a proven track record and even decrease cardiovascular risk even in patients with normal serum lipid levels [62]. There are, however, complications associated with statin therapy. Hepatotoxicity occurs in les than 2% of patients receiving statins [63]. Myositis occurs at a rate of 0.05% [64]. Unfortunately for the medical practitioner, the incidence of abnormal liver enzymes and elevated CPK levels, for reasons unrelated to statin therapy, is quite high. It is also important to note some patients have been shown to have myositis without CPK elevation [65]. An ever more informed patient often refuses statin therapy and an ever more worried practitioner is reluctant to prescribe them. If a patient has an adverse response to the high saturated fat starch avoidance diet, we decrease dietary cholesterol by eliminating eggs and shellfish from the diet. We have seen modest responses to this but then suggest statin therapy. We now have limited experience prescribing ezetimibe as a solitary agent in patients who had relatively contraindications to statin therapy (Table 5) [3]. It appears that most patients can be treated with statins to achieve acceptable lipid levels and it is intriguing to speculate that ezetimibe may be especially helpful in the subpopulation that "hyperabsorbs" cholesterol from the diet. Combined therapy would be predicted to be even more effective. Limited observations in patients not treated with lipid lowering drugs suggests the high saturated fat starch avoidance diet is lipid neutral (Table 6) but once again, we would predict an adverse response in up to 20%.

Table 5. Serum Lipid Changes During High Saturated Fat - Starch Avoidance Diet (HSFSA)*, Diet + Statins** and HSFSA + Zetia***.

	Diet	Diet + Statins	Diet + Zetia
BMI	29.7±3	26.6±2.5	28±2.5
Serum Cholesterol	252±24	359±37	218±12
Triglyceride	165±51	104±36	86±41
HDL-C	39±6	59±10	59±9
LDL-C	180±20	278±41	142±11
VLDL-C	33±10	21±7	17±8.08

HDL-C = High Density Lipoprotein Cholesterol; LDL-C = Low Density Lipoprotein Cholesterol; VLDL-C = Very Low-Density. Lipoprotein Cholesterol; Values represent mean ± SEM. *Diet = HSFSA; **Diet + Statins = HSFSA + Statins; ***Diet + Zetia = HSFSA + Zetia [1, 2]. The values represent the mean ± S.D. obtained from 3 patients.

But why prescribe a therapy that could have an adverse lipid response in so many even if there is available therapy? The prevalence of obesity or being overweight is increasing rapidly across the United States and presently effects approximately two-thirds of the adult population [66]. Alarmingly we are also observing an increase in obesity among the youth population in this country [67]. Obesity has also become an epidemic in developing countries [68]. Obesity is considered a major health problem because of the increased mortality and diseases associated with excess body fat. A study conducted in 1999 concluded that at least 280,000-325,000 deaths in the United States could be attributed to obesity [69]. This conclusion has also been arrived at by several other studies. Both the American Cancer Society's Cancer Prevention Study I and II and other studies concluded that increased body mass index is associated with increased mortality from all causes and from cardiovascular disease [70-72]. Additional studies such as the Aerobics Center Longitudinal Study and Finnish Heart Study also confirmed an increased mortality rate associated with obesity [73].

Table 6. Showing of High Saturated Fat-Starch Avoidance Diet on Serum Lipids in Patients with Polycystic Ovary Syndrome and Reactive Hypoglycemia

	Polycystic Ovary Syndrome (n=15)		Reactive Hypoglycemia (n=8)	
BMI (Kg/m^2)	36.1±9.7	34.4±8.9*	46.8±10.0	37.5±7.5*
Cholesterol (mg/dL)	215.3±46.4	205.3±38.9	221.8±41.6	208.5±16.8
Triglyceride (mg/dL)	121.4±63.0	99.0±43.1	137.4±79.1	95.0±30.9
HDL (mg/dL)	54.4±15.7	54.6±12.3	46.4±14.7	48.0±8.3
LDL (mg/dL)	136.8±43.1	128.7±39.2	144.3±44.8	140.5±18.7

Results of high saturated fat starch avoidance diet in two groups of patients who did not receive lipid lowering medications. Three patients in polycystic ovary syndrome (PCOS) group took metformin 500 mg BID throughout observation. * = p <0.05 versus baseline [2].

Several diseases are associated with obesity. These include psychological disorders, diabetes mellitus, sleep apnea, hypertension, non-alcoholic fatty liver disease, gall bladder disorders, cancer, heart disease and changes in the endocrine system [74-82]. Overweight subjects appear to have an increased risk of psychosocial dysfunction and this appears to be present more in females patients than male patients [74,75]. Significant weight reduction is associated with improvements in psychological function [75]. Type 2 diabetes mellitus is associated with obesity in both men and women in all ethnic groups [76]. Up to 65% of cases of type 2 diabetes mellitus can be attributed to being overweight [76]. Studies have shown that weight loss reduces the risk of developing diabetes mellitus [77,78]. Overweight associated sleep apnea can often be severe. Hypertension is commonly seen in obese subjects. Control of obesity could reduce hypertension by 48% and 28% in Caucasians and African Americans respectively [78,79]. Elevated liver associated enzymes, hepatomegaly, and abnormal liver histology may occur in obesity. The prevalence of steatosis, steatohepatitis and cirrhosis are approximately 75%, 20% and 2% in obese patients [78,80]. Cholelithiasis is often associated with obesity. This has been attributed to increased concentrations of cholesterol relative to bile acids and phospholipids in bile in overweight subjects [78,80]. There is increased risk of cancer in obese patients [82,83]. The risk of cancer of the colon, rectum and prostate is increased in male obese patients [81]. In contrast in overweight females there is an increased risk of endometrial cancer and gall bladder malignancy [83].

Weight gain is associated with an increase in heart disease. The Nurses Health Study has shown that the risk of coronary artery disease is increased 3.3 fold with a body mass index greater than 29 kg/m^2 [84]. Obesity is associated with several cardiovascular abnormalities [85]. These include increased cardiac weight, cardiomyopathy and heart failure. Abnormalities in serum lipid levels such as low HDL cholesterol levels and elevated serum triglycerides at least partly explain the increased risk of heart disease in this population [86]. Furthermore, obesity may be associated with increased levels of atherogenic small dense, low density lipoproteins rather than large fluffy lipoprotein particles [87]. The incidence of osteoarthritis involving knee jointds and ankle joints is much higher in obese patients. Although this may be related to the trauma associated with excessive weight bearing alterations in cartilage and bone metabolism independent of weight bearing may also contribute to the increased prevalence of degenerative joint disease in the population. Several abnormalities in the endocrine system may also occur in obesity. These include irregular menses, anovulatory cycles, abnormalities in the secretions of various pituitary, thyroid and adrenal hormones [88].

Condemning the food of civilization for causing the diseases of civilization seems logical but also disloyal. Most cultures have a starch like bread, rice or corn at the center of their diet. These foods allowed us to survive at a time when population density excluded a hunter gatherer life style. Now that food is abundant, a strategy to induce satiety that excludes these foods seems odd. It is also troubling to face a continuing need for consumption of animal flesh in humans. It suggests a savage side of us, all to easy to see, which must be overcome for us to live together in peace. Many humans abstain or fast from meat for spiritual reasons. Although many of us would like it otherwise, we may carry with us the desire for meat and may overeat carbohydrates if we don't achieve satiety. For the modern human confronted by constant availability of all types of food, there may be a paradoxical recommendation to, "eat more fat to eat fewer calories"©.

Authors' Note

The opinions and assertions contained herein are the private ones of the authors and are not to be construed as official or as reflecting the views of the Navy Department or the Naval Service at large.

References

[1]   Hays, J.H., Gorman, R., Shakir, K.M. (2002). Results of use of metformin and replacement of starch with standard fat in the diets of patients with type 2 diabetes. *Endocr Pract, 8*:177-183.

[2]   Hays, J.H., DiSabatino, A., Gorman, R.T., Vincent, S., Stillabower, M.E. (2003). Effect of a high saturated fat and no-starch diet on serum lipid subractions in patients with documented atherosclerotic cardiovascular disease. *Mayo Clin Proc, 78*:1331-1336.

[3]   Shakir, S.K., Poremba, J.A., Krook, L.S., Drake III, A.J., Hays, J.H. (2004). Adverse serum lipid (LDL cholesterol) response to high saturated fat diet due to enteric hyperabsorption. *Endocrine Society Abstracts*, pg 148.

[4]   Gau, G.T. (2003). The search for the perfect heart-healthy diet. *Mayo Clin Proc, 78*:1329-1330.

[5]   Paabo, S. (2001). The human genome and our view of ourselves. *Science, 291*:1219-1220.

[6]   Diamond, J.M. (1999). *Guns, Germs, and Steel: The Fates of Human Societies*. New York, NY: WW Norton and Co; 93-104.

[7]   Morris, D. *The Naked Ape*. New York, NY: Dell Publishing Co; 1984:153-163.

[8]   Ibid. [6] Diamond, J.M.

[9]   O'Keefe, J.H. Jr., Cordain, L. (2004). Cardiovascular disease resulting from a diet and lifestyle at odds with our Paleolithic genome: how to become a 21st-century hunter-gatherer. *Mayo Clin Proc. 79*:101-108.

[10]   Krauss, R.M., Winston, M., Fletcher, B.J., Grundy, S.M. (1998). Obesity: impact on cardiovascular disease. *Circulation. 98*:1472-1476.

[11]   Keys A. (ed). Coronary heart disease in seven countries. *Circulation* 1970; (Suppl 1) I-1-I-8.

[12]   Simons, L.A. (1986). Interrelationships of lipids and lipoproteins wit coronary artery disease mortality in 19 countries. *Am J Cardio, 57*:59-

[13]   Anderson, K.M., Castelli, W.P., Levy D. (1987). Cholesterol and mortality: 30 years of follow-up from the Framingham study. *JAMA, 257*:2176-.

[14]   Schonfeld, G., Patsch, W., Rudel, L.L., Nelson, C., Epstein, M., Olson, R.E. (1982). Effects of dietary cholesterol and fatty acids on plasma lipoproteins. *J Clin Invest, 69*:1072-1080.

[15] Denke, M.A., Adams-Huet, B., Nguyen, A.T. (2000). Individual cholesterol variation in response to margarine- or butter-based diet: a study in families. *JAMA, 284*:2740-2747.

[16] American Diabetes Association. (2001). Nutrion recommendations and principles for people with diabetes mellitus [position statement]. *Diabetes Care, 24(Suppl 1)*: S44-S47.

[17] Woodyatt, R.T. (1993). In: *Cecil RL*, ed, Cecil's Textbook of Medicine. *Diabetes mellitus: overindulgence and obesity.* New York, NY: Saunders; 628-659.

[18] Bjeregaard, P., Pedersen, H.S., Mulvad, G. (2000). The associations of a marine diet with plasma lipids, blood glucose, blood pressure and obesity among the Inuit in Greenlannd. *Eur J Clin Nutr, 54*:732-737.

[19] http://www.itk.ca/english/itk/departments/enviro/wildlife/narwhal.htm.

[20] Erickson, B.A., Coots, R.H., Mattson, F.H., Klingman, A.M. (1964). The effect of partial hydrogenation of dietary fats on the ratio of polyunsaturated to saturated fatty acids, and of dietary cholesterol upon plasma lipids in man. *J Clin Invest, 43*:2017-2025.

[21] Ibid. [18] Bjerregaard, P., Petersen, H.S., Mulvad, G. (2000).

[22] Stamler, J., Wentworth, D., Neaton, J.D. (1986). Is the relationship between serum cholesterol and risk of premature death from coronary heart disease continuous and graded? Findins in 356,222 primary screenees of the Multiple Risk Factor Intervention Trial (MRFIT). *JAMA, 256*:2823-2828.

[23] Moss, S.E., Klein, R., B.E.K. (1991). Cause specific mortality in a population-based study of diabetes. *Am J Public Health, 81*:1158-1162.

[24] Grundy, S.M. (1983). Hypertriglyceridemia, atherogenic dyslipidemia, and the metabolic syndrome. *Am J Caradiol, 81*:18B-25B.

[25] Barrett-Connor, E., Wingard, D.L. (2001). Normal blood glucose and coronary risk. *BMJ* 322: 5-6.

[26] Taubes, G. (2001). The soft science of dietary fat. *Science, 291*:2536-2545.

[27] Bonanome, A., Grundy, S.M. (1988). Effect of dietary stearic acid on plasma cholesterol and lipoprotein levels. *N Engl J Med, 318*:1244-1248.

[28] Garg, A., Grundy, S.M., Unger, R.H. (1992). Comparison of effects of high and low carbohydrate diets on plasma, lipoproteins and insulin sensitivity in patients with mild NIDDM. *Diabetes, 41*:1278-1285.

[29] Parillo, M., Rivellese, A.A., Ciardullo, A.V., et al. (1992). A high-monounsaturated-fat/low-carbohydrate diet improves peripheral insulin sensitivity in non-insulin-dependent diabetic patient. *Metatolism, 41*:1373-1378.

[30] Fasmussen, O.W., Thomsen, C., Hansen, K.W., Vesterlund, M., Winther, E., Hermansen, K. (1993). Effects on blood pressure, glucose, and lipid levels of a high-monounsaturated fat diet compared with a high-carbohydrate diet in NIDDM subjects. *Diabetes Care, 16*:1565-1571.

[31] Garg, A., Bantle, J.P., Henry, R.R., et al. (1994). Effects of varying carbohydrate content of diet in patients with non-insulin-dependent diabetes mellitus. *JAMA, 271*:1421-1428.

[32] Lerman-Garber, I., Ichazo-Cerro, S., Zamora-Gonzalez, J., Cardoso-Saldana, G., Posadas-Romero, C. (1994). Effect of a high-monounsaturated fat diet enriched with avocado in NIDDM patients. *Diabetes Care, 17*:311-315.

[33] Low, C.C., Grossman, E.B., Gambiner, B. (1996). Potentiation of effects of weight loss by monounsaturated fatty acids in obese NIDDM patients. *Diabetes, 45*:569-575.

[34] Walker, K.Z., O'Dea, K., Johnson, L., et al. (1996). Body fat distribution and non-insulin-dependent diabetes: comparison of a fiber-rich, high-carbohydrate, low-fat (23%) diet and a 35% fat diet high in monounsaturated fat. *Am J Clin Nutr, 63*:254-260.

[35] Garg, A. (1998). High-monounsaturated-fat diets for patients with diabetes mellitus: a meta-analysis. *Am J Clin Nutr, 67(3 Suppl)*:577S-582S.

[36] Sears, B., Lawren, W. (1995). *Enter the Zone.* NY: Harper Collins.

[37] Westman, E.C., Yancy, W.S., Edman, J.S., Tomlin, K.F., Perkins, C.E. (2002). Effect of 6-month adherence to a very low carbohydrate diet program. *Am J Med, 113*:30-36.

[38] Foster, G.D., Wyatt, H.R., Hill, J.O., et al. (2003). A randomized trial of a low carbohydrate diet for obesity. *N Engl J Med, 348*:2082-2090.

[39] Samaha, F.F., Iqbal, N., Seshardri, P., et al. (2003). A low carbohydrate as compared with a low fat diet in severe obesity. *N Engl J Med, 348*:2074-2081.

[40] Brehm, B.J., Seeley, R.J., Daniels, S.R., D'Alessio, D.A. (2003). A randomized trial comparing a very low carbohydrate diet and a calorie restricted low fat diet on body weight and cardiovascular risk factors in health women. *J Clin Endocrinol Metab, 88*:1617-1623.

[41] Ibid. [26] Taubes, G.

[42] Eades, M.R. (1996). *Protein Power.* NY: Bantum Books.

[43] Agatston, A.S. (2003). *The South Beach Diet.* NY: St. Martin's Press.

[44] Atkins, R. (2002). *Dr. Atkin's New Diet Revolution.* NY: Harper Collins.

[45] Ibid. [44]

[46] Boden, G., Surgrad, K., Honiko, C., et al. (2004). Effecs of the Atkins' diet in type 2 diabetes: metabolic balance studies. *Diabetes, 53(Supple 2)*:A75.

[47] Linden A. (1989). Role of cholecystokinin in feeding and lactation. *Acta Physiol Scand Suppl, 585-I-vii*, 1-49.

[48] Ibid. [27]

[49] Ibid. [47]

[50] Lewis, S.B., Wallin, J.D., Kane, J.P., Gerich, J.E. (1977). Effect of diet composition on metabolic adaptations to hypocaloric nutrition: comparison of high carbohydrate and high fat isocaloric diets. *Am J Clin Nutr, 130*:160-170.

[51] Hegsted, D.M., McGandy, R.B., Myers, M.L., Stare, F.J. (1965). Quantitative effects of dietary fat on serum cholesterol in man. *Am J Clin Nutr* 17:281-295.

[52] Grundy, S.M. Vega, G.L. (1988). Plasma cholesterol responsiveness to saturated fatty acids. *Am J Clin Nutr* 47:822-824.

[53] Havel, R.J. (1995). Postprandial hyperlipidemia and remnant lipoproteins. *Curr Opin Lipidol, 5*:102-109.

[54] Vogel, R.A., Corretti, M.C., Vogel, R.A. (1997). Effect of antioxidant vitamins on the transient impairment of endothelium-dependent brachial artery vasoactivity following a single high-fat meal. *JAMA, 278*:1682-1686.

[55] Friendman, P.J. (1977) In *Biochenistry lipid metabolism and biosynthesis*, 1st Edition, Boston MA: Little Brown and Co., 139-161.

[56] Crespin, S.R., Greenough, W.B. III, Steinberg, D. (1973). Stimulation of insulin secretion by long chain fatty acids: a direct pancreatic effect. *J Clin Invest* 52:1979-1984.

[57] Gordon, D.J. (1990) Role of circulating high density lipoprotein and triglycerides in heart disease: risk and prevention. *Endo Metab Clin of North America* 19:299-309.

[58] Ibid. [56].

[59] Otvos, J.D. 92000). In *Handbook of Lipoprotein Testing*, 2nd Edition, Washington, D.C.:AACC Press, 609-623.

[60] Yancy Jr., W.S., Olsen, M.K., Guyton, J.R., Bakst, R.P. Westman, E.C. (2004). A low-carbohydrate, ketogenic diet versus a low-fat diet to treat obesity and hyperlipidemia: a randomized, controlled trial. *Ann Intern Med, 140*:769-777.

[61] Gagne, C., Bays, H.E., Weiss, S.R. Mata, P., Quito, K., Melino, M., Cho, M., Musliner, T.A., Gumbiner, B. (2002). Efficacay and safety of ezetimibe added to ongoing statin therapy for treatment of patients with primary hyper-cholesterolemia. *Am J Cardiol* 90:1084-1091.

[62] Heart Protection Study Collaborative Group (2003). MRC/BHF heart protection study of cholesterol-lowering with simvastatin in 5963 people with diabetes: a randomized placebo-controlled trial. *Lancet* 361:2005-2016.

[63] Larosa, J.C. (2001). In: Becker K.L., eds. Principles and Practice of Endocrinolgoy and Metabolism. *Treatment of the Hyperlipoproteinemias*. 3rd edition. Philadelphia, PA. Lippincott Williams and Wilkins, 1531-1537.

[64] Phillips, P.S., Haas, R.H., Bannykh, S. Hathaway, S., Gray, N.L., Kimura, B.J., Vladutiu, G.D., England, J.D.F. (2002). Statin-associated myopathy with normal creatinine kinase levels. *Ann Intern Med, 137*:581-585.

[65] Bennett, W.E., Drake III, A.J., Shakir, K.M.M. (2003). Reversible myopathy after statin therapy in patients with normal creatine kinase levels. *Ann Intern Med, 138*:436-a-437.

[66] Flegal, K.M., Carroll, M.D., Ogden, C.L., Johnson, C.L. (2002). Prevalence and trends in obesity among U.S. adults, 1999-2000. *JAMA, 288*:1723-1727.

[67] Ogden, C.L., Flegal, K.M., Carroll, M.D., Johnson, C.L. (2002). Prevalence and trends in overweight among U.S. children and adolescents, 1999-2000. *JAMA, 288*:1728-1732.

[68] Popkin, B.M. (1998). The nutrition transition and its health implications in lower-income countries. *Public Health Nutr, 1*:5-21.

[69] Allison, D.B., Fontaine, K.R., Manson, J.E., Stevens, J., VanItallie, T.B. (1999). Annual deaths attributable to obesity in the United States. *JAMA, 282*:1530-1538.

[70] International Agency for Research on Cancer, World Health Organization 2002 Weight control and physical activity. In: Vainio, H., Bianchini, F., eds. *International Agency*

for Research on Cancer handbooks of cancer prevention. Vol 6. Lyon, France: IARC Press.

[71] Stevens, J., Cai, J., Pamuk, E.R., Williamson, D.F., Thun, M.J., Wook, J.L. (1998). The effect of age on the association between body-mass index and mortality. *N Engl J Med, 338*:1-7.

[72] Calle, E.E., Thun, M.J., Petrelli, J.M., Rodriguez, C., Heath Jr., C.W. (1999). Body-mass index and mortality in a prospective cohort of U.S. adults. *N Engl J Med, 341*:1097-1105.

[73] Wei, M., Kampert, J.B., Barlow, C.E., Nichaman, M.Z., Gibbons, L.W. Paffenbarger Jr., R.S., Blair, S.N. (1999). Relationship between low cardiorespiratory fitness and mortality in normal-weight, overweight, and obese men. *JAMA, 282*:1547-1553.

[74] Carpenter, K.M., Hasin, D.S., Allison, D.B., Faith, M.S. (2000). Relationships between obesity and DSM-IV major depressive disorder, suicide ideation, and suicide attempts: results from a general population study. *Am J Public Health, 90*:251.

[75] Williamson, D.A., O'Neil, P.M. (2004). In: Bray, G.A., Bouchard, C., eds. Handbook of obesity: *etiology and pathophysiology. Obesity and quality of life.* 2nd ed. New York: Marcel Dekker: 1005-1023.

[76] Bray, G.A. (2003). Contemporary diagnosis and management of obesity and the metabolic syndrome. 3rd ed. Newton, PA: Handbook in health care.

[77] Chan, J.M., Rimm, E.B., Colditz, G.A., Stampfer, M.J., Willett, W.C. (1994). Obesity, fat distribution, and weight gain as risk factors for clinical diabetes in men. *Diabetes Care, 17*:961-969.

[78] Bray, G.A. (2004). Medical consequences of obesity. *J Clin Endocrinol Metab, 89*:2583-2589.

[79] Sjostrom, C.D., Lissner, L., Sjostrom, L. (1997). Relationships between changes in body composition and changes in cardiovascular risk factors: the SOS Intervention Study. Swedish Obese Subjects. *Obes Res, 5*:519-530.

[80] Matteoni, C., Younossi, Z.M., McCullough, A. (1999). Nonalcoholic fatty liver disease: a spectrum of clinical pathological severity. *Gastroenterology, 116*:1413.

[81] Ko, C.W., Lee, S.P. (2004). In: Bray, G.A., Bouchard, C., James, W.P., eds. Handbook of obesity: *etiology and pathophysiology.Obesity and gallbladder disease.* 2nd ed. New York, Marcel Dekker; 919-934.

[82] Manson, J.E., Willett, W.C., Stampfer, M.J., Colditz, G.A., Hunter, D.J., Hankinson, S.E., Hennekens, C.H., Speizer, F.E. (1995). Body weight and Mortality among women. *N Engl J Med, 333*:677-685.

[83] Lew, E.A. (1985). Mortality and weight: insured lives and the American Cancer Society studies. *Ann Intern Med,103*:1024-1029.

[84] Manson, J.E., Willett, W.C., Stampfer, M.J., Colditz, G.A., Hunter, D.J., Hankinson, S.E., Hennekens, C.H., Speizer, F.E. (1995). Body weight and mortality among women. *N Engl J Med, 333*:677-685.

[85] National Task Force on the Prevention and Treatment of Obesity (2000). Overweight, obesity and health risk. *Arch Int Med* 160: 898-904.

[86] Krauss, R.M., Winston, M., Fletcher, B.J., Grundy, S.M. (1998). Obesity: impact on cardiovascular disease. *Circulation.* 98:1472-1476.

[87] Ibid. [57].

[88] Rich-Edwards, J.W., Goldma, M.B., Willett, W.C., Hunter, D.J., Stampfer, M.J.H., Colditz, G.A., Manson, J.E. (1994). Adolescent body mass index and infertility caused by ovulatory disorder. *Am J Obstet Gynecol*. Jul;171(1):171-177.

In: Nutrition Research at the Leading Edge
Editors: R. E. Cassady, E. I. Tidswell, pp. 191-201

ISBN: 978-1-60456-053-4
© 2008 Nova Science Publishers, Inc.

Chapter VII

The Effect of an Alpha-Linolenic-Acid-Rich Diet on the Circadian Rhythm of Cardiac Events

Gal Dubnov, Daniel Pella and Ram B. Singh[1]***

Department of Human Nutrition and Metabolism, Hebrew University- Hadassah Medical
School, Jerusalem, Israel
*Faculty of Medicine, Safaric University, Kosice, Slovakia
**Centre of Nutrition and Heart, Medical Hospital and
Research Centre, Moradabad, India

Abstract

Objective. Coronary artery disease events have a circadian rhythmicity, clustering more in the second quartile of the day. n-3 fatty acid supplementation reduces the rate of cardiac events, but its effect on their circadian rhythmicity has not been tested.

Design. The Indo-Mediterranean Diet Heart Study was a single blind randomized study that assessed the effect of a diet rich in alpha-linolenic acid, the parent n-3 fatty acid, on the occurrence of myocardial infarction and sudden cardiac death.

Subjects. One thousand subjects of the Indo-Mediterranean Diet Heart Study, focusing on the 115 patients from both control and intervention groups in which cardiac events occurred.

Intervention. The timing of cardiac events throughout the day was compared between the intervention and control groups. The distribution of cardiac events along the four quartiles of the day was compared between groups as well as against equal distribution.

Results. The risk ratio for a cardiac event was lowest between 4:00 and 8:00 in the morning for the intervention group. The control group had a higher rate of events in the second quartile of the day, which deviated from an equal distribution, as expected

1 Corresponding author: Ram B. Singh, MD. Centre of Nutrition and Heart, Medical Hospital and Research Centre, Moradabad-10 (UP)244001, India. E-mail: icn2005@mickyonline.com.

(P=0.013). In the intervention group, events were equally distributed along the day. No statistically significant difference was found in daily event distribution between the groups.

Conclusion. A diet rich in alpha-linolenic acid may abolish the higher rate of cardiac events, normally seen in the second quartile of the day. Additional studies are needed to identify the underlying mechanism.

Introduction

The classical manifestations of coronary artery disease (CAD), such as angina pectoris, silent ischemia, myocardial infarction (MI) and sudden cardiac death, have a pronounced circadian rhythmicity, tending to cluster in the second quartile of the day [1-10]. This increase in the rate of cardiovascular events in the morning may be due to a hypercoagulable state, consisted of increased platelet aggregation, increased tPA inhibitor levels, and rapid metabolism of heparin in the morning [11-13]. In addition, the morning hours are associated with a decrease in vagal tone and increase in sympathetic activity, resulting in lower levels of acetylecholine and melatonin and increased concentrations of cortisol, aldosterone, catecholamines and angiotensin, which make the atherosclerotic plaques more vulnerable to rupture and thrombosis [14-16]. These circadian manifestations are associated with a decreased heart rate variability (HRV), which is an independent risk factor for cardiovascular events [13-16].

Recent studies indicate that n-3 fatty acids may have a beneficial effect on HRV, platelet aggregation, and endothelial function, and that they are neuroprotectors and may enhance hippocampal acetylecholine levels [15-26]. In randomized controlled trials, treatment with n-3 fatty acids led to a significant reduction in cardiac events, in both patients after a MI and those with risk factors only [27-30]. To our knowledge, no study has examined the effect of n-3 fatty acids on the timing of cardiovascular events. The aim of the present study is to examine the influence of a diet rich in alpha-linolenic acid, the parent n-3 fatty acid, on the circadian rhythm of cardiac events.

Methods

Subjects and Study Design

The Indo-Mediterranean Diet Heart Study was a randomized, single-blind study designed to assess the effect of a diet rich in n-3 fatty acids from plant sources on the occurrence of myocardial infarction and sudden cardiac death [29]. One thousand subjects were randomized to either an intervention or a control group by selection of a card from a pile. The intervention group consisted of 499 patients, and the control group 501. The ethics committee of the Medical Hospital and Research Centre at Moradabad approved the study, and written informed consent was obtained from all participants.

Participants in both groups were advised to eat food elements that would provide a dietary intake similar to that recommended at the time by the National Cholesterol Education

Program (NCEP) step I prudent diet [S31], wherein less than 30% of energy comes from total fat, less than 10% from saturated fat, and less than 300 mg of cholesterol is consumed per day. Patients in the intervention group were advised to verify the intake of at least 250–300 g of fruit, 125–150 g of vegetables, and 25–50 g of nuts. They were also encouraged to eat 400–500 g of whole grains (legumes, rice, maize, wheat) daily, as well as to use mustard seed or soy bean oil in 3 to 4 servings per day, in order to ensure a high intake of alpha-linolenic acid.

Both groups were advised to exercise daily and practice yoga meditation techniques, to abstain from smoking and alcohol consumption, and to continue the use of their regular medications.

Food intake and physical activity were monitored by self-report diaries, first weekly, then monthly, and then every 3 months. Nutrient intakes were calculated using Indian foods composition tables and other sources [32,33].and reinforce adherence. Height, weight, and blood pressure were monitored by standard methods. Blood concentrations of glucose, total cholesterol (TC), high-density lipoprotein (HDL) cholesterol, low-density lipoprotein (LDL) cholesterol and triglycerides were also measured. Clinical data, drug intake, adverse events, blood pressure, blood glucose levels, blood lipid levels, hospital admission and coronary events were recorded by physicians blinded to patient grouping.

At the 2-year follow up in the original study, cardiac events had occurred in 39 subjects from the intervention group and in 76 subjects from the control group.

Cardiac Events

The principal endpoints of the original study were fatal or nonfatal MI, sudden cardiac deaths, and the combined total of these events. Owing to the relatively small number of events in each category, we did not attempt a subgroup analysis and focused only on the combined end-point of total cardiac events.

In hospitalized patients, a diagnosis of nonfatal MI was based on a diagnostic electrocardiograph at the time of the event, or the presence of ischaemic cardiac pain and diagnostic enzyme levels of at least twice the upper limit of normal, or the presence of ischaemic cardiac pain and equivocal enzyme levels and an equivocal electrocardiograph. In patients who had not been admitted to the hospital, the diagnosis of MI was considered if they complained of chest pain, breathlessness, or syncope, combined with a diagnostic electrocardiograph at the time of event or new electrocardiographic changes consistent with MI at routine check-up. The electrocardiographic coding and analysis were performed by a cardiologist blinded to patient grouping.

Fatal MI was diagnosed when a hospital record was consistent with cause of death, and there was either a preterminal hospital admission with a definite MI, or official documentation of a myocardial infarction.

Sudden cardiac death was diagnosed when coronary heart disease had been noted, and death occurred within one hour of symptom onset.

Statistical Analysis

Analyses were performed in two ways. One was determining the risk for cardiac events in specific time frames among the whole study population. Second, we determined the number of events in the four quartiles of the day among only those subjects with events in both groups.

In order to assess the effect of the ALA-rich diet on the timing of cardiac event, we constructed a Cox multivariate model, with cardiac event as outcome variable, stratified into six 4-hour periods (0:01-4:00, 4:01-8:00, 8:01-12:00, 12:01-16:00, 16:01-20:00, and 20:01-24:00). In each model, we examined the risk ratio associated with the intervention diet, with patient's age, gender and BMI as covariates. The last available values served as the final risk factors data for the subjects who had fatal events. The analyses were held using standard statistical package (SPSS 11.0).

When comparing only the subgroups in which events occurred, Student's t test with a Bonferroni adjustment was used to analyze between-group differences of the continuous variables; P values less than 0.005 were considered statistically significant. The distribution of the number of events in each quartile of the day was compared by the chi-square test. Event rates were compared between the control and intervention groups, as well as for each group against equal distribution. Thus, for the latter, the observed event rates in the control group were compared with an expected rate of 19 (76 divided by 4) events in each quartile of the day, and the observed events in the intervention group were compared with an expected rate of 9.75 (39 divided by 4) in each quartile of the day. A two-tailed P value less than 0.05 was considered statistically significant for the parametric variables.

Results

Timing of Events in Total Study Population

Baseline characteristics of the Indo-Mediterranean Diet Heart study population was presented elsewhere [29]. In all strata, the ALA-rich diet was associated with protective effect for cardiac events. The lowest risk ratio (RR=0.05; 95%CI: 0.01-0.24) was calculated for cardiac events between 4:01 and 8:00, while the highest was for events between 0:01 to 4:00 (RR=0.15 (95% CI:0.03 – 0.87) as shown in Figure 1. However, differences between strata did not reach statistical significance.

Dispersion of Events Along Quartiles of the Day

Baseline characteristics of the subjects with cardiac events from both groups is presented in Table 1. Subjects in both groups were comparable for all major baseline variables except for body weight (borderline significance, P=0.006), yet BMIs were comparable between groups. At 2 years, only TC and LDL levels differed significantly between groups, with lower values noted in the intervention group. Nutritional data are presented in Table 2. At baseline, values of all nutrients, including fatty acids, were similar in the two groups. At 2 years, n-3 fatty acid intake was significantly higher in the intervention group, and the n-6/n-3 fatty acid ratio was lower. The number of cardiovascular events of each type in both groups is given in Table 3.

The dispersion of cardiac events along the quartiles of the day is presented in Table 4. In the control group, there was an increased rate of cardiac events clustered in the second quartile of the day, which deviated from an equal distribution (P=0.013). In the intervention group, the events were distributed equally along the day (P=0.49 when comparing observed rates and equal distribution). There was no statistically significant difference in the rate of events in each quartile of the day between the two groups (P=0.54).

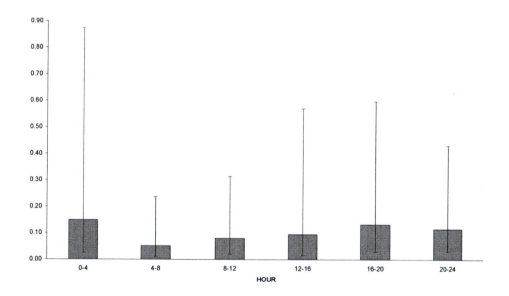

Figure 1. The risk ratio for cardiac events in the intervention group (n=499) compared with the control group (n=501) distributed into 4-hour intervals of the day.

Table 1. Cardiovascular risk factors at baseline and after 2 years in the intervention and control groups. Data presented as means ± SD. BMI- body mass index, BP- blood pressure, TC- total cholesterol, TG- triglyceride, FBG- fasting blood glucose

	Intervention Group A, n = 39			Control Group B, n = 76			P value at 2 years between groups
	Baseline	2 years	P value	Baseline	2 years	P value	
Age (years)	51 ± 10	-	-	49 ± 8	-	-	-
Weight, kg	65 ± 5	62 ± 7	0.0002	68 ± 6	67 ± 6	0.0004	<0.0001
BMI, kg/m^2	24 ± 3	23 ± 3	0.0005	25 ± 2	24 ± 2	0.0005	0.0172
Systolic BP	134 ± 15	129 ± 15	0.0064	133 ± 19	132 ± 17	0.0040	0.2051

Table 1. (Continued)

	Intervention Group A, n = 39			Control Group B, n = 76			P value at 2 years between groups
Diastolic BP	86 ± 6	84 ± 10	0.0931	88 ± 10	87 ± 10	0.0063	0.0532
Cigarettes / day	18 ± 9	19 ± 9	0.0961	21 ± 8	16 ± 5	0.0001	0.1608
TC, mmol/L	232 ± 43	220 ± 39	0.0029	245 ± 34	245 ± 32	0.7507	0.0001
LDL, mmol/L	150 ± 26	137 ± 30	0.0001	156 ± 32	157 ± 31	0.9745	0.0005
HDL, mmol/L	45 ± 15	44 ± 11	0.1319	44 ± 6	43 ± 11	0.3524	0.4414
TG, mmol/L	181 ± 51	169 ± 43	0.0259	176 ± 33	175 ± 35	0.8080	0.1881
FBG, mmol/L	112 ± 28	106 ± 25	0.0001	115 ± 33	109 ± 27	0.0029	0.2661

Table 2. Nutrient data at baseline and after 2 years in the intervention and control groups. Data presented as means ± SD

	Intervention Group A, n = 39			Control Group B, n = 76			P value at 2 years between groups
	Baseline	2 years	P value	Baseline	2 years	P value	0.2589
Energy (kcal.day)	2116 ± 175	2098 241	0.3279	2167 ± 183	2123 ± 163	0.0099	<0.0001
CHO (%en)	57 ± 2	58 ± 3	0.0007	56 ± 2	55 ± 1	<0.0001	<0.0001
Protein (%en)	14 ± 1.7	14 ± 1.3	0.0112	14 ± 1.5	15 ± 0.8	0.1862	0.0241
Fat (%en)	27 ± 3	28 ± 3	0.0206	28 ± 2	30 ± 1.5	<0.0001	<0.0001
Saturated fat (%en)	13 ± 1.8	11 ± 2.3	0.0017	12 ± 1.4	13 ± 1.6	0.0003	<0.0001
MUFA (%en)	7.3 ± 1.6	9.0 ± 2.2	<0.0001	8.1 ± 2.1	8.8 ± 1.3	0.3857	0.01929
PUFA (%en)	7.0 ± 1.0	7.5 ± 1.0	<0.0001	7.5 ± 1.0	7.9 ± 0.8	0.0111	0.0052
n-6 (%en)	6.8 ± 0.9	6.9 ± 1.0	0.4042	7.3 ± 1.0	7.6 ± 0.8	0.0001	<0.0001
n-3 (%en)	0.2 ± 0.1	0.5 ± 0.2	<0.0001	0.2 ± 0.1	0.3 ± 0.1	0.0003	<0.0001

Table 3. Distribution of cardiac events in intervention and control groups. MI – myocardial infarction

	Intervention group (n=39)	Control group (n=76)
Nonfatal MI	21	43
Fatal MI	12	17
Sudden cardiac death	6	16

Table 4. Distribution of cardiac events along the quartiles of the day in the intervention and control groups. In the intervention group, events are near-equally distributed along the day. In the control group, quartile 2 has more events than would be expected assuming equal distribution

Quartile (time range)	Intervention group (n=39) n (% within group)	Control group (n=76) n (% within group)
1 (00:01 – 06:00)	10 (26%)	15 (20%)
2 (06:01 – 12:00)	11 (28%)	29 (38%)
3 (12:01 – 18:00)	8 (21%)	10 (13%)
4 (18:01 – 00:00)	10 (26%)	22 (29%)

Discussion

This study is the first to assess the effect of an ALA-rich diet on the circadian rhythm of cardiac events. We have found that although the intervention diet dramatically lowered the risk for events throughout the day, it nearly abolished it in the early morning hours. The increased rate of events known to occur in the second quartile of the day was eliminated by the diet.

Although n-3-rich diets have been found to be cardioprotective in several randomized controlled trials [27-30], their exact mode of action is still unknown. Our results suggest that dietary supplementation of alpha-linolenic acid may lead to a change in the circadian occurrence of cardiac events. The only major risk factors that differed significantly between the groups at the end of the trial along the trial were the lower levels of total cholesterol and LDL. However, we would expect this change to influence the total rate of events, and not just their distribution during the day, which was the focus of this study.

We are unaware of any other large-scale study that has examined the effect of n-3 fatty acids on the circadian rhythmicity of cardiac events. The Physicians Health Study recorded the number of myocardial infarctions in patients treated with aspirin or not, and found a significant decrease in the rhythmicity of myocardial infarctions in the aspirin group [34]. It is possible that this reduction was the result of the inhibitory effect of aspirin on platelet aggregation, a quality also possessed by n-3 fatty acids [25]. When these findings are combined, it appears that one of the triggers for MI in the morning hours is the increased tendency of platelets to aggregate.

Christensen and coworkers [17] reported a positive correlation between HRV and the platelet content of n-3 fatty acids (docosahexaenoic acid, DHA) in patients with post-MI left ventricular dysfunction. The increase in HRV occurred even after intake of only one fish meal per week, with an increase in standard deviation of normal-normal (SDNN) from 103 to 122ms. Further analysis revealed a negative correlation between the ratio of arachidonic acid/ DHA and the SDNN interval [18], consistent with earlier findings. In a more recent study, of 291 patients referred for coronary angiography that completed a food frequency questionnaire, researchers measured the n-3 fatty acid composition of granulocyte membranes and adipose tissue along with 24-hour HRV analysis [19]. Significant positive correlations were found between HRV indices and the levels of n-3 fatty acids in granulocytes. The positive influence of n-3 fatty acids on HRV suggests that this is indeed a major mechanism of CAD event reduction, as seen even after a few months of treatment [28].

HRV is a manifestation of sympathetic and parasympathetic activity of the heart, and a decreased HRV enhances the risk of circadian rhythmicity of cardiac events. This may well be another mechanism by which n-3 fatty acids reduce coronary events in the morning hours. In one randomized, controlled trial, of 81 patients after MI [17], treatment with n-3 fatty acids was associated with significant increase in HRV compared with controls, indicating an increased vagal cardiac tone. A retrospective analysis of a randomized, controlled intervention trial among 118 (fish oil group) and 122 (control group) patients with acute MI showed that treatment with fish oil (rich in EPA and DHA) was associated with a significant reduction in cardiac events (30% vs 56%, P<0.02) [27]. While the majority of cardiac events in the control group were reported in the second quartile of the day compared to first and third quartiles (35.7% vs 16.0%, 19.6%, respectively, P<0.01), no such association was observed in the fish oil group (unpublished data). These results are consistent with the view that fish oil administration may have a beneficial effect on circadian rhythmicity of cardiac events.

Alpha-linolenic acid is the parent n-3 fatty acid which is converted into long-chain fatty acids such as EPA and DHA in the body, to be later incorporated among phospholipids in cell membranes and adipose tissue. By using a control group which was also given dietary and exercise advice, we were able to isolate and highlight the role of the n-3 fatty acids. A detailed analysis of the role of specific nutrients in our Indo- Mediterranean diet is currently underway. Interim calculations show that the dietary intake of n-3 fatty acids had a major impact on the risk for cardiac events in the intervention group. The main sources of n-3 fatty acids in our diet were plants: walnuts, green leafy vegetables, whole grains, soy bean oil, and mustard oil. Thus, it is not necessary to consume the fish-derived long chain acids, DHA and EPA, in order to reap the benefits of n-3 fatty acids.

The exact mechanism underlying the circadian rhythmicity of cardiac events and its regulation by n-3 fatty acids remains unknown. There is consistent evidence that this rhythmicity is controlled by the suprachiasmatic nucleus [35], a tiny clump of cells in the brain which works as a biological clock and is influenced by daily changes in light and darkness. Brain neurons are rich in n-3 fatty acids, as are cell membranes of cardiomyocytes, endothelial cells and arterial smooth muscle cells. It is there fore possible that a relative deficiency of n-3 fatty acids in these cells enhances their susceptibility to excitation, causing greater neurohumoral and cardiovascular dysfunction, and resulting in a marked increase in the rhythmicity of cardiac events [36]. Increased vagal tone decreases the synthesis of tumor necrosis factor-alpha (TNF-alpha) in the liver and inhibits the release of proinflammatory cytokines such as IL-6 [20-22]. It is possible that low levels of n-3 fatty acids decrease the vagal tone, leading to increased synthesis of TNF-alpha and a greater release of proinflammatory cytokines by increased sympathetic activity. Treatment with n-3 fatty acids may break this cycle, decreasing inflammation and excitation of neurons, cardiomyocytes, endothelial and smooth muscle cells, bringing about a decreased vulnerability for cardiac events. Furthermore, n-3 fatty acids may also enhance brain acetylecholine level and parasympathetic tone, resulting in increased HRV, and hence, protection from pronounced rhythmicity of cardiac events [17-22].

One major limitation of our study is the relatively small number of events both overall and in each quartile of the day, owing to both the concomitant primary prevention arm of our original study (about half of the 1000 subjects had only risk factors for CAD, and were not post-MI patients), and the large reduction in event rate in the intervention group, brought about by the n-3 supplementation. Thus, the statistical analyses can not definitely rule out this factor as the reason for the fairly equal distribution of events in the n-3 group. Given the measured proportion of events in the high risk hours (28%), a power of 80% and 39 participants in the intervention group, allowed the minimal detection of 17% difference compared to control group; the difference observed was 10%. Nevertheless, the many mechanisms by which n-3 fatty acids may influence the circadian rhythm of CAD events cannot be overlooked, and we therefore believe that a biological explanation is plausible. A larger interventional study with more events is needed to confirm our findings.

In summary, our study suggests that an Indo-Mediterranean diet, which is rich in fruits, vegetables, nuts, whole grains, soy and mustard oils, can provide sufficient alpha-linolenic acid, to result in a modulation in the rhythmicity of cardiac events by n-3 fatty acids. Since a high n-6/n-3 ratio may blunt the beneficial effects of n-3 fatty acids, soybean oil should be replaced by more mustard oil. The exact nature of the cardioprotective action of n-3 fatty acids, whether by influencing platelet function or HRV through brain-heart connections, remains to be elucidated.

References

[1]   Pell S, D'Alonzo CA. Acute myocardial infarction in a large industrial population. *JAMA* 1963;185:831-8.
[2]   Arntz HR, Willich SN, Schreiber C, et al. Diurnal, weekly and seasonal variation of sudden death. *Eur. Heart J.* 2000;21:315-20.
[3]   Willich SN. European survey on circadian variation of angina pectoris (ESCVA): design and preliminary results. *J. Cardiovasc. Pharmacol.* 1999;34(suppl 2):s9-13.
[4]   Singh RB, Pella D, Neki NS, et al. Mechanism of acute myocardial infarction study (MAMY Study). *Biomed. Pharmacother.* 2004;57:in press.
[5]   Rocco MB, Barry J, Campbell BAS, et al. Circadian variation of transient myocardial ischemia in patients with coronary artery disease. *Circulation* 1987;75:395-400.

[6]   Muller JE, Stone PH, Turi ZG, et al. Circadian variation in the frequency of onset of acute myocardial infarction. *N. Engl. J. Med.* 1985;313:1315-22.

[7]   Goldberg R, Brady P, Chen J, et al. Time of onset of acute myocardial infarction after awakening. *J. Am. Coll. Cardiol.* 1989;13:133A [abstract].

[8]   Davies MJ, Thomas A. Thrombosis and acute coronary artery lesions in sudden cardiac ischemic death. *N. Engl. J. Med.* 1984;310:1137-41.

[9]   Muller JE, Ludmer PL, Willich SN, et al. Circadian variation in the frequency of sudden cardiac death. *Circulation* 1987;75:131-8

[10] International Study of Infarct Survival-2 (ISIS-2) Collaborative Group. Morning peak in the incidence of myocardial infarction: experience in the ISIS-2 trial. *Eur Heart J* 1992;13:594-608.

[11] Toffler GH, Brezinski D, Schaefer A, et al. Concurrent morning increase in platelet aggregability and the risk of myocardial infarction and sudden cardiac death. *N. Engl. J. Med.*1987;316:1514-8.

[12] Chasen C, Muller JE. Cardiovascular triggers and morning events. *Blood Pressure Monit.* 1998;3:35-42.

[13] Deedwania PC. Hemodynamic changes as triggers of cardiovascular events. Cardiol. Clin. 1996;14:229-38.

[14] Singh RB, Cornelissen G, Siegelova J, et al. About half-weekly (circasemiseptan) pattern of blood pressure and heart rate in men and women of India. *Scripta Medica* (Brno) 2002;75:125-8.

[15] Singh RB, Weydahl A, Otsuka K, et al. Can nutrition influence circadian rhythm and heart rate variability? *Biomed. Pharmacother.* 2001;55 (suppl 11):s115-24.

[16] Singh RB, Niaz MA, Cornelissen GS, et al. Circadian rhythmicity of circulating vitamin concentrations. *Scripta Medica* (Brno) 2001;74:93-6.

[17] Christensen JH, Gustenhoff P, Komp E, et al. Effect of fish oil on heart rate variability in survivors of myocardial infarction. *Br. Med. J.* 1996;312:677-8.

[18] Christensen JH, Komp E, Aaroe J, et al. Fish consumption, n-3 fatty acids in cell membranes and heart rate variability in survivors of myocardial infarction with left ventricular dysfunction. *Am. J. Cardiol.* 1997;79:1670-2.

[19] Christensen JH, Skou HA, Fog L, et al. Marine n-3 fatty acids, wine intake, and heart rate variability in patients referred for coronary angiography. *Circulation* 2001;103:651-7.

[20] Chin JPF. Marine oils and cardiovascular reactivity. *Prostaglandins Leukot Essent Fatty Acids* 1994;50:211-22.

[21] Borovikova LV, Ivanova S, Zhang M, et al. Vagus nerve stimulation attenuates the systemic inflammatory response to endotoxin. *Nature* 2000;405:458-62.

[22] Das UN. The brain-lipid-heart connection. Nutrition 2001;17:260-3.

[23] Lauritzen I, Blondeau N, Heurteaux C, et al. Polyunsaturated fatty acids are potent neuroprotectors. *EMBO J.* 2000;19:1784-93.

[24] Minami M, Kimura S, Endo T, et al. Dietary docosahexaenoic acid increases cerebral acetylcholine levels and improves passive avoidance performance in stroke-prone spontaneously hypertensive rates. *Pharmacol. Biochem. Behav.* 1997;58:1123-9.

[25] Goodnight SH Jr, Harris WS, Connor WE. The effects of dietary omega-3 fatty acids upon platelet composition and function in man: a prospective controlled study. *Blood* 1981;58:880-5.

[26] Pella D, Singh RB, Otsuka K, et al. Nutritional predictors and modulators of insulin resistance. *J. Nutr. Environ. Med.* 2004;14:3-16

[27] Singh RB, Niaz MA, Sharma JP, et al. Randomized, double blind, placebo controlled trial of fish oil and mustard oil in patients with suspected acute myocardial infarction. The Indian Experiment of Infarct Survival. *Cardiovasc. Drug Ther.* 1997;11:485-91.

[28] Marchioli R, Barzi F, Bobma E, et al. Early protection against sudden death by n-3 polyunsaturated fatty acids after myocardial infarction, time-course analysis of the results of the Gruppo Italiano per lo Studio della Sopravvivenza nell'Infarto Miocardico (GISSI)-Prevenzione. *Circulation* 2002;105:1897-903.

[29] Singh RB, Dubnov G, Niaz MA, et al. Effect of an Indo-Mediterranean diet on progression of coronary artery disease in high risk patients (Indo-Mediterranean Diet Heart Study): a randomised single-blind trial. *Lancet* 2002;360:1455-61.

[30] de Lorgeril M, Salen P, Martin JL, et al. Mediterranean diet, traditional risk factors and the rate of cardiovascular complications after myocardial infarction. Final report of the Lyon Diet Heart Study. *Circulation* 1999; 99: 779–85.

[31] National Cholesterol Education Program. Second report of the expert panel on detection, evaluation, and treatment of high blood cholesterol in adults (adult treatment panel II). *Circulation* 1994;89:1333-445.

[32] Narasinga Rao BS, Deosthale YG, Pant KC. Nutrient composition of Indian foods. Hyderbad, India: National Institute of Nutrition, *Indian Council of Medical Research.* 1989.

[33] Goodhart RS, Shils ME, eds. *Modern nutrition in health and disease.* Philadelphia, PA: Lea and Febiger, 1980.

[34] Ridker PM, Manson JE, Buring JE, et al. Circadian variation of acute myocardial infarction and the effect of low dose aspirin in a randomized trial of physicians. *Circulation* 1990;82:897-902.

[35] Ralph MR, Foster RG, Davis FC, et al. Transplanted suprachiasmatic nucleus determines circadian period. *Science* 1990;247:975-8.

[36] Yehuda S. Omega-6/omega-3 ratio and brain related functions. *World Rev. Nutr. Diet* 2003;92:37-56.

Index

B

C

D

F

G

H

I

N

O

T

U

V